Complications of Contact Lens Wear

Complications of Contact Lens Wear

ALAN TOMLINSON, PH.D, F.B.C.O.

Professor and Head
Department of Optometry and Vision
Science
Glasgow Polytechnic
Glasgow, United Kingdom
Formerly
Director of Research
Professor
Southern California College of Optometry
Fullerton, California

Mosby
Year Book

St. Louis Baltimore Boston Chicago London Philadelphia Sydney Toronto

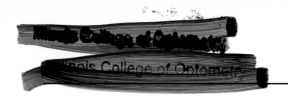

**Mosby
Year Book**

Dedicated to Publishing Excellence

Sponsoring Editor: David K. Marshall
Assistant Editor: Julie Tryboski
Assistant Director, Manuscript Services: Frances M. Perveiler
Production Manager: Nancy C. Baker
Proofroom Manager: Barbara Kelly

1 2 3 4 5 6 7 8 9 0 CL/CL/WA 96 95 94 93 92

Library of Congress Cataloging-in-Publication Data

Complications of contact lens wear / [edited by] Alan Tomlinson.
    p. cm.
  Includes bibliographical references and index.
  ISBN 0-8016-6309-1
  1. Contact lenses—Complications. I. Tomlinson, Alan, Ph.D.
  [DNLM: 1. Contact Lenses--adverse effects. 2. Cornea-
-physiopathology. 3. Eye Injuries--physiopathology. WW 355
C7368]
  RE977.C6C54 1992
  617.7'523--dc20   92-16488
  DNLM/DLC   CIP
  for Library of Congress

To the memory of my father, Arthur Tomlinson, who taught me to work obsessively enough to complete a book project.

Contributors

CAROLYN G. BEGLEY, O.D., M.S.
Assistant Professor
Indiana University School of Optometry
Bloomington, Indiana

EDWARD S. BENNETT, O.D., M.ED.
Associate Professor
School of Optometry
USML
St. Louis, Missouri

JAN P.G. BERGMANSON, O.D., PH.D.
Associate Professor
School of Optometry
University of Houston
Houston, Texas

JOSEPH A. BONNANNO, O.D., PH.D.
University of California at Berkeley
School of Optometry
Berkeley, California

JEFFREY DOUGAL, O.D.
Assistant Professor
Southern California College of Optometry
Fullerton, California

MICHEL MILLODOT, O.D., PH.D.
Optometry Section
Department of Diagnostic Sciences
Hong Kong Polytechnic
Hung Hom, Kawloon
Hong Kong

BARTLY J. MONDINO, M.D.
Professor of Ophthalmology
Jules Stein Eye Institute
UCLA Medical Center
Los Angeles, California

KENNETH A. POLSE, O.D., M.S.
School of Optometry
University of California at Berkeley
Berkeley, California

JOEL A. SILBERT, O.D.
Associate Professor
Pennsylvania College of Optometry
Philadelphia, Pennsylvania

CRISTINA M. SCHNIDER, O.D.
Assistant Professor
College of Optometry
Pacific University
Forest Grove, Oregon

ALAN TOMLINSON, PH.D., F.B.C.O.
Professor and Head
Department of Optometry and Vision Science
Glasgow Polytechnic
Glasgow, United Kingdom

BARRY WEISSMAN, O.D., PH.D.
Professor of Ophthalmology
Jules Stein Eye Institute
UCLA Medical Center
Los Angeles, California

Contents

Preface   *ix*

PART I: ANOXIA   *1*

1 / Oxygen Requirements of the Cornea   *3*
  Alan Tomlinson

2 / Hypoxic Changes in the Corneal Epithelium and Stroma   *21*
  Joseph A. Bonanno and Kenneth A. Polse

3 / Hypoxic Changes in Corneal Endothelium   *37*
  Jan P.G. Bergmanson and Barry A. Weissman

4 / Contact Lens-Induced Changes in Corneal Topography and Refractive Error   *69*
  Edward S. Bennett

5 / Corneal Anesthesia Following Contact Lens Wear   *89*
  Michel Millodot

PART II: ABRASION   *103*

6 / Keratitis   *105*
  Cristina M. Schnider

7 / Abrasions Secondary to Contact Lens Wear   *123*
  Jeffrey Dougal

PART III: XEROSIS   *157*

8 / Tear Film Changes With Contact Lens Wear   *159*
  Alan Tomlinson

9 / Contact Lens-Induced Dry Eye   *195*
  Alan Tomlinson

PART IV: INFLAMMATION   *219*

10 / Ocular Inflammation and Contact Lens Wear   *221*
  Joel A. Silbert

11 / Giant Papillary Conjunctivitis   *237*
  Carolyn G. Begley

PART V: INFECTION   *253*

12 / Corneal Infection Secondary to Contact Lens Wear   *255*
  Barry A. Weissman and Bartly J. Mondino

Index   *275*

Preface

Contact lenses, an intimate form of vision correction, have been fitted for the past 100 years. Since their advent, they have passed through the *ages* of glass, PMMA, hydrogel, and rigid gas permeable materials. Each successive *age* has been shorter than the last as material developments in the field have rapidly advanced. These developments have led to improvements in physiological compatibility of materials to the extent that some patients are now able to wear lenses for several days at a time and, on removal, to dispose of them. But the intimate relationship of lens material to biological tissue requires practitioners to continue to critically challenge the safety of this modality of care.

The growth in the field of contact lenses has been chronicled in many specialist journals and textbooks. Most of the latter are dedicated to the principles and practices of lens fitting; the consequences of wear have received limited attention. In the light of much recent research on the physiological impact of lenses on the eye (particularly those worn for extended wear), it is appropriate that a single textbook be devoted to this topic. It is the intention of this text to provide practitioners and students with a comprehensive clinical guide to the etiology, appearance, course, and management of complications of contact lens wear. These complications are discussed under five section headings of anoxia, abrasion, xerosis, inflammation, and infection which reflect the general categories of the clinical manifestations. In spite of the impression that can arise from descriptions of the negative effects of any procedure, the reader should maintain a balanced view and remember that contact lenses are a generally safe form of vision correction.

There are a number of individuals that I am indebted to for their invaluable assistance in the preparation of this book. Foremost are the contributors, Carolyn Begley, Ed Bennett, Jan Bergmanson, Joe Bonanno, Jeff Dougal, Michel Millodot, Bart Mondino, Ken Polse, Cris Schnider, Joel Silbert, and Barry Weissman, whose knowledge and clinical expertise is expressed in the content of their chapters. I also thank Bob Grohe for his expert clinical review of the material on abrasions of the cornea. All of the contributors are indebted to the many clinicians who have provided illustrative material for this book. Finally, I would like to thank Judy Higgins for making all of those alterations to the manuscript and David Marshall, the Executive Editor, and the production staff at Mosby–Year Book for their encouragement and advice in the preparation of the text.

ALAN TOMLINSON, PH.D., F.B.C.O.

Anoxia

Oxygen Requirements of the Cornea

Alan Tomlinson, Ph.D., F.B.C.O.

The most frequent complications of contact lens wear occur as a direct result of lack of oxygen supply to the cornea (relative corneal anoxia or hypoxia). In addition a series of indirect effects of oxygen deprivation have also been reported. The first section of this book deals with the oxygen requirements of the cornea and the effects of deprivation on the corneal epithelium, stroma, and endothelium, corneal sensitivity, and ocular refraction. In later sections, the less direct, but important, role of anoxia in epithelial keratitis, overwear abrasions, corneal infiltration, neovascularization, and infection is described.

The short- and long-term changes in the tissues of the cornea resulting from insufficient oxygenation are shown in Table 1–1. This information has been reviewed by many authors.[7, 18, 55, 56, 85]

OXYGEN AND CORNEAL METABOLISM

The cornea requires nutriments in the form of glucose, amino acids, and oxygen to perform its normal metabolic functions. In view of the cornea's avascular structure, the principal source of these nutriments is from the aqueous humor and the atmosphere via the tears, the latter providing oxygen and the former the glucose and amino acids.[83, 84] In the absence of adequate oxygen supply, the cornea loses its ability to maintain aerobic glycolosis, the glycogen stores within the cornea become rapidly broken down, and lactic acid accumulates in the corneal tissue. Other metabolic disturbances that may take place include disturbed levels of succinic[52] and lactate dehydrogenase[63] and other enzyme concentrations.[97] This, in turn, leads to the development of edema in the epithelium and stroma of

the cornea because of the additional osmotic load on these tissues.[64] It is clear that the health of the cornea is intimately connected with the availability of oxygen to this tissue.[20]

Forty years ago, Smelzer and Ozanics[95] and Smelzer and Shen[96] showed that oxygen deprivation as a result of polymethylmethacrylate (PMMA) contact lens wear produced marked structural and optical changes in the cornea. Many of the complications of contact lens wear discussed in subsequent chapters arise from the relative anoxia (hypoxia) that the cornea experiences as a result of being covered by a contact lens. The actual amount of oxygen required for the various layers of the cornea to carry out normal respiration has been measured by various investigators. The rate of oxygen consumption of the epithelium has ranged from 1 to 10 μL/hr/cm^2.[30, 62, 69, 71] According to Freeman,[36] the oxygen consumption rate for individual layers of the cornea is 3.83 μL/hr/cm^2 for the epithelium, 3.68 μL/hr/cm^2 for the stroma, 2.03 μL/hr/cm^2 for the endothelium, and 9.54 μL/hr/cm^2 for the whole cornea.

The ability of the cornea to obtain an oxygen supply to satisfy these consumption rates at the various levels will depend on the oxygen available at the atmospheric surface (in the tears), at the aqueous surface from the aqueous fluid itself, and the permeability of the tissue to the transfer of oxygen. In the the open eye situation (uncovered by a contact lens), it is assumed that the tears are fully saturated with the oxygen component of the air, which is equivalent to an oxygen tension level of 155 mm Hg.[21] Measurements from the rabbit eye have shown the oxygen tension of the aqueous humor to be in the range of 25 to 77 mm Hg, and a value of 55 mm Hg is the best estimate of the oxygen tension at the posterior surface of the cornea. With the eye closed, the oxygen tension at the anterior corneal surface is assumed to be equal to that of the

TABLE 1–1.

Corneal Sequelae of Contact Lens–Induced Relative Anoxia (Hypoxia)*

Structure	Short-Term Change	Long-Term Change
Epithelium	Erosians	Microcysts
	Edema	Bullae
	Ulceration	Vacuoles
	Warpage	Thinning
		Vascularization
		Reduced oxygen consumption
		Increased fragility
		Reduced sensitivity
		Reduced cell mitosis
Stroma	Edema	Thinning
	Striae	Infiltrates
		Vascularization
Endothelium	Bleb	Polymegathism
	Folds	Bedewing
		Guttatae

*Adapted from Efron N, Brennan NE: *Aust J Optom* 1985; 68:27.

palpebral conjunctiva that lies adjacent to the surface. This has been found to be in approximately 55 mm Hg,[26, 66, 73] the oxygen tension at the aqueous surface of the closed eye remaining the same as that of the open eye. From this information, Fatt et al.[28] have developed a model of the steady-state distribution of oxygen in the open and closed eye (Fig 1–1).

This model has been validated by passing a fine oxygen sensor through the rabbit cornea.[67] It has been noted that the oxygen tension of the endothelium is dependent solely on the aqueous supply and is therefore independent of the oxygen tension at the atmospheric surface.[22, 70] The stroma obtains oxygen from both the epithelium and endothelial sides because the tension is lower in the posterior epithelium than in either of these two tissues (see Fig 1–1). The epithelium, on the other hand, is solely dependent on the atmosphere for its oxygen supply and receives no meaningful quantity from the aqueous. Clearly, in the non–contact lens wearing eye, the epithelial supply will be directly dependent on the atmospheric supply. This may vary with the altitude above sea level. At sea level the oxygen tension of the atmosphere is 155 mm Hg. However, as altitude increases, this tension reduces. For instance, at a height of 5,000 ft in a city such as Denver, the tension will drop to 134 mm Hg, in Mexico City, it will be down to just over 118 mm Hg, and at the top of Mt. Everest, it will be 52 mm Hg.[40] As the oxygen tension of the anterior corneal surface drops, the ability for the cornea to perform its normal metabolic functions is severely reduced. Some have provided evidence that the cornea is able to adapt to states of relative hypoxia,[78] whereas others have suggested that this apparent adaption is produced by a decrease in epithelial thickness.[57]

The oxygen tension profile of the cornea just described is obviously affected by the presence of the contact lens covering the anterior corneal surface. In most cases this significantly reduces the oxygen tension level. The oxygen available will vary dependent on characteristics of the contact lens material. These include the oxygen trans-

FIG 1–1.
Corneal oxygen tension profiles for values at the anterior corneal surface. The upper curve represents the open eye; the third curve from the top represents the closed eye (the oxygen tension of the palpebral conjunctiva is taken as 55 mm Hg). (From Fatt I, Freeman RD, Lin D: *Exp Eye Res* 1974; 18:357. Used by permission.)

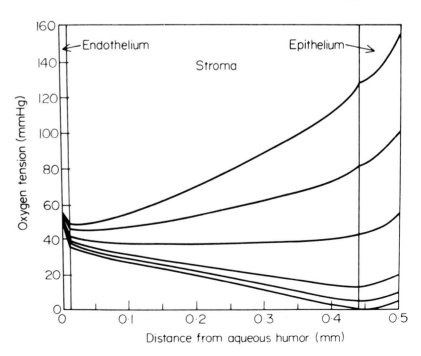

missibility of the material and whether the lens is made from a nonmoving hydrogel or from a hard lens that moves on the cornea. In addition to oxygen supply by transmissibility, hard lenses provide tear pumping under the contact lens and extra oxygen from this source. Finally, the mode of wear of the contact lens will dramatically affect the oxygen experience of the cornea, that is, whether lenses are worn only for daily wear (in an open eye situation) or for extended wear (under a closed lid).

Fatt et al.[27] have reexamined the oxygen tension distributions of the cornea in the open and closed eye situations with contact lenses of differing oxygen permeabilities. The profile for the cornea in an open eye situation when covered by oxygen permeable lenses 0.1 mm thick and with permeabilities of 500 to 5.7×10^{-11} may be seen in Figure 1–2 and for the closed eye situation when the same thickness lenses are worn in oxygen permeabilities of 500 and $13 \times 10^{-11} \dfrac{cm^2 \times \mu L}{sec \times \mu L \times mm\ Hg}$ in Figure 1–3.

Materials currently available provide some of the permeability levels illustrated in this original paper.[27] Although, as shown later, the ideal contact lens material providing the highest levels of permeability has not yet been developed.

The correlate of the oxygen availability to the cornea under various conditions (open eye, closed eye, contact lens wear) is the rate at which metabolic waste products, specifically carbon dioxide, accumulate. Fatt et al.[23] dismissed this as a factor affecting corneal physiology in view of the very high CO_2 permeability (20 times that of oxygen) of the corneal tissue. However, others[14] disagree, linking hypercapnia (CO_2 buildup) in the cornea with changes in corneal and endothelial morphology during lens wear (see Chapters 2 and 3). Although the CO_2 permeability of current contact lens materials is greater than that for oxygen, namely, 21 times for hydrogel lenses, and 7 times for rigid gas-permeable (RGP) lenses,[1] it has been maintained that significant retardation of CO_2 efflux from the deeper layers of the cornea can occur, particularly under conditions of extended wear.[7]

HOW MUCH OXYGEN DOES THE CORNEA NEED?

Exactly what level of oxygen tension is required at the anterior epithelial surface so that the corneal tissue has an amount of oxygen available for normal respiration, nutriment, and cellular activity has received considerable attention from corneal and contact lens researchers. In the nor-

mal oxygen environment, at sea level, where the cornea is not covered by a contact lens, 21% of the air mixture is oxygen at a tension level of 155 mm Hg. This amount, at the anterior corneal epithelial surface, provides the cornea with enough to avoid swelling and other physiochemical and physiological changes. In the closed eye, or where the cornea is covered by a contact lens, the availability of oxygen is reduced. The question then is to what "critical level" the oxygen supply at the anterior epithelial surface can be reduced before corneal dysfunction results. The definition of the critical oxygen level will depend to some degree on the criterion applied to determine this function and the exposure of the cornea (open or closed lid). Several workers have used the criterion of corneal swelling or edema,[17, 59, 61, 79, 91] whereas others have used cell mitosis rates[57] or loss of corneal sensitivity[86] to determine the critical level.

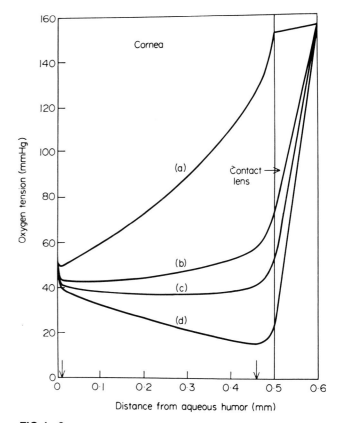

FIG 1–2.
Oxygen tension profiles in the cornea of an open eye covered by an oxygen-permeable contact lens 0.1 mm thick. The left- and right-hand arrows point to the endothelium, stroma, and stroma-epithelium interfaces, respectively. Letters on the curves refer to the oxygen permeability of the contact lenses; *(a)* 500×10^{-11}, *(b)* 13.1×10^{-11}, *(c)* 9.4×10^{-11}, *(d)* 5.7×10^{-11} [in units of mL O_2 cm^2 (mL tiss)$^{-1}$ sec^{-1} mm Hg^{-1}]. (From Fatt I, Freeman RD, Lin D: *Exp Eye Res* 1974; 18:357. Used by permission.)

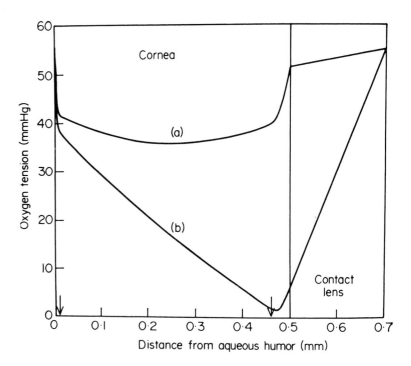

FIG 1-3.
Oxygen tension profiles in the cornea of a closed eye covered by an oxygen-permeable contact lens 0.1 mm thick. The left- and right-hand arrows point to the endothelium, stroma, and stroma-epithelium interfaces, respectively. Letters on the curves refer to the oxygen permeability of the contact lenses; (a) 500×10^{-11}, (b) 13.1×10^{-11}, [in units of mL O_2 cm^2 (mL tiss)$^{-1}$ sec^{-1} mm Hg^{-1}]. (From Fatt I, Freeman RD, Lin D: *Exp Eye Res* 1974; 18:357. Used by permission.)

CRITERIA FOR CRITICAL CORNEA OXYGEN TENSION LEVELS

Corneal Swelling

The first classic experiment in this field was carried out by Polse and Mandell[91] in the late 1960s. This study revealed that when gas of varying oxygen concentrations was passed across the eye with the subject wearing goggles, the cornea required 1.5% to 2.5% oxygen to prevent edema. This result was surprising, however, because the cornea obtains as much as 8% oxygen[17] during eye closure, yet slight corneal swelling (3%–4%) occurs during sleep. This increase is probably not explained by tear osmolarity, temperature, or pH differences with the lids closed.[41] Indeed, it has been shown that some hydrogel contact lenses that transmit more oxygen than the 2% criterion level of Polse and Mandell[91] actually induce corneal edema.[59] A later experiment by Mandell and Farrell[79] raised the minimum oxygen tension level to 3.1% oxygen and found significant intersubject variability in corneal swelling response.

Two major problems, however, existed with these studies.[19] First, only low levels of oxygen were available in the goggle, thus extrapolation of the results was required to obtain the oxygen level needed to give zero swelling. Because the mathematical form of the relationship between edema and precorneal oxygen tension is unknown, this procedure is difficult. In addition, relatively short exposure times (<3 hours) were used in these early experiments. This did not take into the account the possibility that it may take longer for steady-state levels of edema to occur in response to hypoxia. Later experiments by Holden and Mertz[59] and Holden et al.[61] used a wide range of oxygen concentrations within the goggle (1%–21% oxygen) and exposure times up to 8 hours. These experiments indicated that the steady-state edema takes approximately 4 to 5 hours to develop (Fig 1–4), confirmed the very wide subject variability in edema response, and suggested a much higher level than previously reported for the critical oxygen tension level. An average of 10% oxygen was advocated to prevent edema, although individual subject variability showed requirements from 7.5% to as high as 21% oxygen concentration to avoid all corneal swelling (Fig 1–5). This high variability in edema response confirms population distribution of corneal oxygen consumption, which Larke et al.[71] and Quinn and Schoessler[92] found to be widely distributed. Later work by Mandell[74] provided a consensus on the minimum average oxygen requirements of 10% to avoid corneal swelling in daily wear, but this should be heavily qualified with the caveat that other factors may be induced by the contact lens wear. It is of interest, as Mandell[75] has observed, that at zero oxygen levels (100% nitrogen), the cornea swells approximately 8% in 3 hours. A contact lens that is worn overnight under experimental, extended wear conditions shows corneal swelling of about 12% to 13%. Therefore, factors other than hypoxia alone must operate when the eyes are closed during sleep. Throughout these discussions of critical oxygen tension levels, care must be taken to dis-

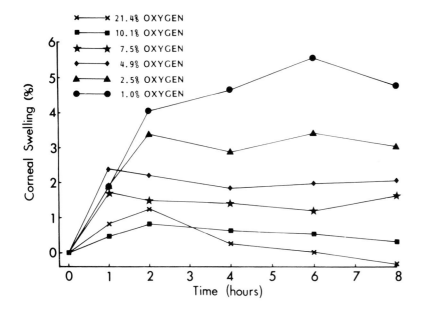

FIG 1–4.
The average corneal swelling for a group of eight subjects exposed for different time intervals to various oxygen concentrations within a gas goggle. (From Holden BA, Sweeney DS, Sanderson G: *Invest Ophthalmol Vis Sci* 1984; 25:476. Used by permission.)

tinguish between corneal effects from low precorneal oxygen tension levels with gas mixtures and corneal effects when a contact lens is worn. The latter do not necessarily show the critical oxygen tension level for normal corneal physiology but the critical oxygen level for normal physiology under contact lenses. Moreover, they do not differentiate factors, other than oxygen, that may influence corneal physiology with the lens in situ.[76]

Other Criteria

If other criteria are used to determine the critical oxygen tension level for the cornea, the line may be drawn at a different point. Hamano et al.[39] confirmed that the cornea requires 13% oxygen to avoid suppression of epithelial mitosis and accumulation of lactate in the anterior chamber. Millodot and O'Leary[86] confirmed that the cornea shows a reduced touch sensitivity after epithelial hypoxia induced

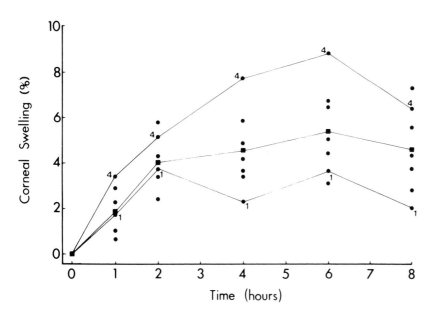

FIG 1–5.
The corneal swelling recorded at various time intervals for individual subjects exposed to a 1.0% oxygen environment. Results for individual subjects are seen in filled circles and the group mean values as filled squares. (From Holden BA, Sweeney DS, Sanderson G: *Invest Ophthalmol Vis Sci* 1984; 25:476. Used by permission.)

by the eyelid closure, indicating that a precorneal oxygen tension of at least 8% is required to avoid corneal sensitivity loss. This is discussed in Chapter 5.

Effect of Altitude

In all of these discussions of critical oxygen tension levels, the literature uses the terminology "percentage of oxygen." One should remember that in the normal atmosphere at sea level, approximately 21% of the air is oxygen. This means that the partial pressure of oxygen in terms of millimeters of mercury is effectively 21% × 760 mm Hg, or 159 mm Hg of oxygen. In general, the actual oxygen available is slightly below this level, and therefore a figure of 155 mm Hg of partial oxygen pressure is taken to be that available at sea level. At levels above sea level, the actual proportion of oxygen in the gaseous mixture remains the same, at 21%, but the partial pressure of oxygen decreases because the pressure of the gaseous mixture as a whole decreases (Fig 1–6). For example, in Denver at 5,000 ft if the air pressure is 638 mm Hg, the actual partial pressure of oxygen at this altitude would be 134 mm Hg. It is this partial pressure of oxygen available to the anterior corneal surface that is the driving force for the gas entering the corneal tissue. Thus, at altitudes above sea level, the cornea receives less actual oxygen. A contact lens that transmits to the cornea just under one half, or 10%, of the actual oxygen available at sea level, at an altitude of 5,000 ft, the same lens would give only 64 mm Hg of oxygen tension. At this altitude, a lens that gives sufficient oxygen for edema-free daily wear[59] at sea level would produce corneal swelling. Therefore, the difficulty of determining oxygen available under a lens in percentage terms arises if values at altitudes above sea level are considered. Practitioners should be aware that the critical or minimum oxygen requirement

of various forms of contact lens wear[59, 61] need to be increased if a patient is to habitually wear a lens at an altitude significantly above sea level.

Effect of Eyelid Closure

The critical oxygen tension level that has been discussed up to this point is that required to produce no edema during open eye wear of a contact lens. However, in the situation of lid closure, the situation is dramatically changed. Under a closed lid, the environment under a contact lens is quite different. The oxygen supply is reduced, the lid action on the lens is eliminated, there is a decrease in tear and stromal pH, and there is an increase of the cornea temperature and tear osmolarity. In this section, the discussion is restricted to the consideration of oxygen tension levels in a closed eye environment. In the extended wear situation, the supply of oxygen to the cornea is confined to that from the palpebral conjunctiva. The oxygen tension available from this source is approximately 55 mm Hg, or in percentage terms (at sea level), just above 7%. It has been established that the minimum standard to avoid corneal edema in the open eye situation is about 10%. Therefore, it is inevitable in the closed eye situation, without the presence of a contact lens, that the cornea should swell. Mandell and Fatt[80] observed that the cornea swelled 3% to 4% on normal eye closure without the presence of a contact lens. In an attempt to define the critical oxygen tension level required in a closed eye situation during extended contact lens wear, Holden and Mertz[59] considered the oxygen availability necessary to avoid any swelling beyond the physiological amount observed by Mandell and Fatt[80] during normal eye closure (Table 1–2). This oxygen availability was found to be 18%, a level difficult to achieve with any current contact lens materials. In consequence, a

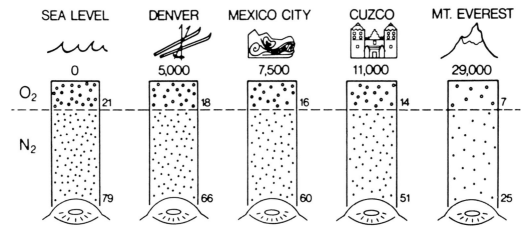

FIG 1–6.
Schematic model of the progressive reduction of oxygen available to the eye at different altitudes (values for oxygen and nitrogen are given in percentages). (From Hill RM: *Int Contact Lens Clin* 1976; 3:49. Used by permission.)

TABLE 1–2.

Critical Oxygen Levels and Lens Thicknesses for Low and High Water Content Hydrogel Lenses.*

Criteria	Critical O$_2$ Levels		Critical Average Lens Thickness (μm)	
	Dk/L$_{avg}$†	EOP‡	Poly-Hema (Dk = 8 × 10^{-11})§	Duragel 75 (Dk = 40 × 10^{-11})§
Zero day 1 corneal swelling	24.1 ± 2.7 × 10^{-9}	9.9	33	166
≤4% overnight corneal swelling	87.0 ± 3.3 × 10^{-9}	17.9	9	46
Zero day 2 residual swelling	34.3 ± 5.2 × 10^{-9}	12.1	23	117

*From Holden BA, Mertz GW: *Invest Ophthalmol Vis Sci* 1984; 25:1161. Used by permission.
†Oxygen transmissibility units: (cm × mL O$_2$)/(sec × mL × mm Hg). D = diffusion coefficient of material; k = solubility coefficient of material; L = thickness.
‡EOP = equivalent oxygen percentage (% atmospheric O$_2$).
§Oxygen permeability units: (cm^2 × mL O$_2$)/(sec × mL × mm Hg).

compromise standard for extended wear oxygen tension level of 12% was suggested. In their group of subjects, this is a level at which no *residual corneal swelling* remained during the daily wear phase of the extended wear cycle. This is the currently accepted, practical standard of oxygen availability for extended wear.

OXYGEN AVAILABILITY DURING CONTACT LENS WEAR

To determine if, during contact lens wear, the cornea has sufficient oxygen supply to meet the critical levels described earlier, one must measure the oxygen availability with lenses. This topic has received a considerable amount of attention over the past 25 years. Two approaches have been taken to answer the question. In one, the physical ability of a contact lens material to pass oxygen gases is measured.[29, 103] The other approach is to determine the end point response of the cornea to contact lens wear, that is, the corneal thickness is measured to determine if edema occurs during contact lens wear. The presence of edema after lens wear indicates inadequate oxygenation.[79, 81] An alternative to this technique considers the impact of contact lens wear on rabbit and human corneas in terms of the resulting oxygen debt of the cornea.[50, 51] This debt is measured by the oxygen uptake from a membrane reservoir in close contact with the corneal tissue. This technique, which provides a measure of equivalent oxygen percentage (EOP), is widely accepted by practitioners as an indication of the oxygen tension of the precorneal tear film resulting from the transmission of contact lens materials. A derivative of the EOP measurement, the hypoxic stress unit (HSU),[53] has recently been introduced to classify corneal response to lens wear.

Measurement of the Oxygen Transmissibility of Contact Lens Materials: Dk/L

Fatt[24] developed a technique for measuring the oxygen transmissibility of various contact lens materials. The transmissibility is defined in terms of physical parameters of the material and expressed as Dk/L. D is the diffusion coefficient of the material, k is the solubility coefficient of the material, and L is the thickness. The terms D and k are independent of altitude. The value of L will vary between different contact lens materials such that the thicker the material, the less transmission of oxygen will take place. In reality, it is not the center thickness of contact lenses that must be considered for this calculation but the average thickness of the material. The contact lens material is placed over an oxygen-sensitive (polargraphic) electrode, which is arranged over a chamber so that only oxygen that passes through the lens material can reach the electrode.[29] A steady-state value recorded by this instrument after a short period of time is known as the transmissibility of the material and defined as Dk/L. The technique for determining oxygen transmissibility of materials is limited by the range of thicknesses over which measurements can be taken,[16, 34] by boundary layer effects, by edge effects,[4] and by other assumptions inherent in the methodology.[2, 3] The conflicting methodologies for measurement of Dk/L have recently been resolved.[58]

In essence, practitioners should remember that the oxygen available with a contact lens will vary with the material itself, the thickness of the lens (integrated over a large area of the lens),[99] the temperature during measurement, and whether the lens moves on the eye. In the case of soft lenses, availability will be lower with thicker and higher-powered lenses (Fig 1–7), with lower water content (the Dk/L varying inversely in a semilogarithmic manner with water content),[87] after lens dehydration on the eye[41, 47]

FIG 1–7.
Calculated oxygen performances across four different soft contact lenses. The three minus series lenses all have power of −3.00D and the high plus lens (+12.0D). All lenses are of the same 38% water content hydroxyethylmethacrylate (HEMA) material, and their normal center thickness is 0.07 mm for the U4, 0.12 mm for the B4, and 0.50 mm for the H4 lens. Dramatically different amounts of oxygen are available at different points under each of these lenses. (From Hill RM: *Int Contact Lens Clin* 1983; 10: 299. Used by permission.)

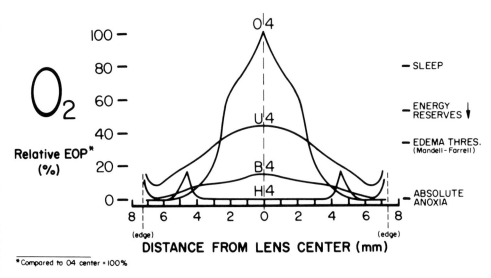

(Fig 1–8), and because the lens has a poor mechanism for oxygen supply by tear pumping under the lens.[90, 102]

Efron and Brennan[15] have described a technique for measuring, in-office, the Dk/L of any soft contact lens. This requires measurement of lens thickness with the electronic thickness gauge and lens water content with a hand refractometer. For RGP lenses, the transmissibility is again material and thickness dependent, but a significant contribution to corneal oxygen supply may be obtained from the tear flow under the lens because of the pump mechanism during blinking (Fig 1–9).[28] This contribution from tear pumping can be equivalent to about one third[8] of the cornea's average requirement of oxygen necessary to avoid edema in daily contact lens wear.[59] An effective rigid lens tear pump can replace 10% to 20% of the postlens tear volume with each blink.[11, 12] The magnitude of the exchange is influenced by the contact lens design[9, 33, 54] and lid geometry.[13, 31] More efficiency in pumping is obtained with smaller-diameter lens designs (Fig 1–10) and greater edge lift and for patients with larger palpebral apertures. In addition, vertical lens movement,[6, 8] the thickness of the tear film,[65] and the dynamics of the blink[32, 37, 89, 93] can be instrumental in providing increased bulk-flow volume exchange and stirring beneath

FIG 1–8.
Oxygen transmissivities of four lens types associated with three different hydration levels for each lens. The lens center thicknesses in mm are shown in brackets, and the measured saturated water values are given as a percentage of total lens weight in each case. (From Hill RM, Andrasko GA: *J Am Optom Assoc* 1981; 52:225. Used by permission.)

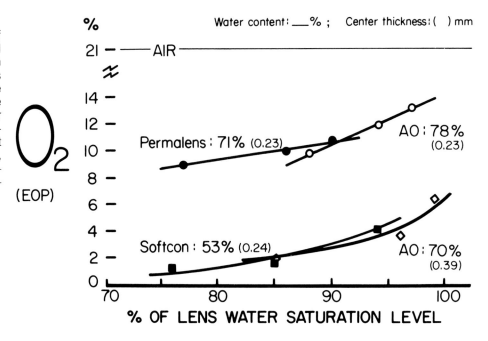

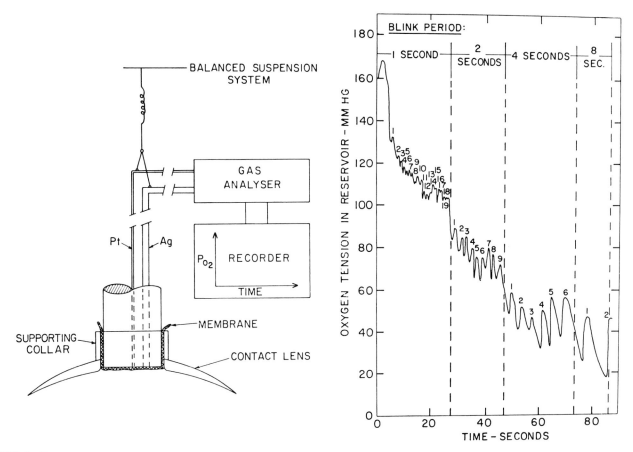

FIG 1–9.
Left, oxygen sensor assembly used to measure oxygen tension under a contact lens during blinking. The platinum *(Pt)* and silver *(Ag)* wires form the sensor electrons. The gas analyzer is an electronic device to convert sensor current to a signal that will operate the recorder. *Right,* oxygen tension recorded from the tear reservoir between a human cornea and a contact lens. (From Fatt I, Hill RM: *Am J Optom Am Acad Optom* 1970; 47:50. Used by permission.)

the contact lens. These aid in supplying the cornea with part of its oxygen requirement and in clearance of metabolic waste and debris from beneath the lens.[100–102]

The choice of RGP materials can be based on oxygen transmissibility of the material. This information can be derived from published nomograms[102] if the mode of lens wear, together with the thickness of the proposed lens design, is known (Fig 1–11).

In most cases practitioners make the oxygen-related choice of materials for hard and soft lenses from published data on Dk/L provided by manufacturers.[104] One should remember that comparisons between materials should be based on data determined at the same measurement temperature. For instance, a lens of Dk of 40 measured at room temperature will have a Dk in the upper fifties at the temperature of the eye. If possible, data measured by an independent source under uniform conditions for a whole group of materials should be available (Table 1–3) to aid practitioners in their clinical decision making.

Measurement of Oxygen Flux Through Contact Lens Materials

Turnbull et al.[103] described another in vitro technique for oxygen measurement through contact lens materials. It allows a direct measurement of oxygen flux through dry and wet RGP contact lenses using a radiometer. This method has the advantage of being a direct measurement of the actual amount of oxygen that diffuses through the contact lens material and that is available in the tear film beneath the lens. The technique is relatively new in its application to contact lenses and has not been widely used. Therefore, it is not the accepted reference standard in terms of corneal physiology that is provided by measurements of Dk/L or EOP.

Corneal Swelling Response

Corneal swelling, an end point response to oxygen deprivation, has been widely used as a means of detecting the

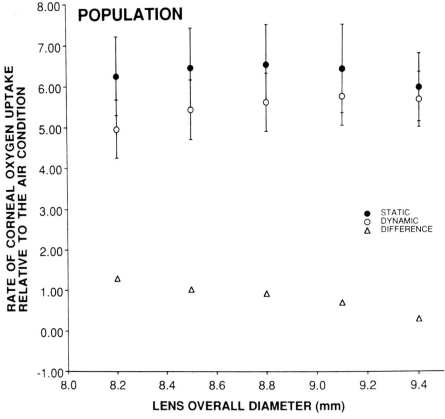

FIG 1–10.
The mean corneal oxygen demands of six human eyes are shown relative to the mean non–lens wearing eye condition, associated with each of five lens overall optic zone diameter combinations (ranging from 8.2/6.8 to 9.4/8.0 mm). Results are shown for the static condition, dynamic condition, and difference data. Each point is a mean of 48 measurements, 8 on each of 6 corneas. One standard deviation above and below each mean is indicated. (From Fink BA, Carney LG, Hill RM: *Optom Vis Sci* 1990; 67:641. Used by permission.)

level of oxygen supply of the cornea under contact lenses.[42, 59, 61, 72, 79, 81, 82, 91, 92, 100] When the cornea's oxygen needs are not provided by the contact lens, corneal swelling takes place. This response has been found to vary depending on the time of measurement (Fig 1–12) and the state of adaptation of the patient when wearing PMMA lenses.[77] The initial reaction to hard lens wear[77] will also depend on changes in tear chemistry (osmolarity) induced by contact lens wear. This topic is discussed in Chapter 8.

In addition, factors such as eye opening and closure will have a marked effect on the cornea swelling response in view of its effect on available atmospheric oxygen supply.[58] The critical oxygen tension levels recommended for daily and extended wear by Holden and Mertz[59] and Holden et al.[61] were derived by extrapolating the curves of corneal edema against lens oxygen transmissibility to the point at which no corneal swelling occurred (Fig 1–13). In extended wear, because of the lack of available materials that reach the optimum oxygen transmissibility levels required, levels of overnight corneal edema with most ap-

proved soft hydrogel extended wear lenses exceed 10% and with RGP extended wear lenses vary anywhere from 2% to 16%.[68]

The swelling response of the cornea will differ widely between individuals wearing the same contact lens material. This is particularly so during overnight wear of contact lenses. The wide variety of physiological response levels for any available oxygen tension underneath the contact lens has been reported by several workers (see Fig 1–5).[60, 61, 80] Of course, it may be possible to place contact lenses of different oxygen transmissibilities on a patient's cornea and measure the corneal swelling response. From those measurements the individual patient's minimum oxygen requirements for daily and extended wear could be calculated by the technique employed by Holden and Mertz[59] and Holden et al.[61] In clinical situation this is not feasible, and the use of the average values for oxygen availability with contact lenses in daily and extended wear have been developed.

In addition to the variability from one individual to

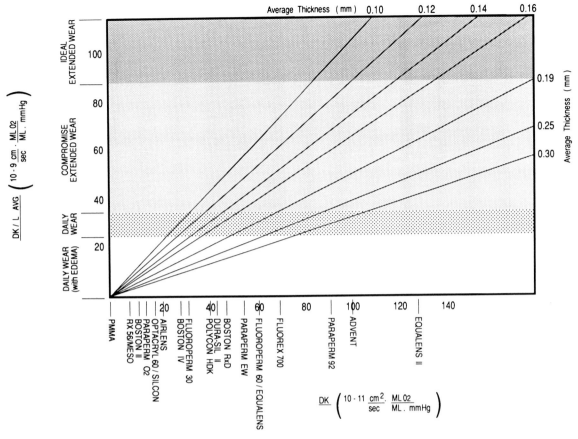

FIG 1–11.
Procedure to determine the appropriate gas-permeable materials for daily and extended wear. (1) Estimate the average lens thickness by *adding* to the center thickness in the case of minus lenses 0.01 mm for −2D, 0.2 for −4D, 0.04 for −6D, and 0.05 for −8D and *subtracting* from the center thickness in the case of plus lenses, 0.03 mm for +2D, 0.05 for +4D, and 0.07 for +6D. (2) Find the diagonal line corresponding to the average lens thickness. (3) Follow line down into "wearing zone" for the patient. (4) Draw a vertical line from the intersection of the diagonal line and the lower boundary of the "wearing zone" to the Y axis. (5) Any lens material to the right of the Y axis intersect provides enough oxygen by transmission for the average patient's corneal physiological requirements as described by Holden and Mertz. (From Tomlinson A: *Contact Lens Spectrum* 1990; 5:27. Used by permission.)

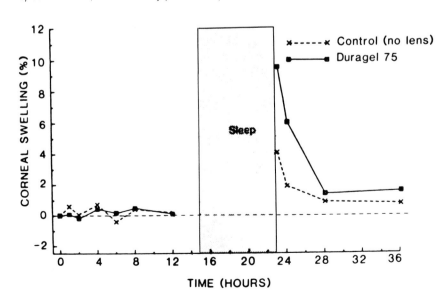

FIG 1–12.
Corneal swelling response as shown for five unadapted subjects wearing a −3D Duragel 75 contact lens continuously for 36 hours on one eye and no lens on the opposite eye. (From Holden BA, Mertz G: *Invest Ophthalmol Vis Sci* 1984; 25:1161. Used by permission.)

TABLE 1–3.

Oxygen Transmissibility of Hydrogel and Rigid Gas-Permeable Contact Lenses*

Lens	Manufacturer	Water Content (%)	BVP† (D)	L_{avg}‡ (μm)	Dk§	Calculated Dk/L‖
U3	Bausch & Lomb Pharmaceuticals	42.0	−3.00	73	9	12
O4	Bausch & Lomb Pharmaceuticals	40.5	−3.00	43	9	20
Hydrocurve II	Barnes-Hind Pharmaceuticals	53.5	−3.50	78	16	21
Permaflex	Coopervision	72.5	−3.25	165	34	21
Boston IV	Polymer Technology Corp.		−2.62	183	18	10
Equalens	Polymer Technology Corp.		−2.75	182	44	24
Paraperm EW	Paragon Optical		−3.25	193	39	20
Fluoropolymer	3M		−3.50	187	78	42

*From Bruce AS, Brennan NA: *Surv Ophthalmol* 1990; 35:25. Used by permission.
†BVP = back vertex power.
‡Average lens thickness for the central 4-mm diameter.
§Material permeability [units of × 10^{-11} (cm^2 × mL O_2)/(sec × mL × mm Hg)].
‖Lens oxygen transmissibility [units of × 10^{-9} (cm × ml O_2)/(sec × mL × mm Hg)].

another, variability will also occur with different lens powers in the same contact lens material. Holden et al.[60] found that high-powered minus lenses produce significantly more central swelling than lower-powered minus power lenses, indicating that the greater average thickness of the former (because of thicker periphery) was a major factor in determining the relative response. Hill[43] has shown that the oxygen available under a contact lens varies from the center to the edge, depending on the profile of the lens. Although the adaptation to extended wear, overnight edema suggested by Mandell[77] may be in question as an artifact of a decrease in epithelial thickness as a result of lens wear,[58] it is true that the number of striae noted in this mode of wear

shows a reduction and suggests some true reduction in corneal edema. Cox et al.[10] have noted that experienced extended contact lens wearers show less overnight swelling response to new materials than new wearers.

Equivalent Oxygen Percentage Measurements

Another technique that measures the effect of contact lens wear on living tissue (either in the rabbit or the human eye) is the measurement of EOP employed by Hill.[46] Based on the original work of Hill and Fatt,[50] this technique compares living eye responses with lens wear to the eye's response to oxygen environments up to 21% (the

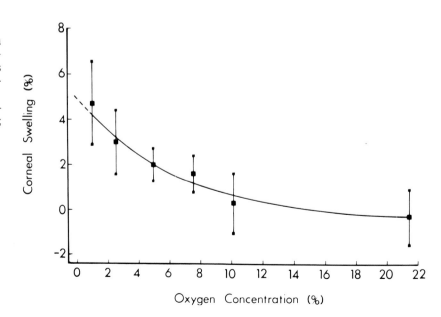

FIG 1–13.
Mean corneal swelling response for a group of subjects after 8 hours of exposure to various oxygen concentrations within a gas goggle. The curve is an exponential fit. The error represents ±1 S.D. (From Holden BA, Sweeney DS, Sanderson G: *Invest Ophthalmol Vis Sci* 1984; 25:476. Used by permission.)

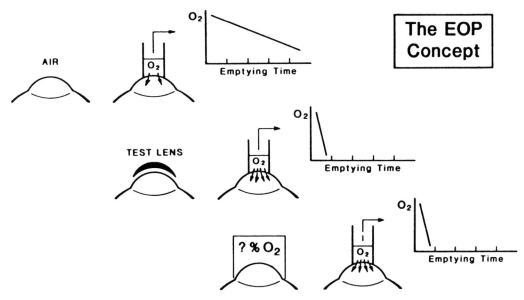

FIG 1–14.

The general concept of equivalent oxygen percentage *(EOP)* determination. *Top,* corneal oxygen uptake from a standard volume (probe) reservoir after stabilization in air (21% O$_2$); *middle,* corneal oxygen uptake rate just after stabilization under a (test) contact lens; *bottom,* searching for that particular oxygen percentage (held over the cornea in a goggle) that produces the same (equivalent) response from the cornea as did the contact lens. That matching oxygen percentage is then taken as the EOP response value of that material for that thickness that resided immediately over the corneal site measured. (From Hill RM: *Contact Lens Spectrum* 1988; 3:34. Used by permission.)

EOP). The values obtained refer strictly to measurements taken in Columbus, Ohio (altitude 235 m above sea level); for all other altitudes, corrections should be made.

The basic principles of the technique are shown in Figure 1–14. For any one material, measurements are taken as follows: First, the cornea's oxygen demand from a standard volume probe reservoir placed in contact with the cornea is measured after the cornea's exposure to nor-

mal atmospheric oxygen (21%). The oxygen debt or demand in millimeters of mercury per second is illustrated as a graph, the shallow slope showing relatively low oxygen demand in these circumstances. A contact lens made from the test material is placed on the cornea for 5 minutes. It is then removed, and the oxygen demand is measured in terms of the time taken for the oxygen within the reservoir to become depleted. This rate of decay is compared with a

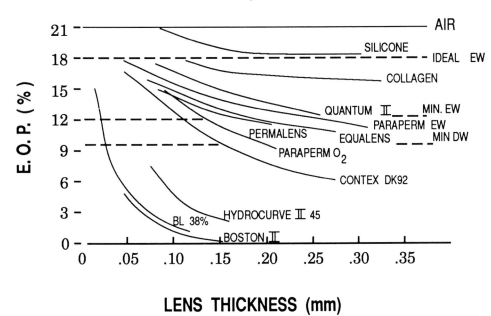

LENS THICKNESS (mm)

FIG 1–15.

Equivalent oxygen percentages *(EOPs)* for various thicknesses of hydrogel and gaspermeable contact lens materials. The values shown on this graph are derived from a number of sources.[5, 35, 41, 43, 48, 94]

FIG 1–16.
Empirically based model for relating equivalent oxygen percentage *(EOP)* to DK (material permeability) for lenses of various thicknesses at eye temperature, 36° C. The minimum EOP levels below which expenditure of corneal energy reserves and the development of corneal edema occurs have been indicated. (From Hill RM: *Int Contact Lens Clin* 1984; 11:118. Used by permission.)

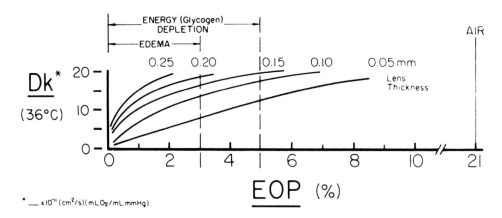

series of standardized curves obtained in known gas environments (≤21% oxygen). By this comparison of "decay" curves, it is possible to determine the EOP underneath the contact lens material.

There are certain advantages to this technique. First, the technique has the benefit of being an on eye (end point response) of the cornea to contact lens wear. Second, it is an in situ technique taken in normal eye conditions, allowing the influence of blink, tear chemistry, eye temperature, and atmospheric effects on contact lens materials (e.g., hydrogel lens dehydration) to contribute to the response of the cornea. Finally, it has the benefit of not being susceptible to some of the measurement errors inherent in other techniques.[29]

Hill has used the EOP technique extensively on contact lens materials that are currently in use.[59,61] The benefit of this technique is that it gives practitioners a means of seeing the thicknesses in which contact lenses may be cut

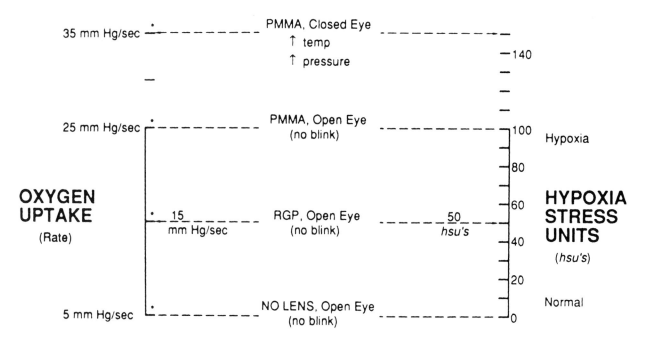

* *Absolute rates may vary slightly, but a relative scale of 100 hsu's always spans the NO LENS (Open Eye) response to the PMMA (Open Eye) response range.*

FIG 1–17.
Relationship of the patient's oxygen uptake rates under open eye nonwearing (0 hypoxic stress units *[HSUS]*), and open eye static polymethylmethacrylate (PMMA)–wearing (100 HSU) conditions. Also illustrated is the effect of closing the lid over the PMMA lens on driving the hypoxic stress level to a value greater than 100 HSUs. The HSU provides an alternative unit to EOP or Dk in describing the effect of a contact lens on corneal physiology. (From Hill RM, Szczotka L: *Contact Lens Spectrum* 1991; 6:31. Used by permission.)

to provide the currently accepted minimum standards of oxygenization for daily and extended wear.[59, 61] Figure 1–15 shows a composite figure derived from the literature on measurements of EOP for the various contact lens materials.[5, 35, 41, 45, 48, 49, 94] The figure shows commonly used contact lens materials, as well as those that define the limits of current technology.

Resolution

There are correlations between the measurements of oxygen availability with contact lenses obtained by the three techniques just described. Lenses with higher Dk and thinner average thicknesses will produce less corneal swelling and a higher EOP measurement. It should be stressed, however, that Dk/L and EOP are different measurements that, though correlated, are not exactly the same. Correla-

tions of the measurements of Dk/L and EOP have been found to be high at around 0.95.[38, 105] It is interesting that the graph of EOP vs. Dk/L shows a plateau at around 16% EOP.[25] This suggests that increasing oxygen supply to the cornea through a contact lens beyond this level would not benefit physiology. This 16% value correlates well with the oxygen transmissibility index between 75 and 100 reported by O'Neill et al.[88] and Holden et al.[60] required to obviate adverse effects on corneal metabolism (edema) during extended contact lens wear.[25] Similar correlations are found between the EOP performance measurements of Hill[46] and corneal swelling responses.

The temptation is great to directly equate Dk/L and EOP measurements in view of their frequent appearance in the literature describing the oxygen availability beneath contact lenses. Hill[44] has described an empiric model relating the two measurements from the same group of lenses

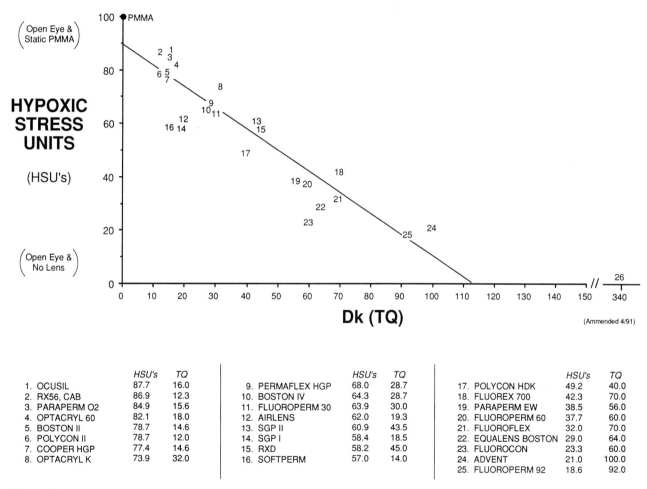

	HSU's	TQ			HSU's	TQ			HSU's	TQ
1. OCUSIL	87.7	16.0		9. PERMAFLEX HGP	68.0	28.7		17. POLYCON HDK	49.2	40.0
2. RX56, CAB	86.9	12.3		10. BOSTON IV	64.3	28.7		18. FLUOREX 700	42.3	70.0
3. PARAPERM O2	84.9	15.6		11. FLUOROPERM 30	63.9	30.0		19. PARAPERM EW	38.5	56.0
4. OPTACRYL 60	82.1	18.0		12. AIRLENS	62.0	19.3		20. FLUOROPERM 60	37.7	60.0
5. BOSTON II	78.7	14.6		13. SGP II	60.9	43.5		21. FLUOROFLEX	32.0	70.0
6. POLYCON II	78.7	12.0		14. SGP I	58.4	18.5		22. EQUALENS BOSTON	29.0	64.0
7. COOPER HGP	77.4	14.6		15. RXD	58.2	45.0		23. FLUOROCON	23.3	60.0
8. OPTACRYL K	73.9	32.0		16. SOFTPERM	57.0	14.0		24. ADVENT	21.0	100.0
								25. FLUOROPERM 92	18.6	92.0

FIG 1–18.
Relationship of HSU values measured for a collection of rigid-gas permeable lenses, all 0.16 mm thick, and their commonly cited Dk values. The linear best fit shown here serves reasonably well for a low and moderate Dk cases, but high Dk materials may require a curvalinear fit, indicating that greater increments of Dk would be required to relieve the last vestiges of hypoxic stress. Material 26 is Silsoft (HSUs = 3, Dk = 340). (From Hill RM, Szczotka L: *Contact Lens Spectrum* 1991; 6:31. Used by permission.)

(Fig 1–16). If the EOP is known for a contact lens, say, 0.05 mm thick, the number can be used to determine a Dk estimate for the material. For example, if the EOP = 7%, Dk = 17×10^{-11} (cm^2/sec) $(mL\ O_2/mL \times mm\ Hg)$, and when divided by L (in centimeters), a Dk/L of 34×10^{-9} (cm/sec) $(mL\ O_2/mL \times mm\ Hg)$ is found.

Hypoxic Stress Measurement of Oxygen Availability Under Contact Lenses

Recently, Hill and Szczotka[53] described the oxygen performance of contact lens materials on the cornea by a new rating system for corneal response to lens transmissivity. This is based on the relative scale of 0 to 100 HSUs where zero represents the cornea's normal (open eye, non–lens wearing oxygen uptake rate, i.e., no hypoxic stress) and 100 represents the cornea's oxygen demand associated with an immobile, impermeable (PMMA) lens sitting on an open eye (i.e., severe hypoxic stress).

Figure 1–17 summarizes the relationship of corneal oxygen uptake rates to the relative scale of HSUs. Because any given lens tends to evoke a similar HSU response from different eyes,[53] the relative scale is a convenient index for clinicians to make comparisons between lenses. More than 100 HSUs will be achieved in the presence of an impermeable, static hard lens worn under closed lid. In such circumstances, the closed eye environment with its higher temperature and consequent higher metabolic rate will create a greater oxygen demand in the cornea.

Figure 1–18 summarizes the HSU-rated performances of 25 RGP materials in 0.16-mm thicknesses; the common Dk values are listed for the same materials.[53] A good linear relationship is found between HSU and Dk scales for low and moderately permeable hard contact lens materials. In the future this new system of comparing the physiological performance of contact lens materials could receive wide acceptance by clinicians.

CONCLUSION

Patients have benefitted from the work of many researchers in corneal physiology and the efforts of the practitioners and the contact lens industry in producing new designs and materials that have dramatically improved the health of the eye during contact lens wear. The signposts erected by researchers and the new directions forged by industry and practitioners are testaments to the collaborative efforts of many in reducing the anoxia-related complications of lens wear. All of the problems have not been solved, as may be evidenced by later chapters, but our understanding is much greater than 20 years ago. The contact lens field, like many other areas of clinical science, has experienced an information explosion in recent times; it is up to practitioners to use this information to the maximum benefit of their patients.

REFERENCES

1. Ang JHB, Efron N: Carbon dioxide permeability of contact lens materials. *Int Contact Lens Clin* 1989; 16:48.
2. Brennan NA, Efron N, Holden BA: Further developments in the RGP Dk controversy. *Int Eye Care* 1986; 2:508.
3. Brennan NA, Efron N, Holden BA: Methodology for determining the intrinsic oxygen permeability of contact lens materials. *Clin Exp Optom* 1987; 70:42.
4. Brennan NA, Efron N, Newman SD: An examination of the "edge effect" in the measurement of contact lens oxygen transmissibility. *Int Contact Lens Clin* 1987; 14:407.
5. Brezinski SD, Hill RM: The new superpermeables. *Contact Lens Forum* 1986; 11:22.
6. Brown SI, Dervichian DG: Hydrodynamics of blinking. *Arch Ophthalmol* 1969; 82:541.
7. Bruce AS, Brennan NA: Corneal pathophysiology with contact lenses. *Surv Ophthalmol* 1990; 35:25.
8. Burger RE: Effect of contact lens motion on the oxygen tension distribution under the lens. *Am J Optom Physiol Opt* 1974; 57:441.
9. Conway HD: The motion of a contact lens over the eye during blinking. *Am J Optom Physiol Optics* 1982; 59:770.
10. Cox I, Zantos S, Osborne GN: The overnight swelling response of long wearing daily wear and extended wear lens patients. *Int Contact Lens Clin* 1990; 17:134.
11. Cuklanz HD, Hill RM: Oxygen requirements of corneal contact lens systems. *Am J Optom Arch Am Acad Optom* 1969; 46:228.
12. Cuklanz HD, Hill RM: Oxygen requirements of corneal contact lens systems: 1. Comparison of mathematical predictions with physiological measurements. *Am J Optom Arch Am Acad Optom* 1969; 46:662.
13. Doane NG: Interaction of eyelids and tears in corneal wetting and the dynamics of the normal human eye blink. *Am J Ophthalmol* 1980; 89:507.
14. Efron N, Ang JHB: Corneal hypoxia and hypercapnia during contact lens wear. *Am J Optom Physiol Opt* 1990; 67:512.
15. Efron N, Brennan NE: Simple measurement of oxygen transmission. *Aust J Optom* 1985; 68:27.
16. Efron N, Brennan NA, Holden BA: The oxygen permeability of rigid gas permeable contact lens materials: Reaching a consensus. *Trans Br Cont Lens Conf* 1987, p 62.
17. Efron N, Carney LG: Oxygen levels beneath the closed eyelid. *Invest Ophthalmol Vis Sci* 1979; 18:93.
18. Efron N, Holden BA: Review of some common contact lens complications, part 2. *Optician* 1986; 192(5062):17.

19. Efron N, Swarbrick H: How much oxygen does the cornea really need? *Int Eye Care* 1986; 2:154.

20. Fatt I: *Physiology of the Eye. An Introduction to Vegetative Functions.* Stoneham, Mass, Butterworth, 1978, p 123.

21. Fatt I: *Physiology of the Eye. An Introduction to Vegetative Functions.* Stoneham, Mass, Butterworth, 1978, p 131.

22. Fatt I: *Physiology of the Eye. An Introduction to Vegetative Functions.* Stoneham, Mass, Butterworth, 1978, p 161.

23. Fatt I: *Physiology of the Eye. An Introduction to Vegetative Function.* Stoneham, Mass, Butterworth, 1978, p 164.

24. Fatt I: Gas permeability and corneal integrity maintenance. *Contact Lens Forum* 1979; 4:99.

25. Fatt I: The superpermeable rigid lens for extended wear. *Contact Lens Spectrum* 1986; 1:53.

26. Fatt I, Bieber MT: The steady state distribution of oxygen and carbon dioxide in the in vivo cornea: I. The open eye in air and the closed eye. *Exp Eye Res* 1968; 7:103.

27. Fatt I, Freeman RD, Lin D: Oxygen tension distributions in the cornea: A re-examination. *Exp Eye Res* 1974; 18:357.

28. Fatt I, Hill RM: Oxygen tension under a contact lens during blinking—a comparison of theory and experimental observations. *Am J Optom Am Acad Optom* 1970; 47:50–61.

29. Fatt I, Rasson JE, Melpolder JB: Measuring oxygen permeability of gas permeable hard and hydrogel lenses and flat samples in air. *Int Contact Lens Clin* 1987; 14:389.

30. Ferris RL, Rakahashi GH, Donne A: Oxygen flux across the in vivo rabbit cornea. *Arch Ophthalmol* 1965; 74:679.

31. Fink BA, Carney LG, Hill RM: Influence of palpebral aperture height on tear pump efficiency. *Optom Vis Sci* 1990; 67:287.

32. Fink BA, Hill RM, Carney LG: Corneal oxygenation: Blink frequency as a variable in rigid contact lens wear. *Br J Ophthalmol* 1990; 74:168.

33. Fink BA, Hill RM, Carney LG: Influence of rigid contact lens overall and optic zone diameters on tear pump efficiency. *Optom Vis Sci* 1990; 67:641.

34. Fitzgerald JK, Jones DP: Oxygen flux data can be misleading. *Int Contact Lens Clin* 1978; 5:61.

35. Flynn WJ, Hill RM: The oxygen performance of hard gas permeables. *Contact Lens Forum* 1984; 9:61.

36. Freeman RD: Oxygen consumption by the component layers of the cornea. *J Physiol* 1972; 225:15.

37. Gilman BG: Eye and contact lens movement measurement. *Am J Optom Physiol Opt* 1982; 59:602.

38. Grecko A: On oxygen, EOP vs. Dk vs. Dk/L. *Int Eye Care* 1985; 1:216.

39. Hamano H, et al: Effects of contact lens wear on the mitosis with corneal epithelium and lactate content in aqueous humor of rabbit. *Jpn J Ophthalmol* 1983; 27:451.

40. Hill RM: Perils of the pump. *Int Contact Lens Clin* 1976; 3:49.

41. Hill RM: Behind the closed lid. *Int Contact Lens Clin* 1977; 4:68.

42. Hill RM: Oxygen insights. *Contact Lens J* 1983; 11:3.

43. Hill RM: Topping up the oxygen. *Int Contact Lens Clin* 1983; 10:299–300.

44. Hill RM: Defining a Dk: *Int Contact Lens Clin* 1984; 11:118.

45. Hill RM: Hydrophilic "horse trades." *Int Contact Lens Clin* 1984; 11:190.

46. Hill RM: What is EOP? *Contact Lens Spectrum* 1988; 3:35.

47. Hill RM, Andrasko GA: Oxygen and water. *J Am Optom Assoc* 1981; 52:225–226.

48. Hill RM, Brezinski SD: The great water race. *Contact Lens Spectrum* 1986; 1:21.

49. Hill RM, Brezinski SD: The superpermeables. *Contact Lens Spectrum* 1987; 2:60.

50. Hill RM, Fatt I: Oxygen uptake from reservoir of limited volume by a human cornea. *Science* 1963; 142:1295.

51. Hill RM, Fatt I: Oxygen measurements under a contact lens. *Am J Optom Arch Am Acad Optom* 1964; 41:382.

52. Hill RM, Rengsdorf RH, Petrali JP, Critical oxygen requirement of the corneal epithelium as indicated by succinic dehydrogenase. *Am J Optom* 1974; 51:331.

53. Hill RM, Szczotka L: Hypoxic stress units: Another look at oxygen performance of RGP lenses on the cornea. *Contact Lens Spectrum* 1991; 6(4):31.

54. Hill RM, Uniacke NP: Lacrimal fluid and lens design. *Contacto* 1968; 12:59.

55. Holden BA: Adverse effects of contact lenses: A brief review. *J Br Contact Lens Assoc* 1988; 5:69.

56. Holden BA: The ocular response to contact lens wear. *Am J Optom Physiol Opt* 1989; 66:717.

57. Holden BA, et al: Recovery of the human cornea following long-term extended wear of hydrogel contact lenses. Proceedings of the Seventh Congress of the European Society of Ophthalmology, Helsinki, 1984, p 273.

58. Holden BA, et al: The Dk project: An interlaboratory comparison of Dk/L measurements. *Optom Vis Sci* 1990; 67:476–481.

59. Holden BA, Mertz GW: Critical oxygen levels to avoid corneal edema for both daily and extended wear contact lenses. *Invest Ophthalmol Vis Sci* 1984; 25:1161.

60. Holden BA, Mertz G, McNally J: Swelling response to contact lenses worn under extended wear conditions. *Invest Ophthalmol Vis Sci* 1983; 24:218.

61. Holden BA, Sweeney DS, Sanderson G: The minimim pre-corneal oxygen tension to avoid corneal edema. *Invest Ophthalmol Vis Sci* 1984; 25:476.

62. Jaurigi MJ, Fatt I: Estimation of the in vivo oxygen consumption rate of the human corneal epithelium. *Am J Optom Arch Am Acad Optom* 1972; 49:507.

63. King JE, Augsburger A, Hill RM: Quantifying the distribution of lactic acid dehydrogenase in the corneal epithelium with oxygen deprivation. *Am J Optom* 1971; 48:1016.

64. Klyce SD, McCarey BE: Physiology of the cornea, in *Contact Lenses: CLAO Guide to Basic Science and Clinical Practice,* vol I, Chapter 5. Philadelphia, Grune & Stratton, 1986, p 1.

65. Knoll HA, Conway HD: Analysis of blink induced vertical motion of the contact lenses. *Am J Optom Physiol Opt* 1987; 64:153.

66. Kwan M, Fatt I: A non-invasive method of continuous arterial oxygen tension estimation from measured palpebral conjunctival oxygen tension. *Anesthesiology* 1970; 35:309.

67. Kwan M, Niinikoski J, Hunt TK: In vivo measurements of oxygen tension in the cornea, aqueous humor, and anterior lens of the open eye. *Invest Ophthalmol Vis Sci* 1972; 11:108.

68. La Hood D, Sweeney BF, Holden BA: Overnight corneal edema with hydrogel, rigid gas permeable and silicone elastomer contact lenses. *Int Contact Lens Clin* 1988; 15:149.

69. Langham N: Utilization of oxygen by the component layers of the living cornea. *J Physiol* 1952; 117:461.

70. Larke J: The eye in contact lens wear. Stoneham, Mass, Butterworth, 1985, p 106.

71. Larke JR, Parish ST, Wigham CG: Apparent human corneal oxygen uptake rate. *Am J Optom Physiol Opt* 1981; 58:803.

72. Lowther GE, Tomlinson A: A study of the corneal response to the wear of low water content soft lenses. *Am J Optom Physiol Opt* 1979; 56:674.

73. Mader TH, et al: Conjunctival oxygen tension at high altitude. *Aviat Space Environ Med* 1987; 58:76.

74. Mandell RB: What is the minimal corneal oxygen requirement? *Invest Ophthalmol Vis Sci* 1985; 26(suppl):181.

75. Mandell RB: *Contact Lens Practice,* ed 4. Springfield, Ill, Charles C Thomas, Publisher, 1988, p 84.

76. Mandell RB: *Contact Lens Practice,* ed 4. Springfield, Ill, Charles C Thomas, Publisher, 1988, p 87.

77. Mandell RB: *Contact Lens Practice,* ed 4. Springfield, Ill, Charles C Thomas, Publisher, 1988, p 98.

78. Mandell RB: *Contact Lens Practice,* ed 4. Springfield, Ill, Charles C Thomas, Publisher, 1988, p 689.

79. Mandell RB, Farrell R: Corneal swelling at low atmospheric oxygen pressures. *Invest Ophthalmol Vis Sci* 1980; 19:697.

80. Mandell RB, Fatt I: Thinning of the human cornea upon awakening. *Nature* 1965; 208:292.

81. Mandell RB, Polse KA: Corneal thickness changes as a contact lens fitting index—experimental results and a proposed model. *Am J Optom* 1969; 46:479.

82. Mandell RB, Polse KA, Fatt I: Corneal swelling caused by contact lens wear. *Arch Ophthalmol* 1970; 83:3.

83. Maurice DM: The use of fluorescein in ophthalmological research. *Invest Ophthalmol Vis Sci* 1967; 6:464.

84. Maurice DM, Watson PG: The distribution and movement of serum albumin in the cornea. *Exp Eye Res* 1965; 4:355.

85. McMahon TT: Comments on the incidence of ocular complications of contact lens wear. *Int Eye Care* 1985; 1:304.

86. Millodot M, O'Leary DJ: Effect of oxygen deprivation on corneal sensitivity. *Acta Ophthalmol* 1980; 58;434.

87. Ng CO: Doctoral dissertation, Birmingham, England, University of Aston, 1974.

88. O'Neill M, Polse KA, Sarver M: Corneal response to rigid and hydrogel lenses worn during eye closure. *Invest Ophthalmol Vis Sci* 1984; 25:837.

89. Piffaretti JM: A study of the movements of the eyelids during normal closure of the palpebral aperture. *Orbit* 1985; 4:53.

90. Polse KA: Tear flow and hydrogel contact lenses. *Invest Ophthalmol Vis Sci* 1979; 18:409.

91. Polse KA, Mandell RB: Critical oxygen tension at the corneal surface. *Arch Ophthalmol* 1970; 84:505.

92. Quinn TG, Schoessler JP: Human corneal epithelial oxygen demand—population characteristics. *Am J Optom Physiol Opt* 1984; 61:386.

93. Riggs LA, Kelly JP, Manning KA, et al: Blink related eye movements. *Invest Ophthalmol Vis Sci* 1987; 28:334.

94. Schoessler JP, Hill RM: The B and L high Dk RGP material: Pilot studies. *Contact Lens Spectrum* 1987; 2:39.

95. Smelzer G, Ozanics V: Structural changes of corneas of guinea pigs after wearing contact lenses. *Am J Ophthalmol* 1953; 88:543.

96. Smelzer G, Shen D: Physiological changes in the cornea induced by contact lens. *Arch Ophthalmol* 1955; 53:676.

97. Thoft RA, Friend J: Biochemical aspects of contact lens wear. *Am J Ophthalmol* 1975; 80:139.

98. Tomlinson A: Choice of materials—a material issue. *Contact Lens Spectrum* 1990; 5:27.

99. Tomlinson A, Bibby MM: Determination of the effective diameter for the calculation of equivalent thickness of soft contact lenses. *Am J Optom Physiol Opt* 1985; 62:398.

100. Tomlinson A, Haack C: Physiological response of the cornea to the fit of CAB contact lenses. *Int Contact Lens Clin* 1982; 9:347.

101. Tomlinson A, Soni PS: Effect of the design and fitting of soft lenses on corneal physiology. *J Br Contact Lens Assoc* 1980; 3:161.

102. Tomlinson A, Soni SP: Peripheral curve design and tear pump mechanism of soft contact lenses. *Am J Optom Physiol Opt* 1980; 57:356.

103. Turnbull DK, et al: Oxygen flux through dry and wet hard gas permeable contact lenses. *J Br Contact Lens Assoc* 1986; 9:75.

104. White P, Scott C: Contact lenses and solutions summary. *Contact Lens Spectrum* 1990; 5(suppl 8).

105. Wilson GS, Roscoe WR: Equivalent oxygen percentage (EOP) technique: A standard calibration curve. *Am J Optom Physiol Opt* 1984; 61:601–604.

Hypoxic Changes in the Corneal Epithelium and Stroma

Joseph A. Bonanno, O.D., Ph.D.

Kenneth A. Polse, O.D., M.S.

Studies by numerous investigators spanning the last 40 years have solidly established that wearing a contact lens can reduce the corneal oxygen tension. Hypoxia has been implicated, either directly or indirectly, as the cause of many complications associated with contact lens wear (see Chapter 1). Many of the problems seen in the early days of contact lens use, such as overwear syndrome, corneal clouding, and warping, can be virtually eliminated by the use of gas-permeable (GP) soft or hard lenses. The advances in lens technology, which allow greater oxygen diffusion to the cornea, has given the clinician much more flexibility in patient management. However, these same improvements have in some cases pushed wearing times to the extreme limit and given us a new set of problems, such as corneal infection, potentially more devastating to the patient. This transition from non-GP lens use (i.e., polymethylmethacrylate [PMMA] lenses) to GP (soft and rigid) lenses has also focused our attention on the chronic effects of hypoxia because with proper management the acute effects can be reduced considerably.

Chronic hypoxia may have both morphological (e.g., endothelial polymegathism) and functional consequences. The concept of "hypoxic dose," a parameter that takes into account the level of hypoxia and years of oxygen reduction, has been recently introduced.[52] Individuals who have had a significant hypoxic dose have slightly poorer corneal hydration control as measured in a corneal stress test when compared with nonlens wearers; however, clinical examination would not reveal any apparent disfunction. Because these patients are not having any problems, should we be concerned? One fear is that these patients may be at greater risk for corneal decompensation after the stress of cataract surgery. Although no hard evidence can be provided showing that as the population ages lens wearers will tend to have more problems, it seems prudent at this point to provide contact lens patients with lenses and wearing schedules that will minimize the hypoxic dose.

This chapter reviews some of the basic corneal physiology related to contact lens–induced hypoxia. Glucose is "burned" by oxygen to supply energy for cell function. In that the cornea is avascular, how does it get its oxygen and glucose? Why is oxygen necessary? What happens when the supply is insufficient? How are the physiological effects of hypoxia related to what is seen clinically? What are the mechanisms by which mild long-term hypoxia causes morphological or functional changes in the cornea? How can the hypoxic changes be prevented or reversed? The goal is to provide the reader with sufficient background for (1) understanding the known etiologies of hypoxic corneal changes, (2) contemplating the possible etiologies of hypoxic changes that are not understood, and (3) arriving at a proper clinical management.

CORNEAL TRANSPARENCY

The function of the cornea is to provide a smooth, regular, and transparent refracting element for the eye. Most body tissues are more or less opaque because of the net effect of light absorption, reflection, and small particle light scattering (particles smaller than the wavelength of light). During absorption, the energy of a photon is captured and reradiated as heat or fluorescent light. In the cornea, very little visible light is absorbed; however, at less than 310 nm (i.e., ultraviolet [UV]), there is strong absorption by corneal proteins, mainly collagen, and cellular nucleic acids (DNA and RNA). High doses of UV light will damage epithelial DNA, causing severe keratopathy.

Reflection is caused by the interaction of light with particles larger than its wavelength that have an index of refraction different from the surrounding medium. In the stroma only the keratocytes are large enough to reflect light, and because they are between the stromal lamellae, we can observe a fine lamellar appearance to the stroma when it is viewed in the slit lamp. Relatively large differences in refractive index also occur at the surfaces of the epithelium and endothelium and are easily visualized in the slit lamp. Subcellular organelles such as mitochondria are also larger than the wavelength of light and will reflect light traversing the epithelium, keratocytes, and endothelium. The endothelium has a high concentration of mitochondria but is very thin (5 μm), yielding very little net reflection. The epithelium is relatively thick (50 μm), but it contains very few mitochondria. The stromal keratocytes also contain mitochondria, but these cells are relatively diffuse. The lack of mitochondria is thus a strategy used to enhance transparency. The tradeoff is that the epithelium must rely heavily on glycolytic (nonoxygen-using) metabolic pathways to generate cellular energy (see the discussion of corneal cell function and oxygen).

In the cornea, small particle scatter is caused primarily by the collagen fibrils of the stroma. Maurice[44] advanced the hypothesis that the orderly arrangement of the collagen fibrils acts as a perfect crystal lattice, producing destructive interference of the scattered light. Hart and Farrell[25] later showed that a perfect orderly arrangement is not found in electron micrographs of the stroma and went on to demonstrate that a perfect lattice is not necessary for transparency, the main requirement for destructive interference being that the local density of scatterers (collagen fibrils) is uniform. For example, if a small volume of stroma is selected and the number of collagen fibrils is counted in this volume and also in an adjacent area of equal volume, if the numbers are very much the same, destructive interference will predominate. When the stroma becomes edematous, the collagen fibril distance increases, the density of fibrils is less uniform, and more light is scattered.[2, 14] In the opaque sclera, the collagen fibrils do not have a uniform density. However, if the sclera is dried or made very thin (e.g., staphyloma), it will appear transparent because the fibers are compressed into a smaller space and the variation in fiber density decreased. Overall, light transmission through the rabbit cornea is 80% at 400 nm and 98% at 700 nm,[14] which is pretty good considering all of the opportunities for reflection and light scatter.

MAINTENANCE OF TRANSPARENCY: PUMP-LEAK HYPOTHESIS

The corneal stroma is composed mainly of collagen fibrils (a protein), a glycosaminoglycan (GAG; the old term was mucopolysaccharide), and glycoprotein ground substance. The ground substance of the stroma provides the cross-linking braces between collagen fibrils. The GAGS are hydrophilic and will absorb fluid like a gel. This is the basis for the imbibition pressure of the stroma.[45] Bare stroma, without epithelium or endothelium, soaking in isotonic saline solution, will absorb many times its weight in fluid. Edematous corneas show a wide range of collagen fibril density and also the appearance of "lakes," or separations, between stromal lamellae,[2] both of which lead to extensive light scatter. It is the function of the corneal epithelium and endothelium to maintain stromal hydration low enough that light scatter is minimized.

Maintenance of stromal hydration is achieved because of the passive barrier properties of the cell layers and the active fluid pumping of these layers. The barrier function alone, however, simply acts to slow down the rate at which water, driven by the stromal imbibition pressure, will leak across the cell layers. This leak must be exactly offset by active fluid pumping to maintain a constant stromal hydration. "Active" implies the use of energy. Interfering with energy production by use of metabolic poisons[12] or cooling down the cornea[11] causes the cornea to swell. Thus, the presence of this active component, taken together with the stroma's passive tendency to swell, has led to the pump-Leak hypothesis for maintenance of corneal hydration,[45] illustrated in Figure 2–1.

Epithelial cell layers in general do not move fluid directly by "water pumps." Instead they pump ions from one side of the cells to the other so that water can follow these ions by osmosis. Both the corneal epithelium and endothelium contain ion pumps, but the endothelium accounts for at least 90% of the total fluid pump.[36, 45] Damage to the endothelium from trauma (e.g., intraocular surgery) or disease (e.g., chronic high intraocular pressure [IOP] or Fuchs' endothelial dystrophy) will lead to corneal edema, light scatter, and poor vision. In contrast, the epithelium is an important barrier to the outside world. The epithelial resistance to water flow is about twice that of the endothelium.[47] The epithelium is also constantly renewing itself, shedding its superficial cells. Microbes attached to the superficial cells are washed away in the tears, not allowing a

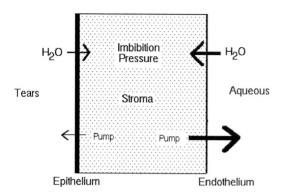

FIG 2–1.
Schematic drawing of an anteroposterior cross-section of the cornea demonstrating the pump-leak hypothesis for maintenance of corneal hydration. The stromal imbibition pressure is the driving force for water to leak across the epithelial and endothelial cell layers. The relatively larger arrow indicating water leak from aqueous to stroma compared with the arrow showing the leak from tears to stroma suggests that the water conductivity across the endothelium is about twice that across the epithelium. This leak must be exactly counterbalanced by a pump mechanism for corneal hydration to remain at a steady state. The relatively large endothelial pump arrow indicates that at least 90% of the cornea's pumping is from this cell layer.

sufficient resident time for microbial penetration. Therefore, interference in epithelial function from either contact lens wear, disease, or trauma increase the likelihood of corneal infection.

OXYGEN PATHWAYS TO THE CORNEA

Oxygen and glucose are typically brought very close to body tissues via the blood. Blood cells and blood vessels, however, will cause significant amounts of light reflection. Therefore, to be transparent, the cornea is avascular and as such must receive its oxygen by diffusion from the adjacent areas: (1) tears, (2) limbus, and (3) aqueous humor. When the eyes are open, the tear oxygen tension is that of the air, 155 mm Hg. When the lids are closed, the tear oxygen tension is determined by oxygen diffusion from the palpebral conjunctival blood vessels and is estimated to be 55 mm Hg.[15] Removing oxygen from the tears by placing a tight fitting goggle over the eye and perfusing the goggle with pure nitrogen produces the effects of contact lens wear.[59, 60] This produces stromal swelling and corneal clouding and demonstrates the importance of oxygen delivery by the tears.

The limbal blood vessels could provide oxygen to the cornea, but because of the long diffusion distance and rapid consumption of oxygen in the cornea, this is probably not significant beyond the peripheral cornea.[45] Calculations of oxygen flux across the endothelial surface for the open eye show a small movement from anterior chamber to cornea.[15] Experimental data, however, have shown oxygen flux in the open eye to be from aqueous to cornea,[41] as well as from cornea to aqueous.[1] Nevertheless, in the closed eye, when tear oxygen tension approximates aqueous oxygen tension, there will be a net flux from aqueous to cornea.[15]

Oxygen delivery to the tears in the lens-wearing eye must be caused by diffusion through the lens, via tear pumping around the lens, or both. The oxygen permeability (Dk) of soft lenses is directly related to lens hydra-

tion.[58] In contrast, rigid GP (RGP) lenses have little or no water content, and their oxygen permeability is determined by the chemical composition of the plastic. The oxygen tension underneath a stationary lens can be predicted from the lens oxygen transmissibility, Dk/L (where O_2 transmissibility is inversely related to the lens thickness, L) (see Chapter 1).[16]

Tear pumping has been recognized as a significant source of oxygen, as well as a pathway for removal of metabolic waste products (e.g., carbon dioxide) and dead epithelial cells. Subjects wearing impermeable polymethylmethacrylate (PMMA) lenses will show substantial stromal swelling within a few hours. Polse and Mandell[54] showed that this swelling could be relieved if the eye was covered by a goggle through which pure oxygen was being passed. Because the lens is essentially impermeable to oxygen, it must be getting underneath the lens by tear pumping. The steady-state oxygen tension behind a PMMA lens was shown to be a function of the blink frequency, percent tear exchange with each blink, and the volume of the tear reservoir behind the lens.[17, 18] The percent tear exchange and tear reservoir volume are much reduced in soft relative to hard lenses.[51] This leads to less stromal edema with hard than soft lenses of the same Dk/L in the open eye.[29] This difference in tear exchange is also apparent in the relative amount of debris often seen trapped behind soft lenses, especially if they are worn continuously.

CORNEAL CELL FUNCTION AND OXYGEN

Cell Homeostatis

All cells precisely regulate their internal environment to maintain viability and preserve function. Ion gradients are established across cell membranes that are responsible for the maintenance of internal pH, calcium concentration, and regulation of cell volume and the ion transport pathways for moving fluid osmotically. Cells have very low internal sodium concentrations and very high potassium concentrations relative to the extracellular fluids. This gradient is established by the Na$^+$/K$^+$ adenosine triphosphatase (ATPase), which pumps Na$^+$ out of cells in exchange for K$^+$ into the cells. This requires energy in the form of adenosine triphosphate (ATP). High Na$^+$ concentrations in the extracellular space and low Na$^+$ concentrations in the cytoplasm constitute a chemical gradient (which can be thought of as a potential energy source) that can drive other molecules into or out of cells against their chemical gradients. For example, cells often need to accumulate glucose and amino acids in concentrations higher than the extracellular fluid. This can be accomplished by tapping the energy in the Na$^+$ gradient to help drive glucose and amino acids into cells against their chemical gradients. Special membrane proteins have evolved, Na$^+$-glucose and Na$^+$–amino acid transporters, which provide this function (Fig 2–2,A).

The Na$^+$ gradient can also be used to regulate the concentrations of other important cytoplasmic ions. Regulation of cytoplasmic pH is very important because many rate-limiting biochemical steps (e.g., the enzyme phosphofructokinase in glycolysis) and cellular functions (e.g., mitotic activity) are pH sensitive. Another important ion is calcium. Calcium modulates many cell functions, such as cell migration during wound healing and ion/water permeability of epithelial cells. The free Ca^{2+} concentration in the cytoplasm is about 10,000 times lower than the extracellular Ca^{2+} concentration. When cells are severely stressed, intracellular Ca^{2+} concentrations can approach the extracellular concentration. At these levels cell membranes and mitochondria are disrupted, and cell death can ensue.[9] To regulate internal pH and Ca^{2+} concentrations, cells contain separate membrane proteins called Na$^+$/H$^+$ and Na$^+$/Ca^{2+} exchangers. That is, Na$^+$ moves into the cell down its chemical gradient, and a proton or Ca^{2+} ion moves out of the cell against its chemical gradients. These functions are summarized in Figure 2–2,A.

Finally, these ion gradients are essential for fluid pumping. For example, in the corneal endothelium, poisoning the Na$^+$/K$^+$ ATPase or reducing the ATP supply by inhibiting metabolism will shut down fluid movement.[20] The exact mechanisms by which fluid transport is coupled to ion transport is only partially understood for the corneal endothelium. The current evidence indicates that the net transport of Na$^+$ and bicarbonate ions from stroma to aqueous humor provides the osmotic gradient for fluid movement across the endothelium.[45] Because HCO$_3^-$ concentrations are intimately tied to the ambient pH, it is likely that one or more of the membrane pH regulators, such as Na$^+$/H$^+$ exchange, will have a role in endothelial fluid transport. A hypothetical model of transendothelial HCO$_3^-$ transport is shown in Figure 2–2,B.

The epithelium and endothelium must also maintain their fluid barrier function. To present a continuous barrier, cells attach to each other by protein seals called *tight*

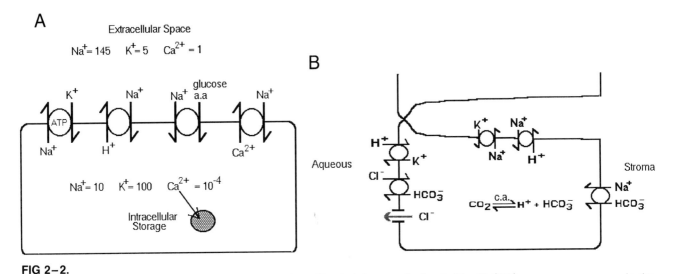

FIG 2–2.
A, extracellular and intracellular ion concentrations (in millimolar) for a typical cell. The Na$^+$/K$^+$ pump uses energy in the form of adenosine triphosphate *(ATP)* to move Na$^+$ out and K$^+$ into the cell. This establishes the chemical gradient for Na$^+$ (145 outside and 10 inside). Other membrane proteins then use this Na$^+$ gradient to pump H$^+$ out, glucose and amino acids in, and Ca^{2+} out of cells. Intracellular Ca^{2+} is further regulated by intracellular storage organelles such as endoplasmic reticulum, mitochondria, and calciosomes. **B,** hypothetical model for corneal endothelial bicarbonate transport. The Na$^+$/K$^+$ pump first establishes the Na$^+$ gradient. An Na$^+$-HCO$_3^-$ cotransport mechanism acts at the basolateral (stromal) side to move HCO$_3^-$ into the cell. Na$^+$/H$^+$ and K$^+$/H$^+$ exchange mechanisms help to maintain intracellular pH at a high level so that intracellular HCO$_3^-$ concentration is kept high. Carbonic anhydrase is present to speed the conversion of CO$_2$ to HCO$_3^-$. At the apical (aqueous) side, a Cl$^-$/HCO$_3^-$ exchanger moves HCO$_3^-$ out into the aqueous. The accumulation of HCO$_3^-$ at the apical side then acts as an osmotic stimulus to draw water out of the stroma.

junctions. Without these seals there would be gaps between the cells through which fluid and ions could easily move. In the case of the endothelium, these seals could be damaged by trauma or degraded by normal wear and tear, and the cells would need to respond by synthesizing new tight junction proteins. In the case of epithelium, however, these tight junctions are constantly broken and lost as superficial cells are sloughed off. Therefore, the proteins making up the tight junctions are constantly resynthesized, they are transported to the cell membrane, and the seals are reformed in the cell layer just below the most superficial layer. This is a very dynamic process, which requires both protein and RNA synthesis.[65] Furthermore, the epithelial thickness and cell number remains constant (completely renewing every 7 days), so there is substantial cell mitotic activity. All of this requires energy, which is provided by cells burning glucose to make ATP. Inadequate energy supply to the epithelium can slow this process, resulting in a fragile epithelium more susceptible to infection.

Adenosine Triphosphate Production

Adenosine triphosphate is the energy currency of the cell. It is produced by a series of complex metabolic pathways located in the free cytoplasm and inside the subcellular organelles, the mitochondria. The ATP-generating steps contained in the mitochondria require oxygen in the very last step of the pathway. If oxygen is not present, these pathways cannot generate ATP, and the cell must rely on the cytoplasmic pathways for all of its ATP. The cytoplasmic pathway is called *glycolysis* and is illustrated schematically in Figure 2–3. Glucose is the fuel for glycolysis. Glucose is changed and broken down to two pyruvate molecules, and in the process two ATP molecules are produced. If oxygen is present, pyruvate will then enter the citric acid cycle, which yields other intermediate molecules used to produce ATP in the oxidative phosphorylation reactions all contained in the mitochondria. A by-product of this oxidative process is CO_2, which is transported by the blood to the lungs and expelled. In the case of the cornea, CO_2 diffuses directly to the air or palpebral conjunctiva. The net ATP production for each molecule of glucose taken through glycolysis, the citric acid cycle, and oxidative phosphorylation is 38 ATP molecules. If oxygen is not present, pyruvate is converted to lactate, and the net production is only two ATP molecules. Of course, the presence of oxygen makes for much more efficient ATP production.

Adenosine triphosphate fuels all of the cell functions that have been mentioned earlier. The actual chemical event for the transfer of energy is the donation of one high energy phosphate group from ATP to the enzyme or substrate reaction that is being fueled. Thus, ATP is changed to adenosine diphosphate (ADP), and a by-product of this reaction is the production of a proton, H^+. The negative log of the H^+ ion concentration is termed pH, for example, pH 7 = 10^{-7} mol/L of H^+. These H^+ ions are later consumed in mitochondrial reactions that make new ATP molecules. Therefore, in oxidative metabolism, if ATP consumption equals ATP production, zero net H^+ ions are produced and cell pH is not affected.

Freeman[21] measured the oxygen consumption rates of the three components of the cornea: epithelium, stroma, and endothelium. The relative O_2 consumption was 40%, 39%, and 21% for epithelium, stroma, and endothelium, respectively. However, if we take into account the cellular volumes, the endothelium consumes O_2 about six times more rapidly than the epithelium. This is not surprising, because, as noted earlier, the epithelium has a relatively low density of mitochondria. Thus, the endothelium, which does most of the fluid pumping, can generate ATP much more efficiently than the epithelium even at the same oxygen tension. In fact, even under normal oxygen conditions, the epithelium converts at least 60% of the glucose it consumes to lactate.[56]

Source of Glucose and Efflux of Lactate

The superficial corneal epithelium is impermeable to glucose,[23] so all of the glucose for the epithelium must come from the limbus and the aqueous. Again, the limbus prob-

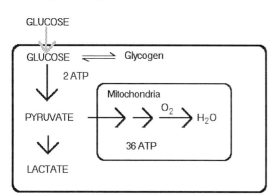

FIG 2–3.
Schematic drawing showing the use of glucose by cells for energy production. Glucose enters cells, usually by facilitated diffusion, and is either stored as glycogen or used. Glycolysis metabolizes glucose to pyruvate and produces a net two ATP molecules. If oxygen is available, some pyruvate can be further metabolized in mitochondria to yield a further 36 ATP molecules. If oxygen is not available, pyruvate is metabolized to lactate, which must then be excreted from the cell.

ably provides glucose only to the very periphery of the cornea, because the consumption of glucose is too rapid and the diffusion distances too long for it to supply much more of the cornea. Therefore, the aqueous is the only source of glucose for most of the cornea. Early experimentation in refractive surgery used PMMA implants into the central stroma of rabbits.[39] These attempts were unsuccessful because the stroma and epithelium anterior to the implant soon degenerated from lack of glucose because the implant was blocking glucose diffusion from the aqueous. So glucose is taken up by the endothelial cells, a small portion is used by these cells, it is then transported out to the stroma where some is used by the keratocytes, and the remainder feeds the epithelium.

Because 60% of the glucose used by the corneal epithelium is converted to lactate even when there is plenty of oxygen available, what happens to all the lactate? Is it a problem? Lactate can be reconverted back to pyruvate, but this will occur only if pyruvate is consumed in the citric acid cycle. Because the epithelium is limited in its citric acid cycle capacity because of the paucity of mitochondria, the lactate must be removed from the cell as a waste product. If lactate is not removed, its concentration builds up, in turn, causing pyruvate concentrations to increase, which slows down the further conversion of glucose to pyruvate, thus slowing glycolysis and ATP formation.

Lactate, like glucose, is also impermeable to the superficial epithelium.[37] Lactate is a charged molecule and thus cannot easily diffuse across the cell's plasma membrane. A recent study[5] has shown that lactate removal from corneal epithelium is facilitated by being coupled to a proton. Lactate and protons move down their chemical concentration gradients from inside the corneal epithelial cell to the extracellular space via a specialized membrane protein, the lactate-proton cotransporter.[5] This cotransporter protein not only removes lactate but also helps to regulate the cytoplasmic pH by removing protons. This is especially helpful because the rate-limiting step in glyco-

lysis is slowed when the cytoplasmic pH drops too low.[62] Figure 2–4 summarizes the movement of lactate and H^+ ions in the cornea.

Once out of the epithelium, lactate must diffuse back to the stroma and out into the aqueous. If oxygen is present, both the keratocytes and the endothelial cells could take up lactate via similar lactate-proton cotransporters and convert it to pyruvate for use in the citric acid cycle. The unused lactate is transported across the endothelium by mechanisms that have not been elucidated and dumped into the aqueous. The high lactate production by the crystalline lens and the cornea account for the relatively high lactate concentrations found in aqueous humor when compared with plasma.[45]

Effect of Hypoxia on Cell Function

Given a sufficient glucose and oxygen supply, ATP production will equal ATP consumption, and cell viability and function will be maintained. What happens to a cell that is using oxygen when the oxygen supply is diminished? Nothing will happen unless the oxygen concentration drops below a level at which the rates of the mitochondrial reactions are affected. If this occurs, the rate of anaerobic glycolysis (glucose to lactate) will increase to compensate for any slowdown in oxidative ATP production. This is called the *Pasteur effect,* named for the person who first described it. For this increase in glycolysis to occur, there must be an increase in glucose consumption. Thus, the supply of glucose must be adequate. The end product of glycolysis, lactate, will also be increased, and because H^+ consumption by mitochondria is reduced, there will be a net production of H^+ ions. Remember that H^+ ions are consumed by the mitochondria to make new ATP molecules. When the mitochondrial reactions slow down, so does the consumption of H^+ ions. Given that the ATP supply is normal and that ATP consumption continues at the same rate, there will be a net production of H^+

FIG 2–4.
Schematic drawing of the cornea showing the fate of lactate and H^+ produced by the epithelium. Lactate and H^+ leave the epithelium via lactate-H^+ cotransporters. Because of the tight superficial epithelium, these molecules must diffuse back toward the stroma and eventually get washed out into the aqueous. Accumulation of lactate between the epithelial cells and in the stroma will osmotically draw fluid into these spaces. In the epithelium, this leads to increased light scatter, and in the stroma, it causes swelling. The metabolic H^+ ions lead to a drop in stromal pH levels and may also change endothelial intracellular pH levels, which may affect its pump function.

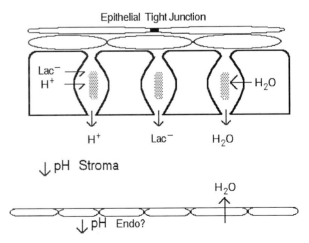

ions because production of H^+ ions now exceeds consumption. If not removed from the cells, these protons will lower intracellular pH, which could slow down glycolytic activity. In the end, given an adequate supply of glucose and the ability to get rid of lactate and H^+ ions, cell viability and function may be maintained in hypoxia.

Numerous studies have shown that the cornea steps up its consumption of glucose[60, 63] and production of lactate[37] and protons[7] when the epithelium is made hypoxic. Both lactate and H^+ ions diffuse to the stroma and then out to the aqueous humor. As a consequence, the added H^+ ions reduce the pH of the stroma (Fig 2–5)[7] and aqueous,[61] which may have a negative effect on endothelial function. The production of lactate and protons will continue at a high rate as long as glucose is available. Of course, the lower the oxygen tension is, the greater the glucose consumption becomes. A point is reached where the glucose consumption rate exceeds the rate that glucose can diffuse from the aqueous. The epithelial cells, however, have stored glucose in the form of glycogen. Glycogen is a complex carbohydrate molecule similar to starch that can be enzymatically broken down to smaller glucose subunits. After about 2 hours of severe hypoxia, however, the corneal epithelial glycogen supply is depleted,[63] and the epithelial cells die.

This discussion has assumed that during hypoxia ATP consumption always proceeds at its normal rate and that when a threshold is reached where ATP production slips behind ATP consumption, there will be a rapidly deteriorating condition that results in cell death. This is probably not the case. More likely there is a concommitant decrease in ATP production and consumption. This would have the action of slowing down cell activity rather than simply

ending it. Evidence that this may occur in the cornea has been given, for example, in studies showing a slowing of mitotic activity in corneal epithelium that has been made hypoxic.[24] This makes sense because mitosis is probably the most energy-consuming activity of the epithelium. The down side to this situation is the slowing of new tight junction formation and superficial cell desquamation, which would have the effect of making the epithelium more susceptible to microbial penetration.

ACUTE COMPLICATIONS OF HYPOXIA

Epithelium

Superficial Punctate Keratitis

Superficial punctate keratitis, or SPK (Fig 2–6), is a common complication of contact lens wear that can often be attributed to hypoxia. If the possibility of a toxic (e.g., solution preservative) or mechanical effect can be eliminated, hypoxic stress is the likely cause. Another "toxic" etiology that should be mentioned occurs mainly with soft lens use. This is the poor-moving lens, which entraps cellular debris and leads to cell death because of the release of epithelial cell hydrolytic enzymes or secondarily from hydrolytic enzymes released from an activated immune response, namely, tight lens syndrome. Treatment in this case is discontinuing lens wear until the SPK is gone and refitting with a better moving lens.

Hypoxic SPK is probably caused by the premature desquamation of stressed superficial cells. This leaves microscopic gaps on the corneal surface where fluorescein is

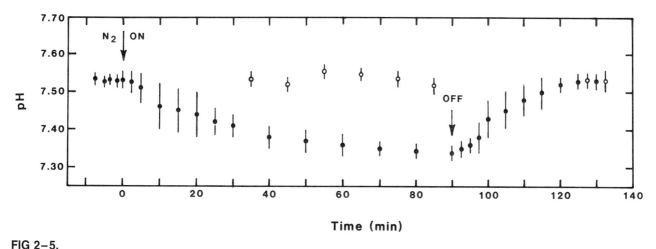

FIG 2–5.
Application of the nitrogen goggle leads to a decrease in stromal pH levels from 7.55 to 7.35 over 60 to 90 minutes *(closed circles)*. N_2 ON indicates nitrogen gas starting; OFF indicates goggle removed. Open circles indicate control eye wearing a goggle with air being perfused (see Bonanno and Polse[7] for details). (From Bonanno JA, Polse KA: *Invest Ophthalmol Vis Sci* 1987; 28:1514. Used by permission.)

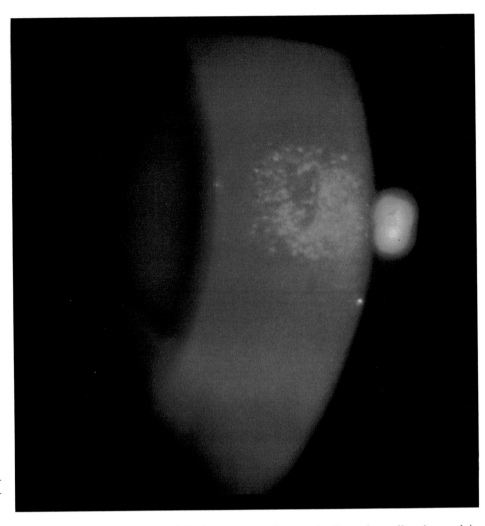

FIG 2–6.
Example of superficial punctate keratitis secondary to contact lens–induced hypoxia.

allowed to pool. Many clinicians believe that the longer SPK is allowed to continue, the greater the likelihood of microbial infection, especially during extended lens wear when the epithelium may not ever have a chance to heal completely. The treatment for SPK is to provide more oxygen by using a lens of higher oxygen transmission, increasing tear pumping, or reducing the wearing time.

Epithelial Edema

Corneal edema accompanying contact lens wear is considered to be the classic sign of hypoxic stress. Although the clinical appearance and location may differ depending on the type of lens worn (hard or soft), the basic mechanism that causes edema is the same. For rigid lens wear, central corneal edema may be seen as edema of the epithelial layer in a proscribed zone corresponding to the area most frequently covered by the contact lens. When the lenses are removed, patients may complain of hazy vision because of increased light scatter within the epithelium. Epithelial edema is best observed by indirect retroillumination or use of the sclerotic scatter technique. When caused by

rigid lenses, central corneal edema is easily observed in the slit-lamp because there is a clear demarcation between edematous central and nonedematous peripheral epithelium.[40] Edema from soft lens wear, however, is more difficult to observe because the edema is spread out across the entire epithelium. Superficial punctate keratitis can be found along with epithelial edema, especially after many hours of lens wear. These breaks in the epithelial surface will allow water to move into the epithelium and contribute to light scatter. However, SPK is often not observed and is not necessary for the patient to experience the hazy vision, sometimes called *Sattler's veil.*[19, 42]

Finkelstein[19] recognized that Sattler's veil was a diffraction phenomenon arising within the epithelium. Work by Lambert and Klyce[42] later showed that epithelial hypoxia in the rabbit produced light scattering sites around the basal cells, which then acted as a large meshwork or diffraction grating. Therefore, if patients with hypoxic epithelial edema fixate on a small pinlight in a darkened room, they will observe diffraction fringes. If a narrow band interference filter is used to observe the pinlight, the diffraction grating size can be estimated by measuring the distance between the first fringe and the pinlight, x, and the distance from the pinlight to the subject, y. The grating size d = wavelength/sin ϕ, where tan ϕ = x/y. Grating size will be around 12 μm, which is the diameter of the basal epithelial cells.

For light to be scattered, the index of refraction around epithelial cells must be different from that of the cells themselves. Studies have shown that the epithelial thickness does not change during acute hypoxia,[64] indicating that epithelial edema occurs without any uptake of water from outside the epithelium. The most likely explanation is that hypoxia, by stimulating lactate production, leads to an increase in lactate concentration between the basal cells.[42] Being osmotically active, lactate will draw water out of the cells, increasing the extracellular space between them. Because this space has very little protein relative to the cells, it has a lower refractive index than the cells (see Fig 2–4), and light will scatter at the interface.

Epithelial Healing

Hypoxia reduces the epithelial healing rate.[68] This is most likely a consequence of a depressed availability of ATP. Two main activities occur during epithelial healing: (1) cells adjacent to the wound will spread into the wound area to try to seal it, and (2) new cells created via mitosis are needed to fill up the gaps created by the initial cell loss. As previously mentioned, mitotic activity is slowed during hypoxia.[24] In addition, cell migration in experimental wounds with rabbits can be completely blocked by severe hypoxia; the rate of cell migration increases with increased oxygen transmissibility of lens worn over the wounded area.[68] These laboratory studies reemphasize the need to modify or discontinue lens wear when the epithelium is compromised. Wearing lenses under these conditions certainly does not guarantee that an infection will occur, but the likelihood is increased especially in individuals who are susceptible or whose immune systems are depressed.

Stroma and Endothelium

Stromal Swelling

Stromal edema will almost always accompany the epithelial edema that occurs as a result of corneal hypoxia. The degree of swelling is inversely related to the oxygen tension of the tears or the Dk/L of the contact lens worn.[48] Stromal edema can occur by either (1) a break in the epithelial or endothelial barriers, (2) a reduction in the "pump," mainly endothelium, or (3) an increase in the osmotic activity (or imbibition pressure) of the stromal compartment. Edema (8%–10% swelling) is easily produced

with the nitrogen goggle technique without causing any cellular breaks. In vitro experiments with isolated rabbit corneas also indicate no change in epithelial resistance during acute hypoxia.[37] It is possible that the stromal acidosis caused by hypoxia[7] inhibits the endothelial pump. Acute decreases in pH within the physiological range, however, could not account for more than 3% to 4% swelling.[33] Klyce[37, 38] has shown that corneal swelling can be predicted based on the osmotic activity of the lactate that is added to the stroma during hypoxia (see Fig 2–4). Other studies[57] that manipulated the lactate production of the cornea during hypoxia are consistent with this "lactate osmotic hypothesis" for hypoxic stromal swelling.

Figure 2–7 shows that vertical lines (corneal striae, folds in Descemet's membrane) can often be seen in the posterior portion of corneas that have swelled 6% to 7%.[53] As the edema increases, the density and number of striae also increase. When the slit lamp is used with direct illumination, striae are relatively easy to observe and can be graded on a 0 to 3 scale, where 0 indicates no striae, 1 indicates one or two faint lines, grade 2 indicates two to six lines, and grade 3 indicates both many lines and black folds.

Hypoxia can also result in corneal distortion or warping. The patient will usually complain of blur with spectacles, and the clinician will be unable to refract the patient to his or her best visual acuity. Keratometric readings usually will be steeper and often distorted. This syndrome was commonly seen in patients wearing PMMA lenses. It is relatively uncommon with RGP lenses and soft lenses even if they produce significant edema. The most likely explanation for the hypoxia-induced distortion is that in rigid lens wear the epithelial and stromal edema is not uniform across the cornea, causing localized curvature changes. The distortion is less likely with soft lenses because the edema is more uniformly spread across the entire corneal surface.[6, 10] Rehabilitation of distorted corneas is often a challenging management problem and is covered in more detail in the last section of this chapter.

Endothelial Blebs and Corneal pH

Zantos and Holden[67] observed that small black spots forming on the endothelial surface within 20 to 30 minutes of inserting a contact lens and that these spots disappeared spontaneously within 1 hour while the lens remained in place. They termed these spots blebs. Blebs could be produced under three conditions: (1) with contact lens wear, (2) with nitrogen gas application through a goggle, and (3) by passing a 10% CO_2, 20% oxygen, and 70% nitrogen gas mixture over the eye. The last condition does not lead to stromal swelling because there is no hypoxia; however, the increased CO_2 concentration reduces the corneal pH. Therefore, hypoxia per se does not cause blebs; rather, it

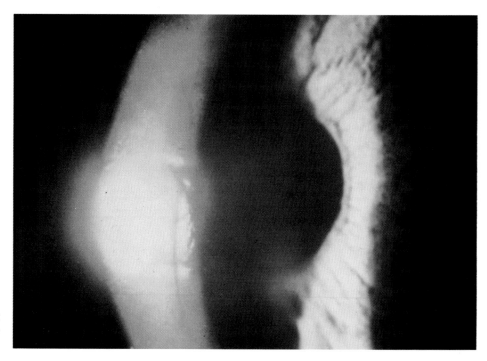

FIG 2–7.
Corneal striae in a contact lens–wearing patient with significant stromal swelling.

is caused by a secondary consequence of hypoxia, stromal acidosis.[32]

Shortly after Zantos and Holden[67] demonstrated the possible effect of pH on bleb formation, Bonanno and Polse[7, 8] produced a series of studies directly measuring reductions of stromal pH in human subjects during hypoxia alone and during lens wear (Figs 2–6, 2–7, and 2–8). Furthermore, it was demonstrated that the drop in pH during lens wear was caused by the sum of hypoxic acidosis and the accumulation of CO_2 in the cornea because of the diffusion barrier properties of the lens. This is illustrated in Figure 2–9. Subsequent studies have concurred that CO_2 can accumulate during lens wear[31] and that the CO_2 transmissibility of contact lenses seems to parallel the oxygen transmissibility.[13] Although the clinical significance of corneal acidosis secondary to contact lens wear is presently not

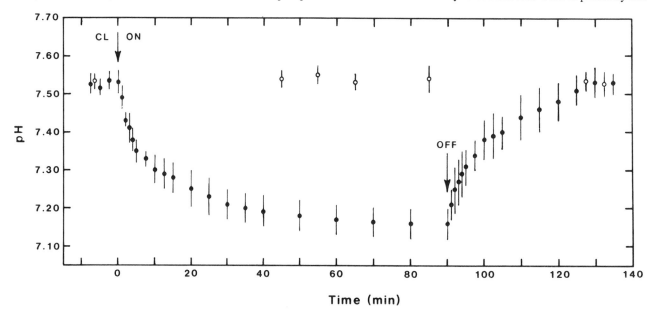

FIG 2–8.
Application of a thick (0.4-mm) low water content (38%) hydrogel lens causes a dramatic decrease in stromal pH level from 7.55 to 7.15 over 90 minutes *(closed circles)*. Open circles indicate non–lens wearing control eye (see Bonanno and Polse[7] for details). (From Bonanno JA, Polse KA: *Invest Ophthalmol Vis Sci* 1987; 28:1514. Used by permission.)

A

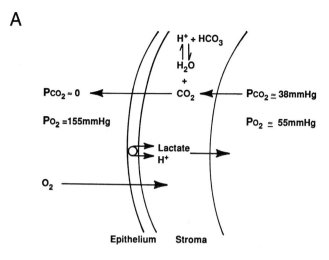

B

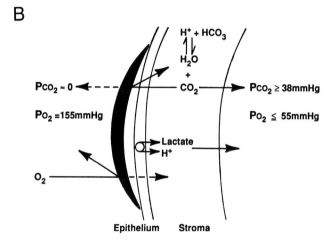

FIG 2–9.

A, the open eye non–lens wearing condition. There is a large gradient for CO_2 to diffuse out of the cornea from the aqueous humor (38 mm Hg) to the tears (0 mm Hg). Oxygen diffuses down its gradient from the air into the cornea. Lactate and protons are being produced by the corneal cells at the minimum metabolic rate. **B,** the lens-wearing condition. The lens will slow CO_2 diffusion, leading to a CO_2 buildup in the cornea. The CO_2 plus water produces carbonic acid, which then quickly dissociates to a proton and an HCO_3^- ion. The lens also prevents oxygen from getting to the cornea, leading to hypoxia and an increase in glycolytic metabolism, with lactate and protons as the final products. The combination of the CO_2 buildup and the glycolytic protons lead to a significant drop in stromal pH levels. (From Bonanno JA, Polse K: *Ophthalmology* 1987; 94:1305. Used by permission.)

well understood, most physiologists and clinicians consider such changes undesirable. Therefore, it is important to choose a lens with a high oxygen Dk/L. This will also minimize CO_2 accumulation and together yield the smallest possible drop in corneal pH during lens wear.

CHRONIC EFFECTS OF HYPOXIA

Epithelium

Microcysts

Epithelial microcyts were first reported in patients using soft lenses on a continual basis.[34, 66] Recently, they have been reported to occur with most RGP extended wear lenses as well. Figure 2–10 shows that the cysts are small (10–15 μm) transparent epithelial inclusions. The cysts usually take 2 to 3 months to occur and begin at the deeper layers of the epithelium. They seem to migrate anteriorly. If they reach the surface, they cause a break in the epithelium that will stain with fluorescein. Suggestions have been made to count the number of microcysts, but this is not very practical; therefore, a grading system based on the density and presence or absence of epithelial staining has been recommended.[35] This grading system is shown in Figure 2–11.

The microcystic response is chronic, and if the patient discontinues wear, it may take several weeks to months for the microcysts to completely disappear. Patients who show a grade 2 or greater microcyst response should return to daily wear. Remission of microcysts can be achieved during day wear of GP lenses; thus, total lens discontinuance is not necessary, but breaking the overnight cycle (i.e., the most severe hypoxia) is essential.

The etiology of microcysts is not known. The persistence of cysts well past the normal epithelial turnover time indicates that either the turnover time in these patients is severely depressed or that the cysts are somehow not tied to the normal migration of cells from basal to superficial layers. Although epithelial mitotic activity is reduced during hypoxia[24] and there is a prolonged cell residence time in contact lens wearers,[43] it is unlikely that turnover time has increased from 1 week to 2 months. This is especially so because patients have discontinued wear and their epithelia are no longer hypoxic.

Biopsy specimens of microcysts suggest that they are degenerated epithelial material.[27] If the basal cell RNA/protein synthesizing machinery is altered by chronic hypoxia, this defect may be passed on to daughter cells and perpetuated until the defect is somehow washed out.[27] Whether the defect is a direct effect of hypoxia or is caused by the chronic hypoxic acidosis will be the subject of further research.

Epithelial Thinning

The Gothenberg study, conducted by Holden et al.,[28] examined many patients who used extended wear hydrogel lenses. In addition to the common occurrence of microcysts, they found that the epithelium was generally thinner

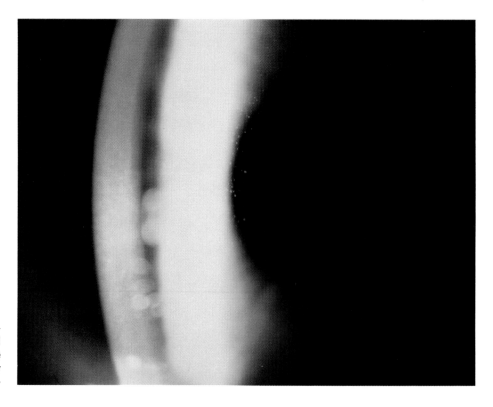

FIG 2–10.
Epithelial microcysts secondary from contact lens–induced hypoxia. (From Kenyon E, Polse KA, Seger RG: *Ophthalmology* 1986; 93:231. Used by permission.)

by 6% and that the oxygen uptake rate was reduced by 15%. The reduction in total cell mass may explain the reduced oxygen uptake rate; nevertheless, this clearly demonstrates that epithelial physiology is significantly altered during chronic hypoxia. This type of epitheliopathy may in part explain the cornea's increased susceptibility to infection during extended wear.

Corneal Sensitivity
Reductions in corneal sensitivity are not uncommon among contact lens wearers. Millodot and O'Leary[46] at-

tribute these observations to hypoxia. Bergenske and Polse[3] later concurred, showing that PMMA lens wearers refitted with GP lenses regained normal touch thresholds. However, in earlier work, Polse[50] had shown little or no reduction in sensitivity in subjects with their epithelium made hypoxic by exposure to nitrogen gas. It could be argued that chronic hypoxia may be needed before nerve deficits can be found.[46] In addition, it must be considered that chronic acidosis may also affect corneal nerve cell conduction. This question is discussed further in Chapter 5.

FIG 2–11.
Microcyst grading system. Because microcysts quickly develop to a point where they can no longer be accurately counted, a grading system based on the density was devised. Higher grades of microcysts are frequently accompanied by light punctate keratitis; when more than two microcysts stained, they were graded a minimum of grade 2. (From Kenyon E, Polse KA, Seger RG: *Ophthalmology* 1986; 93:231. Used by permission.

Grade 1   Grade 2   Grade 3

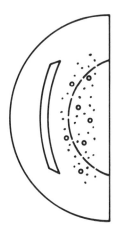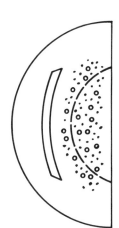

Reduction in sensory nerve function may have an amplifying effect on contact lens–induced epithelial changes. Clinicians have observed that patients with trigeminal denervation have a decreased healing capacity of the skin and cornea. Destruction of the trigeminal ganglion in the rabbit produced an increase in epithelial permeability and a decreased ability to repair epithelial wounds.[4] Also, aphakes who have had 180-degree limbal incisions have reduced corneal sensitivity, reduced hypoxic corneal swelling, and reduced oxygen uptake rates relative to their nonoperated eye,[30] indicating an overall depression in corneal metabolism. Aphakes are also very susceptible to epithelial breaks, infiltrates, and corneal infections during extended wear. These results suggest that corneal nerves transport a substance or substances that influence epithelial cell physiology. Because hypoxia appears to decrease nerve function either directly or indirectly via corneal acidosis, it may also interfere with the axonal transport of this substance.

Stroma and Endothelium

Reduced Stromal Thickness

In the Gothenberg study,[28] after patients discontinued lens wear, the stromal thickness was less than it was before lens wear was started. The authors concluded that the corneas had lost stromal matrix. Maintenance of stromal matrix is the function of the keratocytes. Clearly these cells are also made hypoxic and acidotic during chronic lens wear. The earlier work of Freeman[21] indicated that the oxygen consumption rate of stromal keratocytes was similar to that of endothelial cells. Thus, it would not be surprising that the cells are unable to synthesize collagen and GAGs at the normal rate during chronic hypoxic lens wear.

Neovascularization

Blood vessel growth into the cornea has been observed in lens wearers.[27] Neovascularization was not uncommon during the wear of thick daily wear hydrogel lenses. The use of high Dk/L lenses can reduce vascularization considerably. Neovascularization is particularly problematic if patients have had corneal surgery (penetrating keratoplasty, radial keratectomy, etc.) and are fitted with soft contact lenses. If a patient requires a contact lens for visual rehabilitation following surgery, an RGP lens should be used, if possible.

The biology of new blood vessel formation is very complex and not completely understood. Perilimbal stromal edema seems to be a prerequisite for vessel infiltration, which may explain why vascularization was relatively rare with rigid lenses. It is clear that a cellular distress signal or signals from stressed or dying cells are required. This probably interacts directly with vascular endothelium, inflammatory cells, or both.[26] Inhibition of immune metabolites with corticosteroids, cyclo-oxygenase, or lipoxygenase inhibitors lessens the vessel response in experimental angiogenesis.[26] Prostaglandins, which promote vessel growth, are found in high concentrations after corneal injury.[22] Corticosteroids and nonsteroidal anti-inflammatories thus appear to be useful for slowing neovascularization; however, they can have many known and unknown side effects. The best therapy is to discontinue lens wear. If lens wear is resumed, the patient should be refitted with a lens that allows substantially more oxygen transmission to the cornea, preferably a high DK/L RGP lens, and the vessels should be carefully monitored. Neovascularization is discussed further in Chapter 10.

Endothelial Polymegathism and Reduced Function

The next chapter contains a detailed discussion on the effects of hypoxia on the endothelium. Therefore, we will simply mention that morphological and functional changes occur and are apparently related to epithelial hypoxia. Endothelial polymegathism is an increased variation in the apparent size of corneal endothelial cells. This is a common finding in PMMA and extended lens wearers.[38] Are these morphological changes representing functional alterations? Rao[55] has shown that corneas with polymegathism before cataract surgery were at greater risk to decompensate after surgery. Studies by Polse et al.[52] indicate that corneas with the greatest "hypoxic dose" will have slower corneal thickness recoveries during a corneal stress test. In that study, however, the relation between corneal recovery and polymegathism was not significant, which may simply be a result of the small sample size used.

The etiologies of polymegathism and reduced endothelial function are unknown. Is it chronic hypoxia at the endothelium? Reports indicating no reduction and some reduction of oxygen levels at the endothelium have been equivocal.[1, 41] Is it caused by chronic reductions in corneal pH? Although it has been demonstrated that the stromal[7, 8] and aqueous humor pH[61] are reduced during contact lens wear, the mechanism by which pH could alter cell morphology remains unclear.

CORNEAL REHABILITATION

In cases where severe hypoxic distress is clinically evident, such as neovascularization and chronic SPK, discontinuing lens wear is the most appropriate action. In less severe cases where toxic or mechanical etiologies can be ruled out, enhancing oxygen delivery to the cornea or shortening the wearing time (e.g., extended vs. daily wear) may ameliorate the problem. Persistence of epithelial defects, however, should prompt lens discontinuation until complete healing is achieved, at which time refitting or reevaluation of wearing times can be considered.

The availability of high Dk RGP lenses has allowed the clinician the ability to refit the distorted cornea, which can result from PMMA lenses, without discontinuing lens wear. The most bothersome problem for the patient in this case is the inability to wear spectacles (even on an emergency basis) because of the marked corneal distortion. To the clinician, the most difficult problem is how to prescribe a RGP refitting without seeming to "sell" new lenses to an asymptomatic patient. To resolve the patient management problem, the clinician may demonstrate using trial lenses that it is not possible to prescribe adequate spectacles. It should also be emphasized that this is caused by an irregular cornea, which is a result of altered metabolism. The patient should be made aware that for the long-term health of the eye, this altered physiology is not acceptable and an RGP lens is indicated. Once this management problem has been solved, the clinician can then proceed with the refitting.

How to carry out this refitting has been somewhat controversial among clinicians; however, most contact lens fitters find that it is easier for both practitioner and patient if the refitting is done without interrupting lens wear. This is achieved by ordering new RGP lenses based on a trial fitting. Studies that have monitored PMMA contact lens patients after discontinuing lens wear show that the cornea is stable after about 21 days.[49] It is interesting to note that when PMMA patients are fitted with RGP lenses without interruption of lens wear, the cornea also stabilizes after about 3 weeks.[49] This suggests that the cornea will rehabilitate once sufficient oxygen levels are restored either with total lens removal or by the use of an RGP lens that provides sufficient oxygen. Once the 3-week period is complete, it is usually possible to refract for glasses and also to determine if the lens parameters need to be changed. If the clinician is not completely sure of corneal stability, it might be advisable to take refractive and corneal curvature measurements at the 3-week visit and again at the 5-week visit. In most cases there will be no important measurement differences in this 2-week interval. Usually when the cornea has stabilized, the original refitting does not have to be changed; however, in some cases there may be marked changes in the corneal topography, and a second set of lenses will be required. From the onset of the "refitting" procedure, it is best to indicate to the patient that two pairs may be required. Normal corneal rehabilitation should be achieved after about 3 weeks. If corneal instability persists much beyond this time, a careful diagnostic workup for other corneal disease should be made.

REFERENCES

1. Barr RE, Hennessey M, Murphy VG: Diffusion of oxygen at the endothelial surface of the rabbit cornea. *J Physiol* 1977; 270:1–8.
2. Benedek GB: Theory of the transparency of the eye. *Appl Opt* 10:459–473, 1971.
3. Bergenske PD, Polse KA: The effect of rigid gas-permeable lenses on corneal sensitivity. *J Am Optom Assoc* 1987; 58:212–215.
4. Beuerman RW, Schimmelpfennig B: Sensory denervation of the rabbit cornea affects epithelial properties. *Exp Neurol* 1980; 69:196–201.
5. Bonanno JA: Lactate-proton cotransport in rabbit corneal epithelium. *Curr Eye Res* 1990; 9:707–712.
6. Bonanno JA, Polse KA: Central and peripheral corneal swelling accompanying soft lens extended wear. *Am J Optom Physiol Opt* 1985; 62:74–81.
7. Bonanno JA, Polse KA: Corneal acidosis during contact lens wear: Effects of hypoxia and CO_2. *Invest Ophthalmol Vis Sci* 1987; 28:1514–1520.
8. Bonanno JA, Polse KA: Effect of rigid contact lens oxygen transmissibility on stromal pH in the living human eye. *Ophthalmology* 1987; 94:1305–1309.
9. Bonventre JV, Cheung JY: Effects of metabolic acidosis on viability of cells exposed to anoxia. *Am J Physiol* 1986; 249:C149–C159.
10. Carney LG: Hydrophilic lens effects on central and peripheral corneal thickness and corneal transparency. *Am J Optom Physiol Opt* 1975; 52:521–523.
11. Davson H: The hydration of the cornea. *Biochem J* 1955; 59:24–28.
12. Dikstein S, Maurice DM: The metabolic basis to the fluid pump in the cornea. *J Physiol* 1972; 221:29–41.
13. Efron N, Ang J: Corneal hypoxia and hypercapnia during contact lens wear. *Optom Vis Sci* 1990; 67:512–521.
14. Farrell RA, McCally RL, Tatham PER: Wavelength dependencies of light scattering in normal and cold swollen rabbit corneas and their structural implications. *J Physiol* 1973; 233:589–612.
15. Fatt I, Bieber MI: The steady-state distribution of oxygen and carbon dioxide in the in vivo cornea: I. The open eye in air and the closed eye. *Exp Eye Res* 1968; 7:103–112.
16. Fatt I, Bieber MI, Pye SD: Steady-state distribution of oxygen and carbon dioxide in the in vivo cornea of an eye covered by a gas permeable contact lens. *Am J Optom Physiol Opt* 1969; 46:3–14.
17. Fatt I, Hill RM: Oxygen tension under a contact lens during blinking—a comparison of theory and experimental observation. *Am J Optom* 1970; 47:50.
18. Fink BA, Carney LG, Hill RM: Rigid lens tear pump efficiency: Effects of overall diameter/base curve combinations. *Optom Vis Sci* 1991; 68:309–313.
19. Finkelstein I: The biophysics of corneal scatter and diffraction of light induced by contact lenses. *Arch Am Acad Optom* 1952; 29:185–231.
20. Fischbarg J, Lim JJ: Role of cations, anions and carbonic

anhydrase in fluid transport across rabbit corneal endothelium. *J Physiol* 1974; 241:647–675.

21. Freeman RD: Oxygen consumption by the component layers of the cornea. *J Physiol* 1972; 225:15–32.

22. Fruct J, Zauberman H: Topical indomethacin effect on neovascularization of the cornea and on prostaglandin E_2 levels. *Br J Ophthalmol* 1984; 68:656–659.

23. Hale PN, Maurice DM: Sugar transport across the corneal endothelium. *Exp Eye Res* 1969; 8:205–215.

24. Hamano H, Hori M: Effect of contact lens wear on the mitoses of corneal epithelial cells: preliminary report. *CLAO J* 1983; 9:133–136.

25. Hart RW, Farrell RA: Light scattering in the cornea. *J Opt Soc Am* 1969; 59:766.

26. Haynes WL, Proia AD, Klintworth GK: Effects of inhibitors of arachidonic acid metabolism on corneal neovascularization in the rat. *Invest Ophthalmol Vis Sci* 1989; 30:1588–1593.

27. Holden BA: The Glenn A. Fry Award Lecture 1988: The ocular response to contact lens wear. *Optom Vis Sci* 1989; 66:717–733.

28. Holden BA, et al: Effects of long-term extended wear on the human cornea. *Invest Ophthalmol Vis Sci* 1985; 26:1489–1501.

29. Holden BA, et al: Corneal deswelling following overnight wear of rigid and hydrogel contact lenses. *Curr Eye Res* 1988; 7:49–53.

30. Holden BA, Polse KA, Fonn D, et al: Effects of cataract surgery on corneal function. *Invest Ophthalmol Vis Sci* 1982; 22:343–350.

31. Holden BA, Ross R, Jenkins J: Hydrogel contact lenses impede carbon dioxide efflux from the human cornea. *Curr Eye Res* 1987; 6:1283–1290.

32. Holden BA, Williams L, Zantos S: Etiology of transient endothelial changes in the human cornea. *Invest Ophthalmol Vis Sci* 1985; 26:1354.

33. Huff JW: Contact lens induced stromal acidosis and edema are dissociable in vitro. *Invest Ophthalmol Vis Sci* 1991; 32(suppl):322.

34. Humphreys JA, Larke JR, Parrish ST: Microepithelial cysts observed in extended contact lens wearing subjects. *Br J Ophthalmol* 1980; 64:888–889.

35. Kenyon E, Polse KA, Seger RG: Influence of wearing schedule on extended wear complications. *Ophthalmology* 1986; 93:231–236.

36. Klyce SD: Enhancing fluid secretion by the corneal epithelium. *Invest Ophthalmol Vis Sci* 1977; 16:968–973.

37. Klyce SD: Stromal lactate accumulation can account for corneal oedema osmotically following epithelial hypoxia in the rabbit. *J Physiol* 1981; 332:49–64.

38. Klyce SD, Russel SR: Numerical solution of coupled transport equations applied to corneal hydration dynamics. *J Physiol* 1979; 292:107–134.

39. Knowles WF: Effects of intralamellar plastic membranes on corneal physiology. *Am J Ophthalmol* 1961; 51:1146–1156.

40. Korb DR, Exford JM: The phenomenon of central circular clouding. *J Am Optom Assoc* 1968; 39:223–230.

41. Kwon M, Niimikoski J, Hunt TK. In vivo measurements of oxygen tension in the cornea, aqueous humor and anterior lens of the open eye. *Invest Ophthalmol Vis Sci* 1972; 11:108–114.

42. Lambert SR, Klyce SD: The origins of Sattler's veil. *Am J Ophthalmol* 1981; 91:51–56.

43. Lemp MA, Gold JB: The effects of extended wear hydrophilic contact lenses on the corneal epithelium. *Am J Ophthalmol* 1986; 101:274–277.

44. Maurice DM: The structure and transparency of the cornea. *J Physiol* 1957; 136:263–286.

45. Maurice DM: The cornea and sclera, in Davson H (ed): *The Eye*. New York, Academic Press, 1984, vol I.

46. Millodot M, O'Leary DL: Effect of oxygen deprivation on corneal sensitivity. *Acta Ophthalmol* 1980; 58:434–439.

47. Mishima S, Hedbys B: The permeability of the corneal epithelium and endothelium to water. *Exp Eye Res* 1967; 6:10–32.

48. O'Neal MR, Polse KA, Sarver MD: Corneal response to rigid and hydrogel lenses during eye closure. *Invest Ophthalmol Vis Sci* 1984; 25:837–842.

49. Polse KA: Changes in corneal hydration after discontinuing contact lens wear. *Am J Optom* 1972; 49:511.

50. Polse KA: Etiology of corneal sensitivity changes accompanying contact lens wear. *Invest Ophthalmol Vis Sci* 1978; 17:1202–1206.

51. Polse KA: Tear flow under hydrogel lenses. *Invest Ophthalmol Vis Sci* 1979; 18:409–413.

52. Polse KA, Brand RJ, Cohen SR, et al: Hypoxic effects on corneal morphology and function. *Invest Ophthalmol Vis Sci* 1990; 31:1542–1554.

53. Polse KA, Mandell R: Etiology of corneal striae accompanying hydrogel lens wear. *Invest Ophthalmol Vis Sci* 1976; 15:553–556.

54. Polse KA, Mandell RB: Hyperbaric oxygen effect on edema. *Am J Optom* 1971; 48:197.

55. Rao GN, Shaw EL, Arthur EJ, et al: Endothelial cell morphology and corneal deturgescence. *Ann Ophthalmol* 1979; 11:885–899.

56. Riley MV: Glucose and oxygen utilization by the rabbit cornea. *Exp Eye Res* 1969; 8:193–200.

57. Rohde MD, Huff JW: Contact lens induced edema in vitro: Amelioration by lactate dehydrogenase inhibitors. *Curr Eye Res* 1986; 5:751.

58. Sarver MD, Baggett D, Harris MG, et al: Corneal edema with hydrogel lenses and eye closure. *Am J Optom Physiol Opt* 1981; 58:386–392.

59. Smelser GK, Ozanics V: Importance of oxygen for maintenance of the optical properties of the human cornea. *Science* 1952; 115:140.

60. Smelser GK, Ozanics V: Structural changes in corneas of guinea-pigs after wearing contact lenses. *Arch Ophthalmol* 1953; 49:335–340.

61. Thomas JV, Brimijoin MR, Neault TR, et al: The fluorescent indicator pyranine is suitable for measuring stromal and corneal pH in vivo. *Exp Eye Res* 1990; 50:241–249.

62. Triverdi B, Danforth WH: Effect of pH on the kinetics of frog phosphofructokinase. *J Biol Chem* 1966; 241:4110.

gestation. This membrane is approximately 3 μm thick at birth and will continue to grow throughout life at a rate of approximately 1 μm per decade.[51] It could be argued that this basement membrane should be considered an endothelial structure, but unlike its epithelial counterpart, it has been the custom to describe the former as a separate corneal layer.

Morphology

The purpose of this chapter is to review endothelial morphology with emphasis on its relation to clinical contact lens practice. A number of thorough reviews and descriptions of the anatomy of the human endothelium exist in recent literature, and these may be consulted for further detail.[23, 45, 55, 59]

The corneal endothelium forms the posterior limit of the cornea and faces the aqueous humor in the anterior chamber. Anteriorly the endothelium is lined by its own basement membrane, the posterior limiting lamina, and peripherally it becomes modified to form the trabecular meshes. Within the confines of the cornea, the endothelium is very uniform except for the more extreme periphery, where this layer loses some of its regularity because of the presence of Hassel-Henle warts.[98] The anterior surface of the endothelial cell (facing its basement membrane) is also known as its basal side, whereas the face toward the anterior chamber is sometimes termed the apical side.

The corneal endothelium is comprised of a monolayer with 3.500 to 4.000 cells/mm², or approximately 400,000 cells[55] at birth. The cells are flat and measure approximately 5 by 20 μm (Fig 3–1). They are packed tightly together, leaving no intercellular spaces (Fig 3–2). Anteriorly the endothelial cells closely line the posterior limiting lamina, again allowing no spaces.

The morphology of a structure is to a great extent dictated by its functions. The endothelium has two important functions: an optical and a metabolically driven fluid pump function. The linearly flat anterior and posterior surfaces of the endothelium evolved to meet the optical function of the endothelium. The exception to this general rule are the microvilli along the posterior surface, which are considerably less numerous than those noted along the anterior epithelial surface. They are distributed primarily along the peripheral outline of the cell. The endothelium forms the posterior surface of the corneal "lens," and because of the small change in refractive index between the corneal tissue and aqueous humor, this surface has a negligible effect on the refracting power of the cornea. The lack of spaces between the cells and between the endothelium and the posterior limiting lamina help to facilitate a uniform refractive index for this region. This uniformity of the endothelium with regard to both shape and refractive index is an important factor in explaining its transparency.

In contrast, the lateral sides of the endothelial cell show complex invaginations (Fig 3–3). However, the overall, general orientation of the lateral walls remain perpendicular to the plane of the cornea. The separation between the cells along the lateral sides is, as stated earlier, minimal—in the order of 20 nm.

The shape adopted by cells is often determined by how tightly packed they are in a tissue. In flat section, the

FIG 3–1.
Posterior cornea. The endothelium forms a single, uniform layer of cells covering the posterior cornea. The posterior limiting lamina separates the endothelium from the stromal tissue. Light micrograph. Rhesus monkey. (Magnification approximately ×200.)

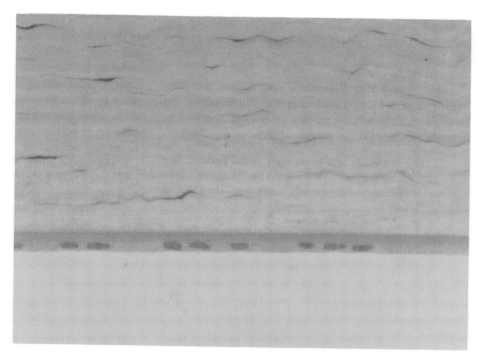

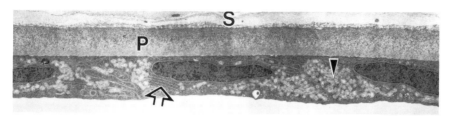

FIG 3–2.
Low magnification transverse section of the posterior cornea. This section shows three consecutive endothelial cells forming a relatively flat posterior and anterior surface of this corneal layer. The endothelial cell contains a large number of mitochondria *(triangle)* and rough endoplasmic reticulum *(open arrow)*. Posterior limiting lamina *(P)*; stroma *(S)*. Transmission electron micrograph. Macaque mulatta monkey. (Magnification ×3,400.)

endothelial cell is classically described as being hexagonal; however, such characterization is strictly inaccurate because it ignores the three-dimensional shape of the cell. The geometrical outline of the cell is found only along its posterior outline, and even in this orientation, not all cells are hexagons. Scanning electron microscopy of the posterior corneal surface demonstrates that normal endothelial cells may have five to seven sides. This endothelial polygonality has been pointed out in previous literature.[24, 105] Figure 3–4 is representative of the endothelial mosaic as seen with the scanning electron microscope.

Given the complexity of the invaginations of the lateral walls, it is hardly surprising that recent studies have found that the basal face of the endothelium does not maintain the geometric mosaic pattern of its apical face.[39, 86, 92] Although none of these studies offers a clear, untraumatized picture demonstrating the cellular outline of the anterior surface of the endothelium, they nevertheless provide good evidence that this surface differs markedly from the posterior one. It appears that the basal endothelium contains numerous small cellular processes, which, by overlapping each other, create a distinctly irregular outline that lacks a semblance to the apical side. Ringvold et al.[86] suggested that the geometric outline of the posterior surface is caused by the presence of tight junctions found only in that location of the cell. It would seem that the uniform mosaic of the apical side is quickly lost because of the invaginations of the lateral wall and is not recovered at the basal side of the cell.

This new information of the three-dimensional appearance of the endothelial cell leads to two conclusions of clinical importance:

1. The image in an endothelial specular microscope (or that obtained in a biomicroscope using specular reflection), showing a uniform, geometric mosaic of predominantly hexagonal cells, arises from the interface between the apical endothelial surface and aqueous humour.

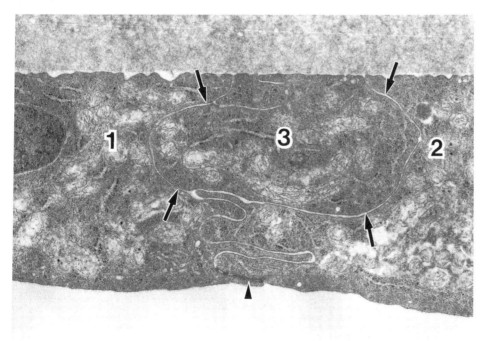

FIG 3–3.
Transverse section through the junction between the lateral sides of neighboring cells. The interdigitated outline of the interface *(arrows)* between two, or possibly three, endothelial cells *(1, 2, 3; 3* is possibly a third cell) may be followed. A zonula occludens *(triangle)* demarkates the posterior limit of this interface. Transmission electron micrograph. Macaque mulatta monkey. (Magnification ×18,500.)

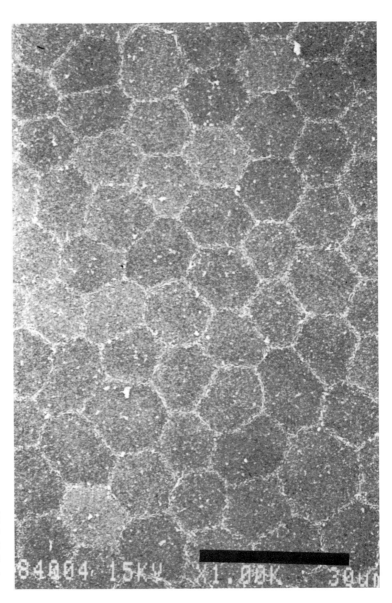

FIG 3–4.
Endothelial mosaic from central cornea prepared after in vitro perfusion with a glucose-bicarbonate-Ringer type of solution. Scanning electron micrograph. Rabbit. Black bar indicates 50 μm (corrected for tissue shrinkage). (Courtesy of M. Doughty.)

2. Although the optical system of these instruments may offer the opportunity to view objects three-dimensionally, the image obtained by specular microscopy is strictly two-dimensional. It follows that assumptions on the three-dimensional size and shape of the endothelial cell when based on such imaging is speculative in nature.

The corneal endothelial intercellular junctions have received relatively little attention. This is somewhat surprising given the known contribution of this tissue to corneal fluid movement. Furthermore, it is well accepted among ophthalmic surgeons that the endothelium may be easily traumatized during surgery by either mechanical means or anterior chamber irrigation solutions.[103] It would therefore be most beneficial to know exactly how the endothelial cells are attached to each other and, above all, what is holding the cells onto the overlying cornea.

Both tight and gap junctions have been documented in the corneal endothelium (Fig 3–5).[39, 55, 58, 73] The tight junctions, or the zonula occludentes, are located on the apical sides of the cells. At the juncture between two neighboring cells, one of them will send a thin protoplasmic flap across the intercellular space and over the edge of the other cell. The zonula occludens located between this flap and the opposing cell will thus seal off the cornea from the anterior chamber (see Fig 3–5). These tight junctions do not, however, appear to constitute an impermeable barrier to fluid passage.[39, 58, 73] Hirsch et al.[39] reported that these cellular junctions were discontinuous and therefore do not provide a beltlike seal along the entire cir-

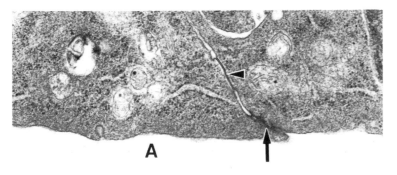

FIG 3–5.
Junctional complex. At the interface with the anterior chamber *(A)*, a zonula occludens *(arrow)* seals the aqueous humour from entry to the endothelium. Slightly anterior to the tight junction is a gap junction *(triangle)*. Transmission electron micrograph. Macaque mulatta monkey. (Magnification ×28,000.)

cumference of the cell. This finding may be a possible explanation to the relative permeability of endothelium.

Gap junctions are important in facilitating cellular exchanges and communications, and they are found along the lateral walls in the endothelium near the apical side of the cells (see Fig 3–5). Here they form discontinuous linear arrays.[39, 58, 73] The gap junctions do not provide a barrier to extracellular fluid, although the intercellular space becomes less than 10 nm at this point.

There are no desmosomal contacts between the endothelial cells, but what is perhaps more interesting is the lack of an anatomical arrangement facilitating the adherence of these cells to the overlying corneal tissue (see Figs 3–2 and 3–3). What is anchoring the endothelium to the posterior limiting lamina? The literature does not provide an answer to this question. Although formed by somewhat delicate cells, this layer nevertheless remains faithfully attached to the cornea throughout life. Thus, some mechanism of adherence is indicated, but it remains to be elucidated. Perhaps the answer to this question may be found in the continuous secretion of basement membrane material,

and this can provide the mechanism for the endothelial adhesion (Fig 3–6).

The cytoplasm of the endothelial cell is packed with organelles, which is a trademark for cells engaged in high metabolic activity. The elevated metabolic rate is necessary for the important physiological functions of this layer. The large nucleus of the endothelial cell is the dominating organelle. In transverse section the nucleus is round or slightly oval, whereas sectioned longitudinally the nucleus has an elongated oval or cigar shape. Sectioned in flat orientation the nucleus is kidney or bean shaped.

The endothelial cell also has a very high count of mitochondria and numerous rough and smooth endoplasmic reticula (see Fig 3–2). In addition, a well-developed Golgi apparatus is found in its cytoplasm. Pinocytotic vesicles have also been noted along the apical face of the cell.[55]

Physiology

To perform its function of transmitting and refracting light, the cornea must, in a teleological sense, maintain its

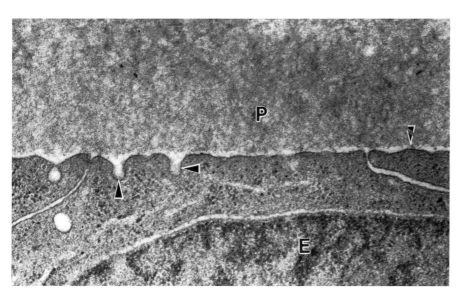

FIG 3–6.
High magnification of interface between the posterior limiting lamina and the endothelium. Electron dense granular basement membrane–like material *(triangles)* bridge the gap between the posterior limiting lamina *(P)* and the endothelium *(E)*. Transmission electron micrograph. Macaque mulatta monkey. (Magnification ×44,800.)

structure. The corneal endothelial cellular layer is intimately involved in this physiological process.

Nutrition

The endothelial cells require nutrients, principally in the form of glucose, amino acids, and oxygen, to perform their metabolic functions. Trace amounts of vitamins and minerals are probably needed as well. Wastes, such as carbon dioxide, must also be removed. As the endothelial layer is isolated from the vascular system, it is clear that most exchanges of metabolites occur either through the overlying stroma or from the aqueous humor that bathes its internal surface. Most current research suggests that all endothelial metabolites (glucose, amino acids, etc.) reach the cornea by diffusion or facilitated transfer from the aqueous humor of the anterior chamber (see Fatt and Weissman[31] for a review).

The oxygen supply of the endothelium, however, is specifically problematic. Some evidence has been presented suggesting that oxygen reaches the endothelium through the corneal epithelium and stroma from the external environment (i.e., the atmosphere under open eye conditions and the palpebral conjunctiva under closed eye conditions) by diffusion and passes on to create a gradient of oxygen tension in the aqueous humor.[3, 4] But this seems most improbable from consideration of the known oxygen consumptions and permeabilities of the corneal layers[32] and because any motion of the eye should homogenize P_{O_2} in the aqueous. Additional data suggest that under normal conditions—with the anterior surface of the cornea at P_{O_2} values ranging from 155 (open eye) to 55 mm Hg (closed eye) and the posterior surface of the cornea at an oxygen tension of about 50 mm Hg—the epithelium receives its oxygen supply from the atmosphere by diffusion through the tears (and any covering contact lens, if present), whereas the endothelium is totally supplied from the circulatory system (in the ciliary body and iris) through the aqueous humor.[109] The two limiting cellular layers of the cornea consume substantial amounts of oxygen, the epithelium more than the endothelium, simply on its greater volume of cells.

Function

The optical properties of the cornea depend on the maintenance of its thickness and hydration in the face of a fluid pressure (called *swelling pressure*), which acts to draw water continuously across the surface cellular layers.[67, 69] Early students of corneal physiology believed that the endothelium and epithelium were so impermeable to water that they were absolute barriers to water flow to maintain corneal dehydration. We now know, however, that these layers are not impermeable to water. Indeed, as discussed earlier, the zonula occludentes have been reported to be discontinuous in the endothelium and may be a contributing factor to the permeability of this layer.[39]

A second hypothesis to explain the maintenance of corneal thickness, hydration and, therefore, optical clarity invoked an osmotic pressure difference between the stromal fluid and other surrounding fluids (tears and aqueous humor). Such a difference would be difficult to physiologically maintain, and later experimentation disproved this hypothesis.

The *temperature reversal experiment* (TRE) of Davson[22] showed that corneal thickness and hydration were instead maintained by cellular metabolism, and so, as the epithelium and endothelium are the cellular layers, it is clear that whatever process is responsible must reside in one or both of these layers.

Although some initial research implicated the epithelium, Maurice[70] clearly demonstrated that primarily the endothelium is responsible for corneal hydration maintenance. His experiment on isolated in vitro endothelium showed that this layer alone could move water at a rate consistent with observed in vivo corneal hydration and also that it was the site of the TRE.

Most corneal biophysicists have now embraced Maurice's results, but how does the endothelium function to maintain corneal hydration? It is unlikely that water itself is directly pumped. Hodson and Miller[43] proposed that the endothelium actively transports bicarbonate ions into the anterior chamber, and water tends to follow osmotically. However, the validity of the HCO_3^- ion theory has recently been questioned.[25, 27] Indeed, Doughty[25] postulated that the stroma is the site for the corneal hydration control, whereas the endothelium merely regulates the HCO_3^- flow into the stroma. The final word on what—if anything— drives the endothelial pump has obviously not been said.

But if the endothelium is responsible for maintaining corneal hydration and thickness (and thus clarity), and if this layer receives all its metabolic needs from the immediately adjacent aqueous humor, and as this source is not interrupted by events on the anterior surface of the eye, why does the cornea swell when a tightly fitted, gas-impermeable contact lens is worn?

One possibility is that anterior hypoxia depresses epithelial metabolism and this layer then becomes secondarily leakier to water. Wilson et al.,[110] however, showed that the hydraulic permeability of the epithelium does not change when it is made anoxic. They also found that stromal swelling begins within a few minutes of the initiation of surface anoxia and that this time interval is consistent with the diffusion of a relatively large molecule "signal" moving across the stroma from the epithelium to the endothelium.

Klyce[54] considered this observation and then experimentally determined that lactic acid was most probably this molecule. His data suggest that excess lactate is produced by hypoxic epithelial cells, and because this molecule is not able to diffuse anteriorly between the tight-bordered epithelial cells, it diffuses back across the stroma to act osmotically and counterbalance the effect of the endothelial pump. This results in stromal swelling. An acid shift may accompany such an increase in stromal lactate.[10]

It is therefore believed that the metabolism of the endothelium is functionally responsible for corneal hydration control. The endothelium maintains itself as a barrier, preventing the free influx of water, and also maintains the pump-leak equilibrium, although Doughty[26] suggests there may not be an obligate coupling between stromal deturgescence and endothelial fluid pump activity as previously proposed by Hodson and Miller.[43] Insult to the endothelium, whether physical or metabolic, is clinically manifested as corneal edema or swelling, such as when oxygen impermeable contact lenses are worn. Severe hypoxic challenge allows the increase in stromal hydration and acidosis to build up to the point where water can accumulate in and under the less water-permeable cellular layers. Clinically this is termed *microcystic edema*. Bullous keratopathy results from more endothelial dysfunction and may be preceded by guttatae, endothelial blebs, or both.[34, 48] If severe and chronic, such events can culminate in corneal decompensation. It should be noted that this is an extreme event; contact lens wear itself has not been shown to cause corneal decompensation, although it may cause edema. Mild corneal edema may not necessarily have a detrimental effect on the cornea, even long term. It occurs every time we close our eyes during sleep and is therefore a frequent and normal experience.

Basement Membrane: Posterior Limiting Lamina

The posterior limiting lamina is the basement membrane of the endothelium, but unlike its counterpart in the epithelium, it is considered a separate corneal layer. Because the posterior limiting lamina truly is an endothelial structure, secreted by the endothelial cells, it will be considered here along with the endothelium.

The posterior limiting lamina is the thickest basement membrane in the body, and it increases in thickness with age (Fig 3–7). During infancy this basement membrane is approximately 3 μm, and during the eighth decade of life it has become up to 17 μm thick.[51] The adult peripheral posterior limiting lamina shows local thickenings known as *Hassell-Henle warts*.[98]

The posterior limiting lamina consists of two portions, an anterior banded portion and a posterior nonbanded portion (Fig 3–8). Only the anterior portion, 3 μm thick, is present at birth, and it remains unchanged during life.[51] The posterior portion, which appears homogenous in histological section, is continuously formed by secretion from the endothelium.

In contrast, the anterior portion shows in transverse section a banded and somewhat granular configuration, whereas a hexagonal array is present in flat section.[55]

This basement membrane is clinically noted for its resilience to physical trauma or disease. For instance, in cor-

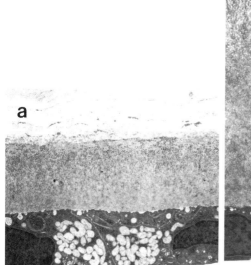

FIG 3–7.
Transverse section through posterior limiting lamina from two humans separated in age by almost 80 years. The older posterior limiting lamina *(b)* is three times thicker than the younger one *(a)*. Transmission electron micrograph. Humans 4 years of age *(a)* and 82 years of age *(b)*. (Magnification ×10,000.)

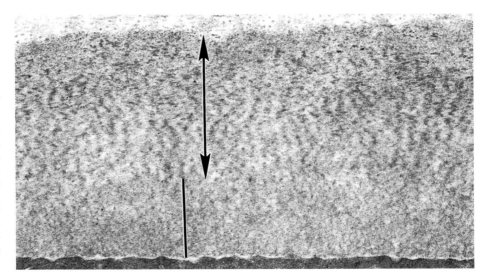

FIG 3–8.
Transverse section through the posterior limiting lamina. The posterior limiting lamina consists of two portions: a posterior, younger, smoother, nonbanded part *(solid line)* and an anterior, older, less uniform, banded part *(solid line with arrowheads).* Transmission electron micrograph. Macaque mulatta monkey. (Magnification ×26,400.)

neal melting from chronic inflammatory disease, the posterior limiting lamina is the last structure to give way before complete corneal perforation; this condition is known as descemetocele.

The attachment apparatus of the epithelial basement membrane does not appear replicated in the case of the posterior limiting lamina. There are no hemidesmosomes between the endothelial cells and its basement membrane, and there appear to be no reticular fibrils from the stroma fusing with this basal lamina as noted with the epithelial basement membrane. In addition to the adhesive effect the continuous secretion of basement membrane material may have, the somewhat irregular interface between the stroma and the posterior limiting lamina may also provide some means for attachment.

EXAMINATION OF THE ENDOTHELIUM

Clinical Techniques

Magnification must be used to directly observe the cells of the corneal endothelium. In addition, because these cells are transparent to visible wavelengths of light, special techniques must be employed.

Vogt first described the use of the biomicroscope in the examination of the corneal endothelium in 1920.[72] He used the technique we term *specular reflection* whereby illumination produced by the instrument's light source is reflected off the posterior corneal surface in a mirrorlike fashion: the angle of incidence is equal to the angle of reflection. This reflection is observed by the clinician through the microscope's eyepiece. Elevations, depressions, and other irregularities (e.g., cell borders) reflect the incident light in directions other than that taken by the

majority of light off the plane of the cellular layer being examined, and, thus, these appear dark to the observer. We presume that the change in optical index from the endothelial cell to the aqueous is greater than the changes in index from the stroma to the posterior limiting lamina or from this layer to the anterior membranes of the endothelial cells; therefore, we believe we are observing the aqueous interface. However, the images obtained in this manner may contain information of other cellular regions because the light will travel twice through the full thickness of the cell and the overlying cornea.

Vogt noted the surface details of the posterior endothelial mosaic and published illustrations of his observations in his *Lehrbuch und Atlas der Spaltlampen Mikroskopie des lebenden Auges* (Fig 3–9). Graves[36] used this technique and then described endothelial layer changes in Fuch's dystrophy (see later discussion). In recent years, both Holm[49] and Zantos and Holden[113] carried this technique one step further and demonstrated that these images, with sufficient magnification, could be photographed directly through the optics of a biomicroscope (see Figs 3–17 and 3–18).

Maurice[68] also extended this specular reflective technique, describing the first laboratory specular microscope. Light was passed down one half of a ×40 water immersion objective to the cornea and, after reflection, was observed through the other half. This device was intended to be used for in vitro research or in the examination of eyebank eyes with the goal of inspecting prospective corneas for corneal transplantation.[44] The examiner would be able to quantitatively and qualitatively judge the potential viability of corneal tissues. Laing et al.[62] estimated that the specular reflection from the aqueous humor–endothelial cell boundary represents only about 0.02% of the incident light in this system.

Others[12, 61] subsequently took an additional step, al-

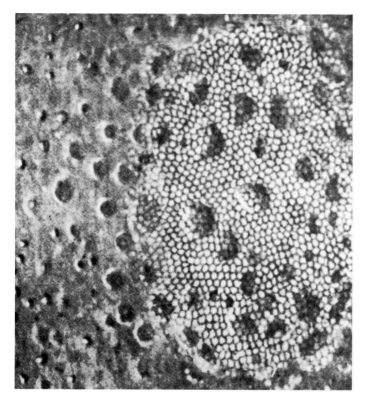

FIG 3–9.
Reproduction of illustration from Vogt's original specular biomicroscopy observation on a human eye. Note the irregularities in the image, probably representing corneal guttatae. (From Duke-Elder S, Leigh AG: *System of Ophthalmology,* Part 2, vol III, in Duke-Elder S (ed): *Diseases of the Outer Eye. St Louis, Mosby–Year Book, 1965. Used by permission.)*

lowing the observation and photographic documentation of corneas in vivo at a magnification of approximately ×50 to 200, first with still photography and eventually with real-time video imagery. A flat-surfaced dipping cone lens in front of the objective lens of the microscope was used to applanate and partially stabilize the cornea under observation.

These devices allow clear observation of only a narrow field of cells. Widening the slit causes an increase in light scatter from the overlying tears, epithelium, and connective tissue, which then decreases contrast and obscures detail of the endothelium.

Koester et al.[56] used the basic principle described earlier by Maurice[71] for a scanning slit microscope to develop a scanning mirror microscope to overcome this limitation. A narrow slit is still used, but the image of the specimen is internally displaced across the film plane so that a wider area is photographed. This technique became clinically available in the Keeler-Konan specular wide-field microscope.

Laboratory Techniques

In vitro and histological observations utilize laboratory techniques. As a rule, laboratory techniques provide superior magnification and resolution over clinical techniques, whereas on the deficit side is the fact that the endothelium is not viewed under natural, in vivo conditions.

In Vitro Techniques

In vitro observation of the endothelium is a standard procedure in all eye banks, which employ specular microscopy for their tissue evaluations. For best results in the in vitro setting, the endothelium needs to be bathed in a physiological medium at 4° C. A common eye bank medium is K-sol, and when placed in this medium, a human cornea stays viable for 10 days.[30] However, bacterial growth is a serious hazard with tissues intended for transplantation, and as a consequence, most storage media have an antibiotic or even a combination of antibiotics, such as gentamicin or gentamicin and vancomycin.[11, 33] The cytotoxicity of the antibiotic together with a reduction in its antibacterial efficacy over a period appear to shorten the time over which a cornea remains useful for transplantation. Of course, in physiological experiments using in vitro corneas, there is usually no need to control antimicrobial activity, and as a consequence, the antibiotic may be left out of the medium.

Histological Techniques

Light microscopy and transmission and scanning electron microscopy are histological techniques that have been used in the study of the corneal endothelium. An excellent review of the histological techniques that have been used to study the corneal endothelium was offered recently by Doughty.[24] Most of the histological studies found in literature have been on corneas that have been exposed to a fixative. As a consequence, the ensuing observations have been made on dead cells. Nevertheless, it is the expectation of these studies that good techniques have caused minimal artefacts. Histological techniques generally reward the observer with greatly enhanced resolution and the option of substantially increased magnification. A further advantage over clinical techniques is that light and transmission electron microscopy offer a view of the internal structures of the tissue or the cells.

Light Microscopy

Histological techniques in conjunction with light microscopy have been used somewhat sparingly on the endothelium. Past studies have often tried to demonstrate the endothelial mosaic, and the preferred technique for this purpose appears to be whole mount of the cornea, because it allows a wider field of view. In such studies it is desirable to use a stain that selectively dyes the cell border. Alizarin red S, orcerin, silver nitrate, and trypan blue have been used as stains to highlight the endothelial mosaic. Other stains, such as toluidine blue, have been employed to show the cytoplasm and the organelles it contains. Vital stains are useful when the viability of the endothelial cells needs to be assessed. This, of course, is an important issue to the eye banks who must assure that their procedures do not lead to an unnecessarily rapid decline of the tissue. Aliizarin red S, trypan blue, Evans blue, and rose bengal are vital stains that have been successfully used to assess the viability of the endothelial cell either individually or in a combination.[87, 94, 99]

Transmission Electron Microscopy

The "light source" in an electron microscope is an electron gun emitting an invisible electron beam that passes through the tissue specimen and then becomes visible on a fluorescent screen placed in its path. The limitation of light microscopy is the relatively long wavelength of visible light. The shorter wavelength of the electron beam is the key to the superior resolution of the transmission electron microscope. A consequence of the different nature of the electron beam over the visible light is the use of electron absorbing stains, which are necessary for best results. Most current studies rely on a dual staining procedure involving exposure of the tissue first to uranyl acetate (3.5%), followed by Reynold lead citrate.

For fixative, most electron microscope studies use glutaraldehyde (e.g., 3% in 0.1M cacodylate buffer at pH 7.2) or Karnovsky's fixative (3% glutaraldehyde combined with 2% paraformaldehyde buffered as previously). To avoid distortion of the tissue from shrinkage, one should excise the cornea after fixation of the tissue has been completed. Optimal preservation of the endothelium—giving a high-contrast, artefact-free view of this layer—is a diffi-

cult task and not always achieved. This technical challenge perhaps best explains the pausity in literature on the ultrastructural response of the endothelium to contact lens wear.[7, 8, 100]

Scanning Electron Microscopy

Scanning electron microscopy (SEM) is the histological variant of specular microscopy of the endothelium. Both techniques offer a view of the same surface, as has been demonstrated by a number of studies.[7, 98, 100] Good correlation between SEM and specular microscope images facilitates the clinical application of the histological findings with SEM. However, it should be recognized that SEM, just like specular microscopy, provides only a two-dimensional view of the posterior surface of the endothelial cell and, as a consequence, offers little or no information about any other aspect or portion of the cell, such as overall volume, size, or cytoplasmic content.

Scanning electron microscopy is a technically demanding technique. For instance, it is very important not only to have an excellent cellular preservation but also to maintain the overall, natural tissue contour. The most useful micrographs are often low-magnification, wide-field illustrations showing, in the case of the corneal endothelium, the mosaic formed by a number of cells. Unfortunately, the past literature is not abundant with such views. The SEM micrograph should show a flat surface contour without wrinkles, and the individual cells should not have a bump at the location of the nucleus. In the peripheral cornea, however, endothelial irregularities, or Hassel-Henle warts,[98] are normal.

Confocal Microscopy

The confocal microscope represents a new technology that shows a great deal of promise in corneal application. It is currently a laboratory instrument but could in its in vivo configuration become a useful clinical tool.

The disadvantage of traditional histology is that it requires the fixation, processing, and sectioning of a tissue that all can lead to artefacts. In addition, conventional histology will present only a static picture of cells, whereas we know that a tissue is a very dynamic entity. The confocal microscope is designed to overcome these drawbacks. The instrument is in its infancy of development, and progress has already been made to overcome the short comings of conventional histology. However, further improvements, especially in the areas of lateral resolution and clinical practicality of the instrument, are necessary before it will break into the clinical setting.

The confocal microscope uses both a light source and an objective lens system that are focused on the same very small point. The light passes through a Nipkow disk containing thousands of pinholes, each 20 μm in diameter.

The pinholes allow for a small field of view to enhance the resolution. By rotating the disc and scanning the image, one can obtain a larger field of view. The light source could be either incoherent light or a laser beam. Because of light losses, which are in the order of 98% or more through a Nipkow disk, a high-intensity source is needed (e.g., 100-W mercury arc lamp). The unique design of this microscope has overcome many of the disadvantages of using a visible light source, and as a consequence, this instrument has an impressive resolution.

The laboratory application of this exciting new technology has been described recently.[50, 66] The instrument offers the opportunity to examine the cornea noninvasively either under in vitro or in vivo conditions. It is hoped that improvement in the optics of the microscope, together with advancements in the electronic accessories such as video attachment, computor enhancement, and computor analysis, will overcome current limitations and make this instrument a valuable addition to the science and clinical practice of eye care.

CHANGES IN THE CORNEAL ENDOTHELIUM

Senescent Endothelium

Cell Density

The human endothelium shows no mitosis after birth, which distinguishes it from that of some other species. For instance, young rabbit endothelium shows cell division postnatally.[78] The loss or death of an endothelial cell in the case of the human, however, is not compensated by cellular reproduction, and, therefore, there is a steady decline in cellular density as a function of age. An age-related decline in endothelial count is not necessarily the trend in every species. For example, in analyzing the cat endothelium, Chan-Ling and Curini[19] found that there was no significant decrease in cell density with age.

Under the age of 1 year the human endothelial cell density is on average 4,252 to 4,425 cells/mm^2.[95, 98] A considerable individual variation in endothelial cell population (2,987–5,632 cells/mm^2) exists already at birth.[95, 98] Individual variations in cell density are manifested in all age groups throughout life, and to further complicate matters, there are also variations between different studies on what is normal for a particular age group. However, most studies seem to agree that during early adulthood (20–30 years), a normal human cell density is approximately 3,000 to 3,500 cells/mm^2.[9, 12, 111, 112] In the middle-aged human (40–50 years), the endothelial cell count has declined to 2,500 to 3,000 cells/mm^2, and on

entering the eighth decade of life, the cell population has decreased to 2,000 to 2,500 cells/mm^2.[9, 12, 112] The rate at which the endothelial cell density declines may slow down with age,[9, 112] and one study arrived at the conclusion that the decline ceased at age 50.[111] Other studies, however, have shown a more linear relationship between age and cell density.[12, 76] Murphy et al.[76] stated that this linear and "age-related decline in cellularity is probably due to the loss of 0.56% cells per year from the endothelial layer."

There appears to be a generous reserve built into the endothelium that can maintain physiological function with fewer than 1,000 cells/mm^2.[55, 85] To uphold its functions, the endothelium needs to offer a complete coverage of the posterior limiting lamina. The endothelial cell has considerable flexibility in achieving this minimum requirement, and this is associated with primarily two factors probably occurring together. The first factor is the ability of the normaly invaginate sides to straighten out, and the second one is the facility the cell has to reduce its thickness to become flatter and, therefore, wider. The limit for corneal coverage appears to be a cell density of 400 to 700 cells/mm^2; once the endothelial population falls below this critical value, corneal edema will follow because of the loss of endothelial function.[55]

Cell Shape

The literature on the endothelium includes a varied terminology that sometimes may be misunderstood or misused. The appropriate definition of some common terms is found in Table 3–1.

The morphology of the endothelium as seen by the specular microscope has been studied in various populations, and it has been shown conclusively that there is an increase in the variation of size of cells and the number of sides forming cells (polymegethism and polygonality), in addition to the age-related decline in cell density, as a function of advancing age.[16, 85, 96, 112] It should be noted that the term polymegethism, which is a phenomenon closely associated with contact lens wear, was introduced by Rao et al.,[84] who evaluated a non–contact lens wearing population. Indeed, it is very important that the clinician recognize that regardless of contact lens wear, it is a natural consequence of aging to have a decrease in endothelial cell count and an increase in polymegethism, pleomorphism, and polygonality. The possible contribution by the

TABLE 3–1.

Definition of Terminology

Polymegethism—variation in cell size
Pleomorphism—variation in cell shape (form)
Polymorphism—variation in cell shape (form)
Polygonal—multiple sides forming the cell

contact lens to further development of these phenomena is discussed below.

Cell Function

Does the functional ability of the surviving endothelial cell decrease with age? If the criterion for normal function is corneal transparence as opposed to edema, there appears to be no deficit linked to the aging of the endothelium, at least as long as there are about 1,000 cells/mm^2.[55, 85] However, studies have shown that corneas first challenged with a hypoxic stress and subsequently measured for the time to return to normal thickness need longer time with increasing age.[79, 82] The ability of the cornea to return from a swollen state to its normal thickness has been termed the *corneal deswelling function*. Using pachometer readings over time does not permit the conclusion that it is an endothelial function that is measured, although an endothelial factor in this corneal function is not an unreasonable assumption. There may be other factors contributing to this function; for instance, Doughty[23] has demonstrated corneal deturgescence in the absence of the obvious participation of the endothelial pump.

Carlson et al.[16] showed an increase in endothelial permeability to fluorescein with increasing age. This may suggest that the endothelial layer becomes leakier with age.

In summary, it is fair to say that the aging characteristics of the endothelium are generally recent knowledge, and their impact on the cornea remains difficult to assess. Except for cell density, none of these characteristics, even in their more severe presentations, appears independently as a threat to either endothelial health or corneal transparency.

Posterior Limiting Lamina

As has been pointed out earlier in this chapter, the posterior limiting lamina increases in thickness as a function of age.[51] This increase in thickness, which amounts approximately to 1 μm per decade of life,[51] is the result of its continued secretion by the endothelium (see Fig 3–7). The overall structure of the posterior limiting lamina and its anterior and posterior relations remain unchanged through life. Therefore, a deterioration of this corneal layer with age is not to be expected. On the contrary, the increased thickness of the posterior limiting lamina may, indeed, make it an even more resilient structure in trauma or disease.

Endothelial and Associated Pathological Conditions

Diseases of the corneal endothelium may be divided into (1) dystrophies, (2) degenerations, and (3) other processes.

Changes in endothelial layer form and function, however, manifest themselves in only three ways regardless of etiology. First, stressed endothelial cells produce excess collagen posterior to the posterior limiting lamina (termed the *posterior collagen layer* by Waring et al.[104]), which can be laminar, nodular (called *corneal guttatae*), or both. Second, the endothelial cells may change in size (polymegethism) and shape (polymorphism or pleomorphism) either acutely, as in Zantos-Holden blebs, or chronically, as in Fuchs' dystrophy. Third, corneal edema, both stromal and eventually epithelial, may occur following abnormalities to both the mechanical fluid barrier provided by the endothelial layer and some degradation in its ability to metabolically maintain normal corneal hydration. Corneal decompensation may follow as a consequence of endothelial dysfunction. Changes caused by contact lens wear may be confused for disease processes in either of these classifications, so it is helpful in this review to consider a few of the more common pathological conditions here.

Dystrophies and Degenerations

Corneal dystrophies are commonly considered to be genetically inherited abnormalities of form, function, or both. Often they are bilateral, isolated to the central portion of the cornea, and noninflammatory. The inheritance pattern is usually autosomal dominant. Degenerations, however, are age on disease related, may be unilateral, and often affect the corneal periphery. Arcus senilus, for example, is clearly a degeneration, whereas granular dystrophy is clearly a dystrophy with an autosomal dominant inheritance pattern. Salzmann's nodular dystrophy, however, is now known to probably be a degeneration secondary to chronic phlyctenular disease. Keratoconus has elements of both dystrophy and degeneration, so its classification is less clear.

Fuchs' Dystrophy.—Fuchs' endothelial dystrophy is a primary disease of the corneal endothelium. It has also been called *combined epithelial-endothelial dystrophy* and *late hereditary endothelial dystrophy,* but the former eponym is the most universally used term and correctly identifies the endothelium as the primary site of the disease. Fuchs' dystrophy is believed to be inherited in an autosomal dominant manner (almost all corneal dystrophies, with the exception of macular dystrophy, are usually reported as autosomal dominant in the literature) and occurs in three stages. First a few corneal guttatae pepper the posterior cornea; this may be a common accompanying feature of aging, and if these changes are restricted to the corneal periphery, they are Hassel-Henle warts. Larger numbers of guttatae, often accompanied by flecks of endothelial pigment and together with edema (Fig 3–10), are termed *endothelial dystrophy;* this probably represents early Fuchs'.

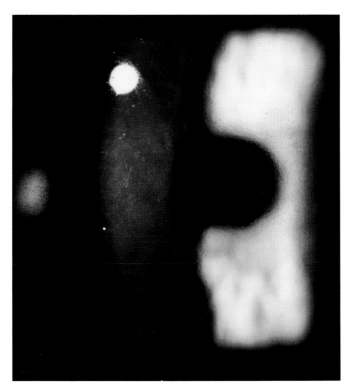

FIG 3–10.
Early Fuchs' dystrophy changes seen in the cornea of an 80-year-old aphakic male patient. Note stromal haze, endothelial pigment, and ground glass appearance seen in retroillumination.

Corneal guttatae in conjunction with stromal and sometimes epithelial edema, including bullae, leading to decreased vision and occasional episodes of pain from ruptured bullae, constitute the full clinical picture of Fuchs' dystrophy (Fig 3–11). The endothelial cells become large and thin and lose the characteristic hexagonal shape of their posterior surface, but they usually maintain an intact covering over the posterior corneal surface. This disease is commonly bilateral, is often asymmetrical, affects women more severely than men, and has a course of 10 to 20 years. Symptoms rarely appear before 50 years of age. It is important to note an association with Fuchs' dystrophy and ocular hypertension and chronic open angle glaucoma.[106]

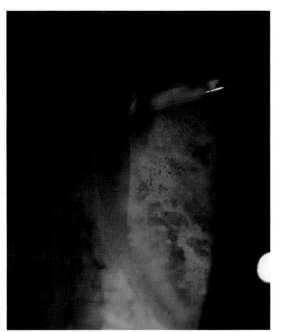

FIG 3–11.
Peripheral epithelial bullae seen in direct illumination by the pooling of fluorescein around the elevated lesions. This patient is an elderly man, aphakic for more than 10 years. These lesions probably represent early aphakic bullous keratopathy and, because of their peripheral location, do not interfere with vision at this point.

Posterior Polymorphous Dystrophy.—A second inherited change is termed posterior polymorphous dystrophy (PPD). It has also been called other names in the past. It represents a large variety of changes in the posterior corneal surface and usually has an autosomal dominant inheritance pattern, although occasional reports of autosomal recessive inheritance have been reported.[106] It is generally considered bilateral but may be asymmetrical or occasionally unilateral. Because this is most commonly an asymptomatic disease, the age of onset is difficult to determine and the changes may be congenital. It is also usually considered stable, but there are reports of slow progression and rare incidents of stromal edema. The clinical picture is one of a wide variety of lesions: clusters of discrete small vesicles surrounded by faint gray halos, larger blisterlike lesions, or even bands or sheets of irregular grayish "stretched cellophane" at the level of posterior limiting lamina (Fig 3–12). Although corneal guttatae are not seen clinically, specular microscopy reveals endothelial pleomorphism and clusters of abnormal epithelial-like cells with indistinct cell boundaries. In the classical literature, PPD has been linked with only a rare posterior form of keratoconus, but more recent reports suggest that this disease may coexist occasionally with keratoconus.[107] Contact lens wear is usually not contraindicated in patients with PPD.

Congenital Hereditary Endothelial Dystrophy.—Congenital hereditary endothelial dystrophy is not likely to be confused with a contact lens–induced complication. Not only is this disease restricted to the pediatric population, but substantial corneal edema is a distinguishing feature and would be noted as a preexisting feature.

Acquired Endothelial Pathological Conditions.—*Keratic Precipitates.*—Keratic precipitates (KPs) have often been termed "mutton fat." As the term KPs implies, it is a condition referring to the deposition of material on the posterior endothelial surface. This material is either cellular or pigmented and may have arrived because of uveitis, trauma, or aging.[1, 18, 28] Keratic precipitates originate primarily from inflammatory cells that have escaped or were released into the aqueous humor in response to an anterior uveitis or trauma, but occasionally these deposits can be erythrocytes or precipitation from neoplasms.[1, 28]

Most patients with KPs are asymptomatic, and only patients with an active iritis or iridocyclitis are likely to have a complaint, which, in such a case, will be exactly that associated with an active anterior uveitis. Precipitates in a quiet eye are usually a sign of what had once occurred but is no longer the case.

Keratic precipitates are distributed over the inferior third of the cornea in an almost triangular shape, with its apex pointing toward the superior cornea. This peculiar distribution of matter is dictated by convection currents of the aqueous humor in the anterior chamber. The deposits may be seen in most slit-lamp illuminations but is perhaps best observed in direct or retroillumination against the

FIG 3–12.
Posterior polymorphous dystrophy lesions seen in retroillumination (with a dilated pupil); in addition, note the persistent pupillary strand as an incidental finding. This 30-year-old male patient also has keratoconus. (From Weissman BA, et al: *Optom Vis Sci* 1989; 66:243–246. Used by permission.)

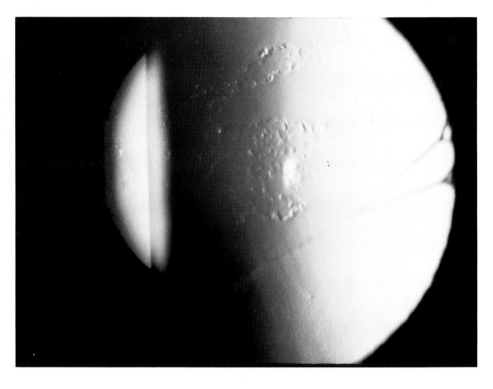

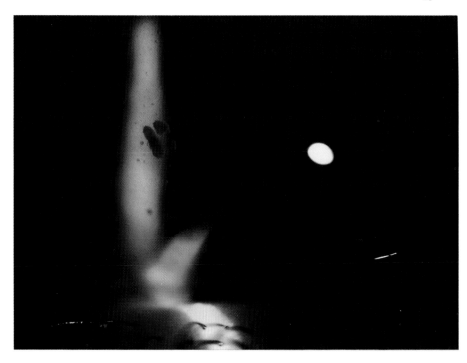

FIG 3–13.
Retroillumination view of "mutton fat" keratic precipitates (KPs) seen in the cornea of a young male patient (age 13 years) with chronic iridocyclitis of unknown etiology.

dark pupil (Fig 3–13). In these two latter illuminations, the inflammatory cells appear bright white or milky white (hence the term mutton fat). Apart from the distribution of the spots, specular microscopy may be helpful in differentiating these deposits from corneal guttatae because the precipitates will not show the characteristic dark holes in the mosaic pattern as is characteristic of guttatae.

It is interesting to note that histopathology of KPs demonstrate that these cells are not adherent to the posterior surface of the cornea but have with time become entrapped intercellularly within the endothelium (Fig 3–14). This seems to explain how KPs remain visible in the same place year after year. Before becoming lodged intracellularly, the inflammatory cells appear to be able to adhere to the endothelial surface by expressing an intercellular adhesion molecule.[29] The presence of KPs in a quiet eye is not a contraindication to wearing contact lenses. However, because this condition involves the endothelium, it would be prudent to monitor a little more closely for stromal edema, especially during the initial visits. Secondary "pigmentary" glaucoma should also be a concern for the clinician seeing a patient with KPs.

Other Diseases.—Other diseases can also occur in the endothelial layer and be confused with contact lens–associated changes. After surgery, especially cataract extraction, epithelial cells can become seeded on the posterior cornea and grow down over the endothelial layer, leading to both functional and anatomical loss. This is called *epithelial downgrowth. Essential iris atrophy*

(Chandler's syndrome) is yet another disease in which the endothelial cells become abnormal, assuming epithelial cell morphology; these abnormal cells grow across the trabecular meshwork and iris, leading to decreased aqueous outflow facility and secondary glaucoma. Rents in the iris and displaced pupils are commonly seen. In contrast, the normal corneal endothelium of the rabbit continues across the entire trabeculum.[6] However, this complete endothelial coverage does not lead to a high intraocular pressure in the rabbit as it does in the human.

Some other less usual changes can also occur. Figure 3–15, for example, shows a rare pigmentation plaque of the endothelial layer after early cataract extraction.

Posterior Mosaic Shagreen.—Posterior mosaic or crocodile shagreen is an involutionary alteration of the posterior cornea. It is a bilateral condition affecting the posterior stroma.[1, 57] Usually occupying the central one to two thirds of the cornea, posterior mosaic shagreen may be mistaken for central corneal clouding in the older contact lens wearer. However, the characteristic polygonally shaped areas of corneal clouding or graying, separated by lines of clear stroma, sets the former apart from the latter. Furthermore, these patients do not have increased corneal thickness or folds of posterior limiting lamina.

Histopathological examination of corneas with posterior mosaic shagreen indicates that alterations to the normal organization of the collagen lamellae have occurred. Some lamellae in the posterior stroma appear perpendicular to the plane of the cornea, and others have adopted a

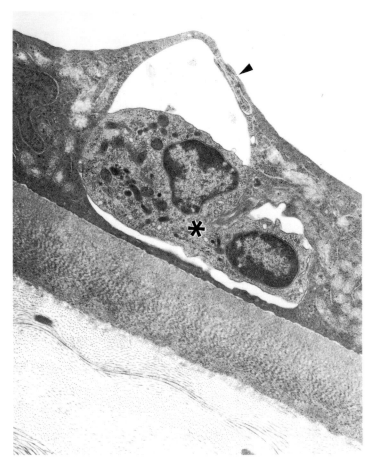

FIG 3-14.
Keratic precipitate. A leukocyte (neutrophil) *(asterisk)* is located in a space formed between two adjacent endothelial cells. This KP is sealed from access to the anterior chamber by a zonula occludens *(triangle)*. Transmission electron micrograph. Macaque mulatta monkey. (Magnification ×12,000.)

sawtooth-like outline.[57] In addition, patches of collagen fibers show a 100-nm banding pattern.[57]

Patients are asymptomatic, and the noninvolvement of the endothelium in this condition allows for normal contact lens wear.

Cornea Farinata.—This corneal entity was named according to its clinical presenting symptoms. Farina is latin for "flour," and in cornea farinata it appears that the posterior stroma immediately anterior to the posterior limiting lamina has become covered by white, flourlike spots. These dots are distributed across the cornea and may be best studied with indirect retroillumination.

Cornea farinata is an asymptomatic, age-related condition, usually manifested in both eyes, and only rarely believed to be inherited.[1, 97] Patients with cornea farinata should be differentiated from those with guttatae and pre-Descemet's dystrophy. Unlike cornea farinata, many of the small whitish opacities found in the posterior stroma in pre-Descemet's dystrophy show distinct spindle shape and, in addition, may be encountered infrequently more anteriorly. When one is differentiating cornea farinata from guttatae, the most important fact to remember is that one condition is stromal and the other is endothelial. Specular reflection of cornea farinata should generate a nice uniform endothelial mosaic. Although cornea farinata in some patients has a dramatic manifestation, it nevertheless does not appear to affect vision.

Histopathologically little is known regarding the characteristics of cornea farinata. It has been suggested that there may be some similarity with pre-Descemet's dystrophy, which affects the posterior corneal keratocytes. The affected keratocytes appear to contain lipofuscin.[21]

Because cornea farinata affects only the extreme posterior stroma and not the endothelium, contact lenses may be fitted on patients with this anomaly.

Pre-Descemet's Dystrophy.—The close clinical and histopathological resemblance between pre-Descemet's dystrophy and cornea farinata has sometimes caused the former abnormality to be regarded as a variant of the latter. However, leading authorities prefer to classify them separately primarily because cornea farinata appears late in life, whereas pre-Descemet's may manifest in the early thirties, thus making this condition more dystrophic than degenerative.[1]

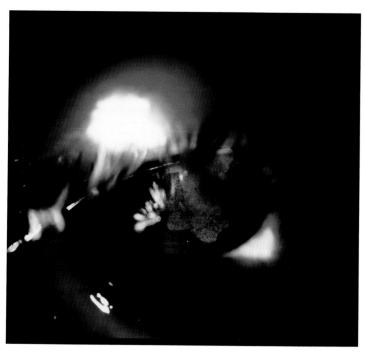

FIG 3–15.
Large pigment plaque on the endothelial surface of the cornea of a 70-year-old male aphakic patient some 35 years after uncomplicated cataract extraction.

As with cornea farinata, pre-Descemet's dystrophy may easily be mistaken for guttatae, but careful observation using high magnification and specular reflection type of illumination will reveal a normal endothelial mosaic. In addition, use of an optical section will show that the minute opacities in pre-Descemet's dystrophy are located predominantly in the posterior stroma and only infrequently in the anterior four fifths of the stroma. The distribution of the opacities may be uniformly across the entire corneal width, annular (sparing central cornea), or axial (sparing peripheral cornea).[37] The red reflex retroillumination biomicroscope setup is particularly useful when one is assessing the distribution of the opacities (Fig 3–16).

The opacities, showing more variations in pre-Descemets dystrophy than in cornea farinata, may follow dentritic, boomerang, circular, comma, linear, and filiform

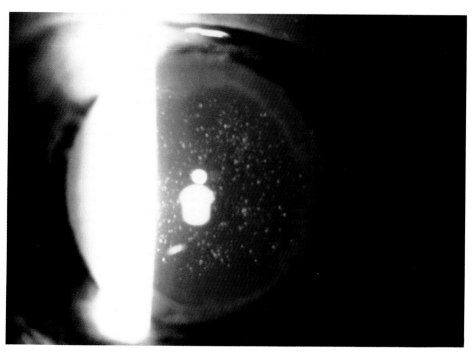

FIG 3–16.
Pre-Descemet's dystrophy. The red reflex through a dilated pupil clearly demonstrates the distribution of the numerous, small opacities in the posterior stroma. Biomicroscope photograph. (Courtesy of W. Jones, Albuquerque, NM.)

patterns.[37] The dendritic or spindle-shaped opacity is a giveaway that the posterior stromal keratocyte is the affected corneal component.

Pre-Descemet's dystrophy is bilateral, is more common in females than males, and may or may not be inherited.[37] Patients with pre-Descemets dystrophy are asymptomatic and do not have a decreased visual acuity because of the anormaly.

Histopathological analysis of pre-Descemet's dystrophy has shown that only the keratocytes in the vicinity of the posterior limiting lamina are affected, leaving the endothelium, posterior limiting lamina, and surrounding collagen normal.[21] The affected keratocytes had become vacuolated, and many of these vacuoles appeared to contain lipofuscin. Because the formation of lipofuscin is associated with age-related degenerative changes, Curran et al.[21] speculated that the pre-Descemet's dystrophy is a degeneration rather than dystrophy and possibly shares its pathogenesis with cornea farinata. However, they cautioned that a primary genetic disorder predisposing the cornea to these changes may be the truly underlying cause.

FIG 3–17.
Endothelial mosaic before insertion of a contact lens in a young human subject who is not a contact lens wearer.
(Courtesy of S. Zantos and Bausch & Lomb, Rochester, NY.)

Pre-Descemet's dystrophy should not deter the practitioner from fitting a contact lens.

HYPOXIC EFFECTS OF CONTACT LENS WEAR ON THE CORNEAL ENDOTHELIUM

Although the majority of contact lens wearers experience a minimum of difficulties, a certain number encounter complications, including epithelial and stromal edema, vascularization, allergies, and the rare but potentially devastating corneal infection. The endothelial layer is not immune to contact lens–induced changes, but the functional consequences of these changes are still debated.

Obrig[77] gave no hint that the endothelial layer is affected at all by contact lens wear; in fact, this layer was basically "terra incognito" to the contact lens practitioner until Zantos and Holden[113] described a method of photographing the in vivo corneal endothelium by specular re-

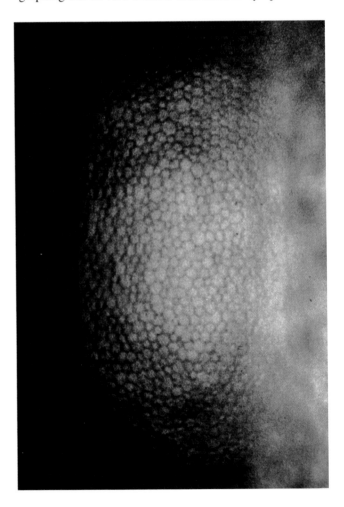

flection through the slit-lamp biomicroscope (see earlier discussion) and detailed the observation of "blebs" in this layer shortly after contact lens application (Figs 3–17 and 3–18). Later, Schoessler and Woloschak[90] described increased polymegethism in contact lens wearers. It follows that the conscientious contact lens practitioner can no longer ignore the endothelium.

Zantos-Holden Bleb Response

These dark areas (see Fig 3–18) in the endothelial mosaic pattern, similar in clinical appearance to Hassel-Henle warts or the corneal guttatae of Fuchs' dystrophy, are now known to reach a maximum in number and relative area about 30 minutes after the application of a rigid or soft contact lens (of relatively low oxygen transmissibility) to the eye of an unadapted subject.[2, 91, 101] Unlike Hassel-Henle bodies or Fuchs' guttatae, however, these changes rapidly (e.g., a few minutes) reverse if lenses are removed. Experienced contact lens wearers show lessened bleb responses, suggesting an adaptive process. Holden et al.[48] found that these changes could be induced in the absence of increased corneal hydration. In addition, they found that the response does not itself acutely compromise endothelial layer pump or barrier functions.

The apparent cause for these dark areas is localized bulging of the posterior endothelial cell membranes, inducing a disruption of the specularly reflected light.[100] Bergmanson[7] suggested that the blebs may represent intercellular edema in the endothelium (see Figs 3–29 and 3–30). Subjects vary greatly in the magnitude of the bleb response, and the blebs will slowly resolve after about 2 hours even if contact lens wear continues. These transient changes have now been observed not only with contact lens wear but also with lid closure and in both nitrogen and CO_2 external ocular environments[48, 53]; Holden et al.[48] theorized that this effect is mediated by a hypoxia-driven stromal pH change. Such a pH change was, in fact, later confirmed,[10] but a direct linkage between increased stromal acidity and the observed morphological change in the endothelium has yet to be demonstrated.

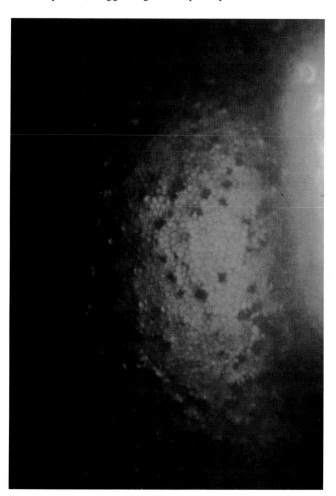

FIG 3–18.
Endothelial mosaic in the same human subject as in Figure 3–16 after 20 minutes of standard-thickness (approximately 0.1-mm) hydroxyethylmethacrylate contact lens wear. Note the numerous blebs that interrupt the mosaic. The blebs involve multiple cells, and many are located near or at the border regions of cells. (Courtesy of S. Zantos and Bausch & Lomb, Rochester, NY.)

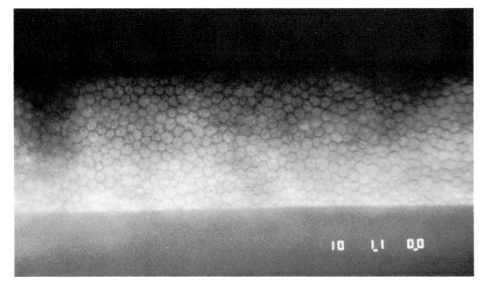

FIG 3–19.
Specular micrograph (Konon-Keeler, original magnification ×40) from the left eye of a 21-year-old subject with no contact lens experience. (Courtesy of J.P. Schoessler, Columbus, OH.)

Endothelial Bedewing

A change in the endothelial cell layer called bedewing has also been reported in association with chronic contact lens intolerance and active inflammation of the anterior segment.[75, 114] This may represent clusters of inflammatory cells, but the exact etiology is undefined.

Cell Density

It is believed that the normal health adult corneal endothelium numbers 2,500 to 3,500 cells/mm^2 (see earlier discussion) and that this figure slowly declines with normal aging.[9, 12, 60, 111, 112] Caldwell et al.[14] reported a decreased endothelial cell density after hard (polymethylmethacrylate, or PMMA) lens wear, exceeding the usual decrease expected with aging, but their data are not convincing because of the lack of an adequate control group. Indeed, other research found no statistically significant reduction in endothelial cell density in wearers of hard, soft, or extended wear contact lenses.[41, 47, 65, 88, 90] These studies, all of which used age-matched control groups, demonstrated that contact lens wear of many forms is not associated with endothelial cell loss other than that expected as a function of age.

Polymegethism

Schoessler and Woloschak[90] were first to show that contact lens wear can induce polymegethism. Further studies have confirmed this important observation beyond a doubt.[41, 47, 65, 88] The degree of polymegethism appears dependent on the level of anterior hypoxia induced by the contact lens. The most hypoxic wearing conditions, such as PMMA and soft extended contact lens wear, produce the most polymegethism.[47, 88, 90] In contrast, the highly oxygen-permeable silicon elastomer lenses[108] do not cause polymegethous changes.[17, 89]

To illustrate these observations, examine Figures 3–19 to 3–28 and Tables 3–2 to 3–5. The photographs are in vivo specular micrographs made with the Konan-Keeler microscope (JP Schoessler, personal communication, 1991), and the histograms show corresponding cell area distributions. The tables provide other analyses, including cell density and coefficient of variation (COV). The COV has become the number most commonly used to mathematically quantify the degree of polymegethism in a sample and is obtained by dividing the standard deviation of the cell areas observed with the arithemetic mean cell area of all of the cells shown in the sample.

Figure 3–19, for example, shows endothelial cells from one eye of a 21-year-old subject who has had no contact lens experience. Presumably because of this subject's relative youth and lack of history of other ocular or systemic diseases that might affect the corneal endothelium, this represents a "normal" corneal endothelium. Table 3–2 shows that the endothelial cell density is about 3,200 cells/mm^2, which is normal for this subject's age, and the COV is about 0.2. The corresponding histogram (Fig 3–20)

TABLE 3–2.

No Contact Lens Wear*

Parameter	Value
Mean cell area	0.000308 mm^2
Cell density	3,243 cells/mm^2
Coefficient of variation	0.228
Coefficient of skewness	0.0291
Hexagonal cells (%)	72.8

*Courtesy of J.P. Schoessler.

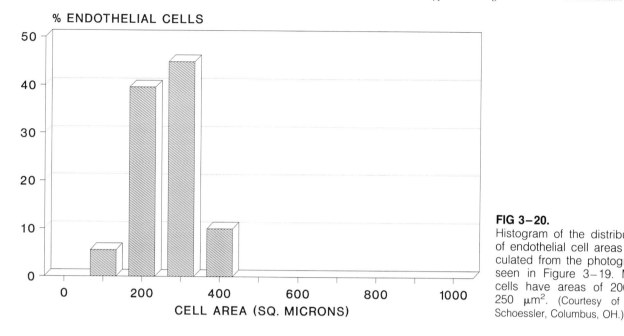

FIG 3–20.
Histogram of the distribution of endothelial cell areas calculated from the photograph seen in Figure 3–19. Most cells have areas of 200 to 250 μm^2. (Courtesy of J.P. Schoessler, Columbus, OH.)

shows that cell areas are relatively uniform at about 250 μm^2.

Figures 3–21 to 3–24 and Tables 3–3 and 3–4, however, show the endothelial cells and corresponding analysis from subjects who have worn contact lenses, presumably daily wear. The hydrogel lens wearer (see Figs 3–21 and 3–22 and Table 3–3) has about 6 years of experience and is 37 years old. The cell density is normal for age at 2,432 cells/mm^2, but the COV has increased to 0.3. Similarly, the rigid lens user (9 years of experience with PMMA lenses; see Figs 3–23 and 3–24 and Table 3–4) has a normal cell density of 2,902 cells/mm^2, but the COV is about 0.4. Both histograms suggest an increase in cell areas for some endothelial cell apical surfaces.

Finally, Figure 3–25 shows the endothelial apical surfaces for another 38-year-old subject; this patient wore a PMMA lens on this eye for 23 years (presumably daily wear). Not only is polymegethism easily apparent in the photograph, but the COV has increased to 0.9 (Table 3–5). The histogram (Fig 3–26) also shows the spread in cell area; some cells have become larger, but also some

TABLE 3–4.

Polymethylmethacrylate Contact Lens Wear*

Parameter	Value
Mean cell area	0.000345 mm^2
Cell density	2,902 cells/mm^2
Coefficient of variation	0.405
Coefficient of skewness	1.0218
Hexagonal cells (%)	52.4

*Courtesy of J.P. Schoessler.

smaller cells are now found. Cell density, however, is still normal for this subject's age at 2,951 cells/mm^2.

Although oxygen, or rather the lack of it, would seem implicated as the stimulus to the formation of polymegethism, it may act only indirectly to achieve this structural alteration. Clements[20] postulated that polymegethism is induced by corneal acidosis, which itself is caused by inhibition of CO_2 efflux from the anterior corneal surface, together with increased lactic acid production.

Polymegethism occurs as a function of age and as a

TABLE 3–3.

Soft Contact Lens Wear*

Parameter	Value
Mean cell area	0.000411 mm^2
Cell density	2,432 cells/mm^2
Coefficient of variation	0.300
Coefficient of skewness	0.8526
Hexagonal cells (%)	65.4

*Courtesy of J.P. Schoessler.

TABLE 3–5.

Polymethylmethacrylate Contact Lens Wear*

Parameter	Value
Mean cell area	0.000339 mm^2
Cell density	2,951 cells/mm^2
Coefficient of variation	0.904
Coefficient of skewness	4.1414
Hexagonal cells (%)	43.1

*Courtesy of J.P. Schoessler.

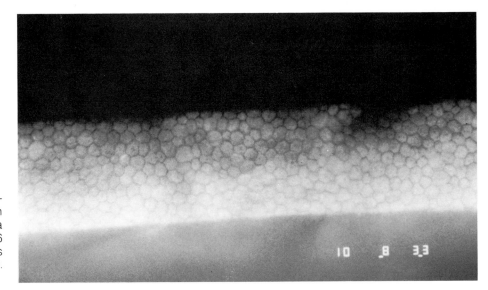

FIG 3–21.
Specular micrograph (Konan-Keeler, original magnification ×40) from the right eye of a 37-year-old subject after 6 years of hydrogel contact lens experience. (Courtesy of J.P. Schoessler, Columbus, OH.)

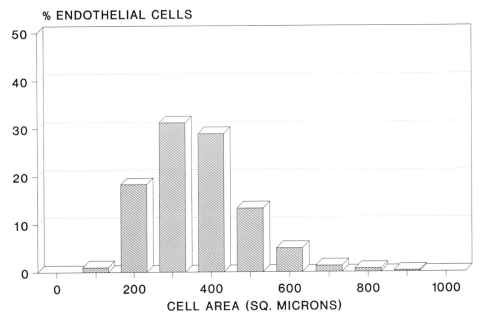

FIG 3–22.
Histogram of the distribution of endothelial cell areas calculated from Figure 3–21. Most cells are still about 200 to 400 μm^2. (Courtesy of J.P. Schoessler, Columbus, OH.)

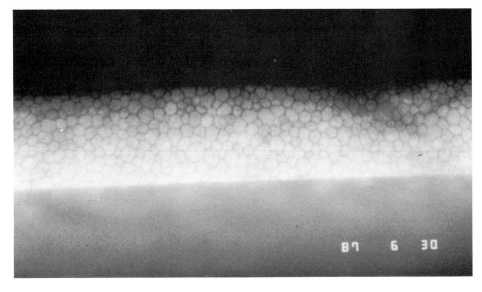

FIG 3–23.
Specular micrograph (Konan-Keeler, original magnification ×40) from the eye of a 45-year-old subject with 18 years of contact lens wear (9 years polymethylmethacrylate [PMMA], 9 years rigid gas permeable [RGP]). (Courtesy of J.P. Schoessler, Columbus, OH.)

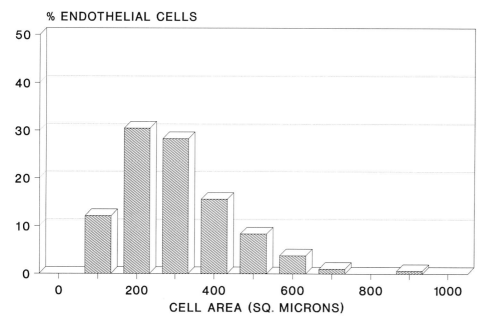

% ENDOTHELIAL CELLS

CELL AREA (SQ. MICRONS)

FIG 3–24.
Histogram of the distribution of endothelial cell areas calculated from Figure 3–23. Note cell areas have increased to 200 to 400 μm^2. (Courtesy of J.P. Schoessler, Columbus, OH.)

result of contact lens wear, as described earlier. In addition, polymegethism may also be induced by trauma, (e.g., surgery) and ultraviolet radiation.[35, 64, 81] Furthermore, endothelial polymegethism has been reported to occur in certain pathological conditions, such as Fuchs' dystrophy, diabetes, and cystic fibrosis.[13, 63] It is quite likely that other diseases are accompanied by endothelial polymegethism, but these have yet to be documented.

It should be noted that an increase in the number of sides forming the endothelial cell has been noted to accompany polymegethism in the contact lens wearer (Figs 3–27 and 3–28). This phenomenon occurs also as a function of aging in the nonlens wearer, as discussed earlier.

The diagnosis of polymegethism in a patient is accomplished clinically using a specular endothelial microscope or by employing specular illumination of the endothelium with the biomicroscope. These techniques, described earlier, visualize the interface between the posterior endothelial wall and the aqueous humor in the anterior chamber. Although COV has become the generally accepted way to quantify the polymegethism in an endothelium, its use has been questioned.[24, 25] The use of COV has a number of limitations. First, the COV, being a ratio derived entirely from a single and perhaps abnormal population, is, therefore, an index most valid for the individual from whom it was obtained. Consequently, COV is less useful for comparisons with other corneas. Second, this ratio does not indicate if cells generally shift toward larger cell areas (as would be expected to occur with aging) or toward smaller cell areas (both of which can occur without affecting

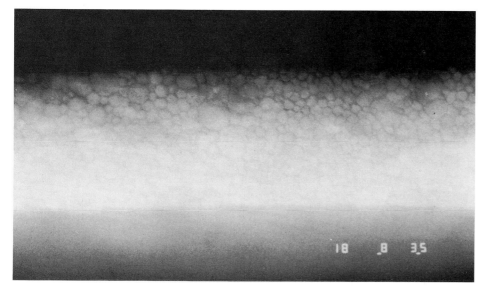

FIG 3–25.
Specular micrograph (Konan-Keeler, original magnification ×40) from the left eye of a 38-year-old subject after 23 years of PMMA contact lens wear. Note pleomorphism and obvious polymegethism. (Courtesy of J.P. Schoessler, Columbus, OH.)

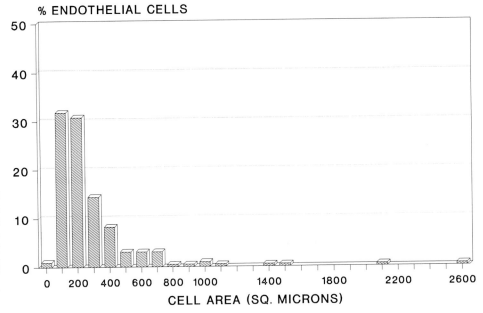

% ENDOTHELIAL CELLS

CELL AREA (SQ. MICRONS)

FIG 3–26.
Histogram of endothelial cell areas calculated from Figure 3–25. Note cell areas, have spread dramatically, both increasing to greater than 1,000 μm² in some instances and decreasing to 100 μm² as well. (Courtesy of J.P. Schoessler, Columbus, OH.)

COV). Because of such shortcomings, Doughty[25] went as far as saying that "the continued use of the coefficient of variations is thus not recommended."

The clinical evaluation of the central and paracentral endothelium using a specular microscope typically yields a sample of 75 to 200 cells from which the COV is calculated. Hirst et al.[42] examined whether this sampling correlates to the index obtained by measuring all cells within the central 4 mm of the same cornea. In this in vivo study, wide-field specular micrographs from the central 4 mm of a cornea were assembled in a montage and, depending on cell density, included between 2,800 and 5,300 cells.

They found that the small clinical sample was "at least 10% from the true mean cell size of all cells of the central 4 mm in any endothelium other than that with the most homogeneous pattern." In other words, when all cells are of the same size, a small sample—in the extreme case, only one cell—will produce a COV representative for the whole cornea (or at least the central 4 mm). On the other hand, in corneas with polymegethism, the clinical small sample will be erronous by a margin of 10% or greater.

It follows that the current method of sampling for COV involves too few cells to provide an accurate COV.[40, 42] To analyze 3,000 or more cells per cornea us-

FIG 3–27.
Histogram of distribution of number of cell sides for the 21-year-old subject (Fig 3–19) with no history of contact lens wear. (Courtesy of J.P. Schoessler, Columbus, OH.)

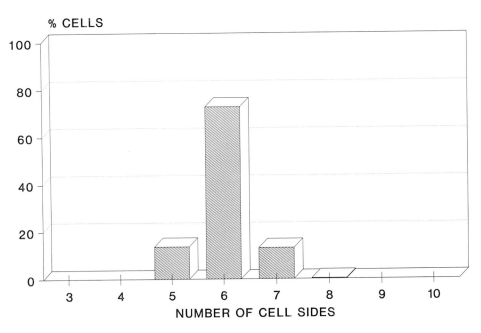

% CELLS

NUMBER OF CELL SIDES

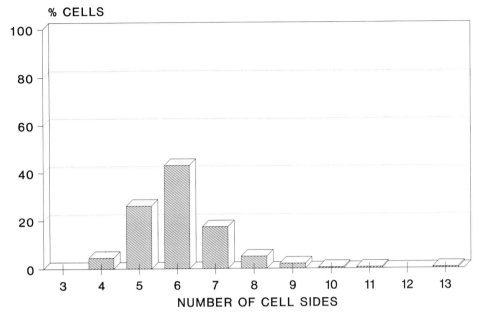

FIG 3–28.
Histogram of distribution of the number of cell sides for the 38-year-old subject after 23 years of experience with PMMA contact lens wear. Note increase in number of cell sides compared with Figure 3–27. (Courtesy of J.P. Schoessler, Columbus, OH.)

ing currently available technology, however, is not feasible for most of the occasions when a COV for a cornea is sought. For lack of a better method, we are in all likelihood going to see COVs being sampled and calculated as they are now. Therefore, it is important that the reader of these data be fully aware of the limitations of this index on cell size variation. It certainly would be helpful if the researchers publishing such data would acknowledge that their method of sampling has an associated error and that this error increases for increasing polymegethism. The current method does not have the resolution to detect small differences in COV.

What are the functional consequences of polymegethism? After a decade of searching, and all too frequently merely speculating, the fact, to everyone's relief, is that no scientifically proven loss of endothelial function has been demonstrated in contact lens wearers with polymegethism. Studies that specifically examined a possible correlation between the altered endothelial morphology and detrimental changes in endothelial function have been unable to demonstrate that such a relationship exists. In a study comparing 40 long-term contact lens wearers with 40 non–contact lens wearers, it was found that the increased polymegethism of the contact lens wearers was not accompanied by reduced corneal transparency, increased corneal thickness, or changes in endothelial permeability when compared with the control group.[16] Yet another study on experienced contact lens wearers found that the correlation between polymegethism and the corneal deswelling function was statistically insignificant.[83]

However, recent studies have shown a decrease in the deswelling function occurring with aging.[79, 82] According

to O'Neal and Polse,[79] the ability to recover from stromal swelling when measured over time is reduced by 10% at the age of 65; the cornea will return to its normal thickness, but it will take 10% longer. Two points should be made here because we also link polymegethism with aging. The first point is that although it is often assumed that the deswelling function is a measurement of an endothelial function, this has never been proved. Doughty,[23] for instance, reported an experiment where corneal deturgescence occurred without the apparent participation of the endothelium. Therefore, there may be other factors involved in corneal hydration control, and as a consequence we should not assume that the endothelium is solely involved in this process.

The second point is that the endothelial mosaic changes associated with aging have a different etiological background than those seen in contact lens wearers. Polymegethism in the older individual occurs with decreased cell density, but in the contact lens wearer these morphological changes are not accompanied by cell loss. The endothelial response to cell loss is to spread out existing cells to cover the space previously occupied by the lost cell. In the contact lens wearer there is no such gap to fill. The different origins to the morphological changes in the endothelia of contact lens wearers and that associated with aging may have different consequences, one of which may be the response to a hypoxic stress. This notion appears substantiated by a study where the correlation between contact lens–induced polymegethism and deswelling function was statistically insignificant.[83] In addition, it is interesting to note that with regard to the endothelial permeability to fluorescein, there is indeed a difference between the contact

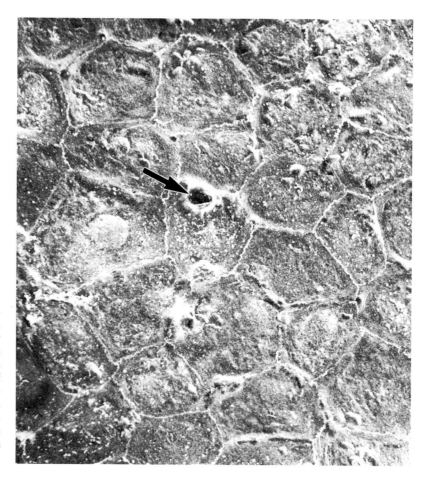

FIG 3–29.
Endothelial mosaic exhibiting polymegethism. The tissue was recovered from a 66-
year-old aphakic soft contact lens wearer
on a daily wear schedule for the previous
8 years. Note the distinct variation in the
area formed by the posterior surface of
the cell, along with pleomorphism and polygonality. An apparently erupted intercellular vacuole *(arrow)* is also present. Scanning electron micrograph. (Magnification
×600.) (From Bergmanson JPG: *Cornea* [in
press]. Used by permission.)

FIG 3–30.
Transverse section through the endothelium of the same
cornea as in Figure 3–29. An intercellular vacuole *(asterisk)* is present, together wtih cellular overlapping because
of the oblique reorientation of the lateral sides *(arrows)* of
two adjacent cells. Organelles are present, but note the
variation in cytoplasmic electron density. Transmission
electron micrograph. (Magnification ×10,000.) (From Bergmanson JPG: *Cornea* [in press]. Used by permission.)

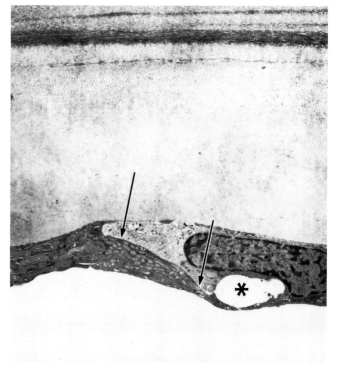

lens–wearing cornea and the aging cornea—permeability increases with age but not from contact lens wear.[15, 16]

Against this background it is perhaps not too surprising that when the endothelium from human long-term contact lens wearers was examined histopathologically, no significant cell degenerative changes were noted.[7] This ultrastructural study of six eyes from contact lens wearers and six eyes from nonlens wearers found that the organelles of endothelial cells were normal in all eyes. There was intercellular edema in the contact lens–wearing group, and, in addition, the endothelial cells in this group had an altered shape (Figs 3–29 and 3–30). Interestingly, the most important structural alteration appeared to have occurred along the lateral walls, which had straightened out from their interdigitated outline and were reoriented obliquely (see Fig 3–30). This, possibly fluid driven, change demonstrated that the specular microscope image of the posterior cell wall cannot be used to predict the total size or volume of the cell. Furthermore, it was hypothesized that cells with a large posterior surface had a small anterior surface and vice versa (Fig 3–31). Consequently, large and small cells, as seen in the specular microscope, are perhaps not different in total volume. If this hypothesis proves to be correct, the fact that cells simply rearranged their sides should appear less alarming than if they have become bloated or shrunken as the current thinking suggests. In addition, it would no longer be necessary to explain the troubling logic of how and why the uniform endothelial cells randomly react by enlarging or shrinking when exposed to the one and same stimulus, namely, anterior hypoxia. Finally, the histopathological results appear to support earlier studies that reported no functional deficit from contact lens–induced polymegethism.[16, 83]

In the absence of distinctly degenerative morphological changes and clinically meaningful functional deficits, are there any other negative consequences of contact lens–induced polymegethism? It has been postulated that endothelial morphology, as opposed to cell density, is a more important factor in the success in corneal surgery; Rao et al.[84] found that when bullous keratopathy developed postoperatively, it was correlated to endothelial morphology and not cell density. However, a later study on postsurgical bullous keratopathy failed to substantiate this relationship.[5] It would seem fairest to conclude that the jury is still out on the consequences of pleomorphism and polymegethism when facing corneal surgery.

Long-term wear of contact lenses impermeable to gases (PMMA) has been said to lead to an entity called *corneal exhaustion syndrome*.[46] Clinical signs of this syndrome are reported to be lens discomfort, periods of edema after 6 to 8 hours of contact lens wear, and a general loss of tolerance to the contact lenses.[46] These symp-

DEVELOPMENT OF POLYMEGETHISM DUE TO ANTERIOR HYPOXIA
A Theory on its Morphologic Presentation

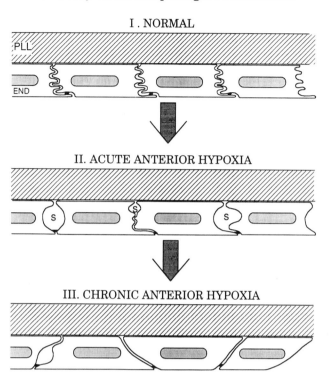

FIG 3–31.
Schematic diagram illustrating a theory on the formation of contact lens–induced endothelial polymegethism. *I*, the normal endothelium show considerable interdigitation of the lateral sides and minimal separations between cells. *II*, acute anterior hypoxic stress causes a water imbalance that leads to the filling up of the potential spaces between the endothelial cells with a resultant straightening of the interdigitated lateral walls of the cells. *III*, chronic anterior hypoxia has caused an oblique reorientation of the lateral walls of the endothelial cell. Therefore, a cell with a large anterior surface may have a small posterior surface and vice versa. As a consequence, cellular volume may remain constant despite a variation of the surface area along the posterior wall of cells. (From Bergmanson JPG: *Cornea* [in press]. Used by permission.)

toms are commonly met in many contact lens wearers, both long-term and newly fitted patients, and may not permit the diagnosis of such a syndrome to the exclusion of other possible causes. Furthermore, the literature at this time is completely devoid of the description of a single case of corneal exhaustion syndrome. Admittedly, to prove such a case to the exclusion of other causes would be a most arduous task. This is especially true when we consider all existing possible causes of polymegethism, stromal edema, discomfort, and lens intolerance. One would have to eliminate all other possible confusing factors such as age, disease, and ultraviolet exposure in a lifetime. Furthermore, other factors leading to nontolerance of contact lenses would have to be eliminated, and these include allergies, dry eye conditions, motivation, and social aspects. Until convincing evidence has been presented and published supporting the existence of the corneal exhaustion syndrome to the exclusion of other factors in contact lens intolerance, one is forced to view this entity as anectdotal rather than scientifically proved.

Where do these conflicting evidence and statements leave the practitioner? What is the appropriate action once polymegetism has been diagnosed in a contact lens wearer? It is obvious that the finding of polymegetism in a, say, young, contact lens wearer signals some change. We know this change originates from anterior hypoxic stress and, furthermore, that once this challenge is removed, there will be minimal or no recovery.[74] In the absence of truly degenerative changes, morphologically or clinically significant functional losses, it would seem prudent to regard these endothelial changes as an adaptation to a changed environment rather than a threat to corneal transparency. Of course, we have yet to obtain all the answers on many of the questions, and subsequent research may indeed prove polymegethism more of a hazard to the health of the endothelium and, as a consequence, corneal health. It would appear realistic to regard polymegethism, especially of the young, as a sign of chronic corneal hypoxic stress.

We know that hypoxic stress affects the corneal epithelium, leading to edema (circular corneal clouding, edematous corneal formations, microcysts, microcystic edema), decreased sensitivity, adhesion, and reduced mitosis. Furthermore, chronic hypoxia may induce corneal vascularization and may even make the cornea less resistant to microbial infection (see Chapter 12). Therefore, it would be prudent for the clinician caring for contact lens patients to concern himself or herself with the management of all forms of corneal response to lower than normal oxygen supply.

It is clinically often easier to detect epithelial and stromal edema than endothelial changes, which require either excellent technique with a high-powered biomicroscope or endothelial specular photography. Observation of any corneal swelling should alert the clinician that not only is the epithelium under stress but most likely the endothelium is being stressed as well. Management of edema requires adjustment of contact lens–wearing time (i.e., reducing hours of lens wear per day or changing from extended to daily wear) as well as lens design modification. Many different contact lens materials are available now, and they have varying oxygen permeabilities (Dk). Lens thickness also plays a role in oxygen delivery, as does the presence or absence of a tear pump. Increasing lens overall oxygen transmissibility (Dk/L), and improving tear pumping when possible will also aid in the reversal of hypoxia and subsequent stress.

SUMMARY

Endothelial photography has not yet and is unlikely to ever become a routine part of contact lens care. Those of us who care for contact lens patients, however, must learn to appreciate the role and delicacy of this important corneal layer; even though the lens rests on the epithelial surface of the cornea, the endothelium certainly plays a role in the maintenance of corneal integrity and in the success or failure of contact lens systems. This is an area in which we may anticipate much advancement in knowledge in the next decade, and much of what we now know—probably much of what has been discussed in this chapter—will be superceded by more advanced understanding of the role of this fascinating tissue.

Acknowledgment

We acknowledge the support of Ms. Yvonne Blocker in the preparation of this manuscript. We sincerely thank Michael Doughty, Ph.D., John P. Schoessler, O.D., Ph.D., and Steven Zantos, O.D., Ph.D., for their courtesy and consideration in sharing both intellectual support and figures for this work.

REFERENCES

1. Arffa RC: *Grayson's Diseases of the Cornea*, ed 3. St Louis, Mosby–Year Book, 1991.
2. Barr J, Schoessler J: Corneal endothelial response to rigid contact lenses. *Am J Optom Physiol Opt* 1980; 57:267–274.
3. Barr RE, Roetman EL: Oxygen gradients in the anterior chamber of anesthetized rabbits. *Invest Ophthalmol* 1974; 13:386–389.
4. Barr RE, Silver IA: Effects of corneal environment on oxygen tension in the anterior chambers of rabbits. *Invest Ophthalmol* 1973; 12:140–144.
5. Bates AK, Cheng H: Bullous keratopathy: A study of endothelial cell morphology in patients undergoing cataract surgery. *Br J Ophthalmol* 1988; 72:409–412.
6. Bergmanson JPG: The anatomy of the rabbit aqueous outflow pathway. *Acta Ophthalmol* 1985; 63:493–501.
7. Bergmanson JPG: Histopathological analysis of corneal endothelial polymegethism. *Cornea* (in press).
8. Bergmanson JPG, Chu L W-F: Corneal response to rigid contact lens wear. *Br J Ophthalmol* 1982; 66:667–675.

9. Bigar F: Specular microscopy of the corneal endothelium: Optical solutions and clinical results. *Dev Ophthalmol* 1982; 6:1–94.

10. Bonanno JA, Polse KA: Measurement of in vivo human corneal stromal pH: Open and closed eyes. *Invest Ophthalmol Vis Sci* 1987; 28:522–530.

11. Bourne WM: Corneal preservation, in Kaufman HE, Barron BA, McDonald MB, et al (eds): *The Cornea.* New York, Churchill Livingstone, 1988.

12. Bourne WM, Kaufman HE: Specular microscopy of human corneal endothelium in vivo. *Am J Ophthalmol* 1976; 81:319–323.

13. Burns RR, Bourne WM, Brubaker RF: Endothelial function in patients with cornea guttatae. *Invest Ophthalmol Vis Sci* 1981; 20:77–85.

14. Caldwell DR, Kastle PR, Dabezies OH, et al: The effect of long-term hard lens wear on the endothelium. *Contact Intraoc Lens Med J* 1982; 8:87–91.

15. Carlson KH, Bourne WM, Brubaker RF: Effect of long-term contact lens wear on corneal endothelial cell morphology and function. *Invest Ophthalmol Vis Sci* 1988; 29:185–193.

16. Carlson KH, et al: Variations in human corneal endothelial cell morphology and permeability to fluorescein with age. *Exp Eye Res* 1988; 47:27–41.

17. Carlson KH, et al: Effect of silicon elastomer contact lens wear on endothelial morphology in aphakic eyes. *Cornea* 1990; 9:45–47.

18. Catania LJ: Primary care of the anterior segment. Norwalk, Mass, Appleton & Lange, 1988.

19. Chan-Ling T, Curini J: Changes in corneal endothelial morphology in cats as a function of age. *Curr Eye Res* 1988; 7:387–392.

20. Clements LD: Corneal acedosis, blebs and endothelial polymegethism. *Contact Lens Forum* 1990; March; 39–46.

21. Curran RE, Kenyon KR, Green WR: Pre-Descemet's membrane corneal dystrophy. *Am J Ophthalmol* 1974; 77:711–716.

22. Davson H: The hydration of the cornea. *Biochem J* 1955; 59:24–28.

23. Doughty MJ: Physiologic state of the rabbit cornea following 4° C moist chamber storage. *Exp Eye Res* 1989; 49:807–827.

24. Doughty MJ: Toward a quantitative analysis of corneal endothelial cell morphology: A review of techniques and their application. *Optom Vis Sci* 1989; 66: 626–642.

25. Doughty MJ: The ambiguous coefficient of variation: Polymegethism of the corneal endothelium and central corneal thickness. *Int Contact Lens Clin* 1990; 17:240–247.

26. Doughty MJ: Evidence for a direct effect of bicarbonate on the rabbit corneal stroma. *Optom Vis Sci* 1991; 68:687–698.

27. Doughty MJ, Maurice D: Bicarbonate sensitivity of rabbit corneal endothelium fluid pump in vitro. *Invest Ophthalmol Vis Sci* 1988; 29:216–223.

28. Duke-Elder S, Leigh AG: *Diseases of the Outer Eye, Part 2*, vol VIII, in Duke-Elder S (ed): *System of Ophthalmology.* St Louis, Mosby–Year Book, 1965.

29. Elner VM, et al: Intercellular adhesion molecule-1 in human corneal endothelium. Modulation and function. *Am J Pathol* 1991; 138:525–536.

30. Farge EJ, et al: Morphologic changes of K-sol preserved human corneas. *Cornea* 1989; 8:159–169.

31. Fatt I, Weissman BA: *Physiology of the Eye,* ed 2. Stoneham, Mass, Butterworths (in press).

32. Freeman RD: Oxygen consumption by the component layers of the cornea. *J Physiol* 1972; 225:15–32.

33. Garcia-Ferrer FJ, et al: Antimicrobial efficacy and corneal endothelial toxicity of Dex-Sol corneal storage medium supplemented with vancomycin. *Ophthalmology* 1991; 98:863–869.

34. Gonnering R, et al: The pH tolerance of rabbit and human corneal endothelium. *Invest Ophthalmol Vis Sci* 1979; 18:373–390.

35. Good GW, Schoessler JP: Chronic solar radiation exposure and endothelial polymegethism. *Curr Eye Res* 1988; 7:157–162.

36. Graves B: A bilateral chronic affection of the endothelial face of the cornea of elderly persons, with an account of the technical and clinical principles of its slit-lamp observation. *Br J Ophthalmol* 1924; 8:502.

37. Grayson M, Wilbrandt H: Pre-Descemet's dystrophy. *Am J Ophthalmol* 1967; 64:276–282.

38. Hay ED: Development of the vertebrate cornea. *Int Rev Cytol* 1980; 61:263–322.

39. Hirsch M, et al: Study of the ultra-structure of the rabbit corneal endothelium by freeze-fracture technique. Apical and lateral junctions. *Exp Eye Res* 1977; 25:277–288.

40. Hirst LW, et al: Quantitative analysis of wide-field endothelial specular photomicrographs. *Am J Ophthalmol* 1984; 97:488–495.

41. Hirst LW, et al: Specular microscopy of hard lens wearers. *Ophthalmology* 1984; 91:1147–1153.

42. Hirst LW, et al: Quantitative analysis of wide-field specular microscopy: II. Precision of sampling from the central corneal endothelium. *Invest Ophthalmol Vis Sci* 1989; 30:1972–1979.

43. Hodson S, Miller F: The bicarbonate ion pump in the endothelium which regulates the hydration of rabbit cornea. *J Physiol* 1976; 263:563–577.

44. Hoefle FB, Maurice DM, Sibley RC: Human corneal donor material: A method of examination before keratoplasty. *Arch Ophthalmol* 1970; 84:741–744.

45. Hogan MJ, Alvarado JA, Weddel JE: *Histology of the Human Eye: An Atlas and Textbook.* Philadelphia, WB Saunders Co, 1971.

46. Holden BA: Suffocating the cornea with PMMA. *Contact Lens Spectrum* 1989; 4(5):69–70.

47. Holden BA, Sweney DF, Vannas A, et al: Effects of long-term extended contact lens wear on the human cornea. *Invest Ophthalmol Vis Sci* 1985; 26:1489–1501.

48. Holden BA, Williams L, Zantos S: Etiology of transient endothelial changes in the human cornea. *Invest Ophthalmol Vis Sci* 1985; 26:1354–1359.

49. Holm O: High magnification photography of the anterior segment of the human eye. *Acta Ophthalmol* 1977; 56:475–476.

50. Jester JV, Cavanagh, Lemp MA: Confocal microscopic imaging of the living eye with Tandem scanning confocal microscopy, in Master BR (ed): *Noninvasive Diagnostic Techniques in Ophthalmology*. New York, Springer-Verlag New York, 1990.

51. Johnson DH, Bourne WM, Campbell RJ. The ultrastructure of Descemet's membrane: I. Changes with age in normal corneas. *Arch Ophthalmol* 1982; 100:1942–1947.

52. Kaufman HE, Capella JA, Roblinson JE: Human corneal endothelium. *Am J Ophthalmol* 1966; 61:835–841.

53. Khodadoust A, Hirst L: Diurnal variation in corneal endothelial morphology. *Ophthalmology* 1984; 91:1125–1128.

54. Klyce SD: Stromal lactate accumulation can account for corneal edema osmotically following epithelial hypoxia in the rabbit. *J Physiol* 1981; 321:49–64.

55. Klyce SD, Beuerman RW: Structure and function of the cornea, in Kaufman HE, Barron BA, McDonald MB, et al (eds): *The Cornea*. New York, Churchill Livingstone, 1988.

56. Koester CJ, Roberts CW, Donn A, et al: Wide-field specular microscopy. Clinical and research applications. *Ophthalmology* 1980; 87:849–860.

57. Krachmer JH, et al: Corneal posterior crocodile shagreen and polymorphic amyloid degeneration. A histopathologic study. *Arch Ophthalmol* 1983; 101:54–59.

58. Kreutziger GO: Lateral membrane morphology and gap junction structure in rabbit corneal endothelium. *Exp Eye Res* 1976; 23:285–293.

59. Kuwabara T: Current concepts in anatomy and histology of the cornea. *Contact Intraoc Lens Med J* 1978; 4:101–132.

60. Laing RA, Sandstrom M, Berrospi A, et al: Changes in corneal endothelium as a function of age. *Exp Eye Res* 1976; 22:587–594.

61. Laing RA, Sandstrom MM, Leibowitz HM: In vivo photomicrography of the corneal endothelium. *Arch Ophthalmol* 1975; 93:143–145.

62. Laing RA, Sandstrom MM, Leibowitz HM: Clinical specular microscopy: I. Optical principles. *Arch Ophthalmol* 1979; 97:1714–1719.

63. Lass JH, et al: A morphologic and fluoreophotometric analysis of the corneal endothelium in type 1 diabetes mellitus and cystic fibrosis. *Am J Ophthalmol* 1985; 100:783–788.

64. Ling T, Vannas A, Holden BA: Long-term changes in corneal endothelial morphology following wounding in the cat. *Invest Ophthalmol Vis Sci* 1988; 29:1407–1412.

65. MacRae SM, et al: The effects of hard and soft contact lenses on the corneal endothelium. *Am J Ophthalmol* 1986; 102:50–57.

66. Masters BR, Kino GS: Confocal microscopy of the eye, in Masters BR (ed): *Noninvasive Diagnostic Techniques in Ophthalmology*. New York, Springer-Verlag New York, 1990.

67. Maurice DM: The structure and transparency of the cornea. *J Physiol* 1957; 136:263–286.

68. Maurice DM: Cellular membrane activity in the corneal endothelium of the intact eye. *Experimentia* 1968; 24:1094–1095.

69. Maurice DM: The cornea and the sclera, in Davson H (ed): *The Eye*. New York, Academic Press, 1969, vol 1.

70. Maurice DM: The location of the fluid pump in the cornea. *J Physiol* 1972; 221:43–54.

71. Maurice DM: A scanning slit optical microscope. *Invest Ophthalmol* 1974; 13:1033–1037.

72. Mayer DJ: *Clinical Wide-Field Specular Microscopy*. London, Balliere-Tindall, 1984.

73. McLaughlin BJ, et al: Freeze-fracture quantitative comparison of rabbit corneal epithelial and endothelial membranes. *Curr Eye Res* 1985; 4:951–961.

74. McLaughlin R, Schoessler J: Corneal endothelial response to refitting polymethyl methaorylate wearers with rigid gas-permeable lenses. *Optom Vis Sci* 1990; 67:346–351.

75. McMonnies CW, Zantos SD: Endothelial bedewing of the cornea in association with contact lens wear. *Br J Ophthalmol* 1979; 63:478–481.

76. Murphy C, et al: Prenatal and postnatal cellularity of the human corneal endothelium. A quantitative histologic study. *Invest Ophthalmol Vis Sci* 1984; 25:312–322.

77. Obrig T: *Contact Lenses*. Philadelphia, Chilton, 1942.

78. Oh JO: Changes with age in the corneal endothelium of normal rabbits. *Acta Ophthalmol* 1963; 41:568–573.

79. O'Neal MR, Polse KA: Decreased endothelial pump function with aging. *Invest Ophthalmol Vis Sci* 1986; 27:457–463.

80. Ozanios V, Jakobiec FA: Prenatal development of the eye and its adnexa, in Tasman W, Jaeger EA (eds): *Duane's Foundations of Clinical Ophthalmology*. Philadelphia, JB Lippincott Co, 1990, vol 1, Chapter 2.

81. Pitts DG, et al: Ultrastructural analysis of corneal exposure to UV radiation. *Acta Ophthalmol* 1987; 65:279–286.

82. Polse KA, et al: Age differences in corneal hydration control. *Invest Ophthalmol Vis Sci* 1989; 30:392–399.

83. Polse KA, et al: Hypoxic effects on corneal morphology and function. *Invest Ophthalmol Vis Sci* 1990; 31:1542–1554.

84. Rao G, et al: Pseudophakic bullous keratopathy: Relationship to pre-operative corneal endothelial status. *Ophthalmology* 1984; 91:1135–1140.

85. Rao GN, Waldron WR, Aquavella JV: Morphology of graft endothelium and donor age. *Br J Ophthalmol* 1980; 64:523–527.

86. Ringvold A, Davanger M, Gronvold-Olsen E: On the spatial organization of the corneal endothelium. *Acta Ophthalmol* 1984; 62:911–917.

87. Ruiz JM, Medrano M, Alio JL: An improved method of vital staining of the corneal endothelium. *Ophthalmol Res* 1991; 23:27–30.

88. Schoessler JP: Corneal endothelial polymegethism associated with extended wear. *Int Contact Lens Clin* 1983; 10:144–148.

89. Schoessler JP, Barr JT, Fresen DR: Corneal endothelial observations of silicon elastomer contact lens wearers. *Int Contact Lens Clin* 1984; 11:337–340.

90. Schoessler JP, Woloschak MJ: Corneal endothelium in veteran PMMA contact lens wearers. *Int Contact Lens Clin* 1981; 8:19–25.

91. Schoessler JP, Woloschak MJ, Mauger TF: Transient endothelial changes produced by hydrophilic lenses. *Am J Optom Physiol Opt* 1982; 59:764–765.

92. Sherrard ES, Ng YL: The other side of the corneal endothelium. *Cornea* 1990; 9:48–54.

93. Sherrard ES, Novakovic P, Speedwell L: Age-related changes of the corneal endothelium and stroma as seen in vivo by specular microscopy. *Eye* 1987; 1:197–203.

94. Singh G, Bohnke M, von Domarus D: Vital staining and corneal endothelium. *Cornea* 1985; 4:80–91.

95. Speedwell L, et al: The infant corneal endothelium. *Arch Ophthalmol* 1988; 106:771–775.

96. Suda T: Mosaic pattern changes in human corneal endothelium with age. *Jpn J Ophthalmol* 1984; 28:331–338.

97. Sugar A: Corneal and conjunctival degenerations, in Kaufman HE, Barron BA, McDonald MB, et al (eds): *The Cornea*. New York, Churchill Livingstone, 1988.

98. Svedbergh B, Bill A: Scanning electron microscopic studies of the corneal endothelium in man and monkeys. *Acta Ophthalmol* 1972; 50:321–336.

99. Taylor MJ, Hunt CJ: Dual staining of corneal endothelium with trypan blue and alizarin red S: Importance of pH for the dye-lake reaction. *Br J Ophthalmol* 1981; 65:815–819.

100. Vannas A, Holden B, Makitie J: The ultrastructure of contact lens induced changes. *Acta Ophthalmol* 1984; 62:320–333.

101. Vannas A, Makitie J, Sulonen J, et al: Contact lens induced transient changes in corneal endothelium. *Acta Ophthalmol* 1981; 59:552–559.

102. Vogt A: *Lehrbuch und Atlas der spaltlampen Microskopie des lebenden Auges*. New York, Springer-Verlag New York, 1930.

103. Waltman SR: Corneal changes from intraocular surgery, in Kaufman HE, Barron BA, McDonald MB, et al (eds): *The Cornea*. New York, Churchill Livingstone, 1988.

104. Waring GO: Posterior collagenous layer of the cornea. *Arch Ophthalmol* 1982; 100:122–134.

105. Waring GO: Corneal structure and pathophysiology, in Liebowitz HM (ed): *Corneal Disorders. Clinical Diagnosis and Management*. Philadelphia, WB Saunders Co, 1984.

106. Waring GO, Bourne WM, Edelhauser HF, et al: The corneal endothelium. Normal and pathological structure and function. *Ophthalmology* 1982; 89:531–590.

107. Weissman BA, Ehrlich M, Levenson JE, et al: Four cases of keratoconus and posterior polymorphous dystrophy. *Optom Vis Sci* 1987; 68:243–246.

108. Weissman BA, Fatt I, Phan C: Polarographic oxygen permeability measurement of silicon elastomer contact lens material. *J Am Optom Assoc* (In press).

109. Weissman BA, Fatt I, Rasson J: Diffusion of oxygen in human corneas in vivo. *Invest Ophthalmol Vis Sci* 1981; 20:123–125.

110. Wilson GS, Fatt I, Freeman RD: Thickness changes in the stroma of an excised cornea during anoxia. *Exp Eye Res* 1973; 17:165–171.

111. Wilson RS, Roper-Hall MJ: Effect of age on the endothelial cell count in the normal eye. *Br J Ophthalmol* 1982; 66:513–515.

112. Yee RW, et al: Changes in the normal corneal endothelial cellular pattern as a function of age. *Curr Eye Res* 1985; 4:671–678.

113. Zantos SD, Holden BA: Transient endothelial changes soon after wearing soft contact lenses. *Am J Optom Physiol Opt* 1977; 54:856–858.

114. Zantos SD, Holden BA: Guttate endothelial changes with anterior eye inflammation. *Br J Ophthalmol* 1981; 65:101–103.

Contact Lens–Induced Changes in Corneal Topography and Refractive Error

Edward S. Bennett, O.D., M.S, Ed.

Contact lens–induced complications are often perceived by clinicians as those *overt* problems (e.g., staining, ulcers, giant papillary conjunctivitis) that are accompanied by patients' symptoms diagnostic of the condition. However, it would be erroneous to exclude more subtle contact lens–induced problems, in particular, changes in refractive error and corneal curvature, which can result in a reduction in wearing time or even discontinuation of contact lens wear. The purpose of this chapter is to describe the etiology and management of contact lens–induced refractive and corneal curvature changes. Essentially these changes can be divided into two categories: (1) accidental and (2) deliberate.

ACCIDENTAL REFRACTIVE AND CORNEAL CURVATURE CHANGES WITH CONTACT LENSES

Polymethylmethacrylate-Induced Changes

Complications

Edema.—As discussed in Chapters 2 and 3, polymethylmethacrylate (PMMA) lens wear can induce numerous hypoxia-related complications, including central corneal clouding, edematous corneal formations, and endothelial polymegethism. Central corneal clouding has been reported in 98% of PMMA wearers[42] and often results in the subjective symptom of blurred vision through spectacles.

Spectacle blur has been defined as good vision through contact lenses with reduced vision with spectacles after contact lens removal. It is caused by the (typically) centralized corneal edema haze and leads to steepening and irregularities of the corneal surface; therefore, it is often accompanied by an increase in myopia, astigmatism, or both.[81]

Corneal Exhaustion Syndrome.—Recently it has been claimed that not only do almost all long-term PMMA wearers exhibit corneal edema accompanied by spectacle blur, but an increasing number are experiencing the so-called *corneal exhaustion syndrome*.[71] This complication includes excessive corneal edema, discomfort, and general loss of tolerance to contact lens wear and appears to be caused by chronic hypoxia. It is possible that the endothelium of these patients is compromised and unable to adequately control corneal hydration.

Corneal Curvature and Refractive Changes.—Several reports have indicated that corneal steepening occurs during initial adaptation to PMMA lenses.[22, 68, 95, 96, 113, 132, 133] After the initial adaptation period, the curvature changes toward the baseline value.[68, 119] After about 1 year, the cornea actually shows flattening beyond the original baseline values.[132, 133] Consequently, an increase in myopia has been reported during the initial adaptation period.[33, 68] After adaptation, the refractive error has been found to return to baseline[68] and then becomes less myopic with long-term wear.[116, 131]

The effect of the base curve fitting relationship on corneal topography has been evaluated by Carney,[31, 32] who found that during adaptation, flat-, steep-, and alignment-fitting lenses all reduced the asphericity of the cornea. After adaptation, the steeply fitted group continued to show a decrease in asphericity; the flat-fitting group, however, actually showed an increase in asphericity, with the alignment-fitting group between the other groups. In some cases the inferior quadrant was more affected, especially in the case of flat-fitting lenses. When the effects of varying oxygen concentration on corneal topography with PMMA lens wear was evaluated, it was found that in the normal hypoxic state, the oxygen distribution is unevenly distributed across the cornea; therefore, the uneven thickening caused by edema can cause unusual topographical changes. When the edema reaction was eliminated by exposing the eyes to 100% oxygen, the steeply fitted eyes showed a steepening of the corneal topography, and the flat-fitting eyes showed a corresponding flattening. It was concluded that these changes are a result of both corneal molding and inadequate oxygen.

There is much evidence to indicate that diurnal variation occurs for both corneal curvature and refractive error during PMMA lens wear. It has been found that myopia increases approximately 1.00D during the first 8 hours of wear and then decreases about 0.25D from 8 to 16 hours of wear.[121, 127] In addition, the diurnal increases in myopia appear to be related to wearing time and the number of years that contact lenses have been worn.[127, 131] The average diurnal increase in myopia for individuals who wore lenses for 6 months was less than 0.75D compared with

about 1.50D for those with more than 3 years of wear. Individuals wearing their lenses only 12 to 14 hours had diurnal increases of less than 1.00D; wearing lenses all waking hours was associated with diurnal increases of more than 1.00D. Diurnal variation has also been found in corneal curvature.[123] Both the horizontal and vertical meridians showed much variation in the amount of steepening resulting from 4, 8, and 16 hours of lens wear. It was concluded that the lens-cornea fitting relationship must vary during the day. The amount of variation appears to be directly related to the number of years of lens wear and the amount of daily wearing time. Control measurements used for nonlens wearers show stable corneal curvature values[124] and refractive error findings.[131]

Corneal Warpage Syndrome.—It has been found that long-term PMMA lens wear can result in corneal distortion in as many as 30% of patients.[115] Patients with corneal distortion but few or no subjective symptoms have specific problems. Often because of the subtle and gradual onset of the syndrome, no problems are noticed. If undiagnosed and untreated, corneal distortion can lead to altered corneal transparency coincident with a decrease in visual acuity and contrast discrimination.[16] The clinician should notice distorted keratometry mires with or without irregular astigmatism and decreased visual acuity on the postwear refraction. This pattern of change is termed *corneal warpage syndrome,* a clinically significant cause for concern. Refitting these patients is a serious problem because the cornea tends to exhibit keratoconus-like changes with inconsistent and unpredictable refractive changes (Figs 4–1

FIG 4–1.
Photokeratograph of PMMA-induced corneal distortion. (Courtesy of R. Kame.)

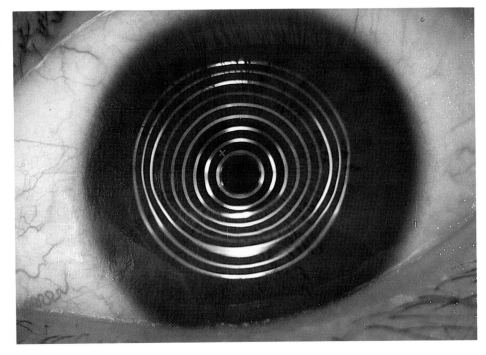

and 4–2). In one retrospective study, 50 patients acquired 1D or more of irregular astigmatism as a result of long-term contact lens wear.[91] This change in astigmatism correlated with the duration of PMMA lens wear.

What causes corneal warpage syndrome? It is evident that long-term corneal hypoxia can result in corneal curvature changes, typically central steepening and irregular astigmatism. These changes are encouraged by the presence of an inflexible foreign body molding the cornea. Eventually a change in the lens-cornea fitting relationship can occur, resulting in decentration. The effects of a decentered rigid lens on the cornea can induce corneal distortion because the shift in position of the lens results in regions of excessive pressure or bearing in regions adjacent to areas of excessive clearance.[150] Typically the corneal distortion is temporary, and the cornea will gradually return to normal with PMMA removal; however, this is dependent on how early the patient is diagnosed and what method of management is selected.

Management

The management of PMMA-induced complications is dependent on both a comprehensive evaluation and selection of the most appropriate lens material and method of refitting.

Patient Evaluation and Communication.—The importance of patient recall cannot be overemphasized. Patients fitted with PMMA lenses should be evaluated, at minimum, every 12 months. At these visits, a thorough case history and evaluation should be performed. The history should include the following questions:

1. Hours/day of lens wear?
2. Years of lens wear?

3. Spectacle blur? If so, how long?
4. Corneal abrasions?

Correlations have been found between the greater number of years and hours per day of lens wear.[120] Spectacle blur, if longer than 30 minutes, is indicative of excessive corneal edema. A history of recurrent corneal abrasions, especially of recent origin, can signal the presence of corneal exhaustion syndrome.

A comprehensive evaluation of the PMMA lenses should be performed, including:

1. Visual acuity. Is it reduced compared with the previous examinations?
2. Spherocylindrical overrefraction.
3. Biomicroscopy evaluation of the current lens fit with fluorescein.
4. Biomicroscopy after lens removal to evaluate lids, corneal integrity, and tear quality.
5. Subjective refraction. Is best visual acuity reduced?
6. Keratometry. Note any steepening, irregular astigmatism, or distortion.
7. Verification of lens parameters. Determine if warpage is present or the surface quality impaired.

In particular, the presence of any edema-related clinical signs, corneal distortion, central corneal staining, or reduced spectacle, visual acuity necessitates a refit.

With few exceptions, these patients would benefit from a refit into a rigid gas-permeable (RGP) lens material. However, it can be difficult to convince relatively asymptomatic patients that a refit would help rehabilitate their corneas. The benefits of RGP lenses, including oxy-

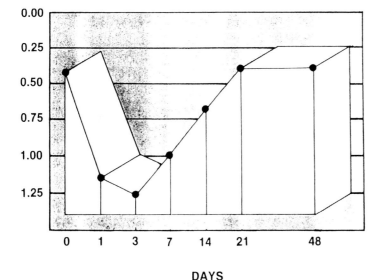

FIG 4–2.
Rengstorff curve. Changes in refractive error after discontinuing PMMA lens wear. (From HOM MM: *Contact Lens Forum* 1986; 11[11]: 16–18. Used by permission.)

gen permeability, healthier eyes, the ability to obtain good vision through spectacles, and being a recipient of the latest technology can be emphasized to these patients. In addition, the verbal message can be reinforced by using pamphlets, photographs or 35-mm slides (showing PMMA-induced complications), videotapes, and other audiovisuals to demonstrate the necessity of a refit.[65] The Contact Lens Manufacturers Association and RGP Lens Institute Video Library provide videos that pertain to these patients.

Methods of Management.—Three methods have been advocated for refitting the previous PMMA wearer: (1) cold turkey, (2) deadaptation, and (3) immediate refitting.

Cold Turkey.—Because the cornea has been compromised from PMMA contact lens wear, a traditional method of managing these patients has been sudden discontinuation of lens wear in an effort to quickly rehabilitate the cornea (i.e., cold turkey). Unfortunately, it has been found that many patients who discontinued lens wear in this way showed wide fluctuations in both the refractive state and corneal curvature.[116, 120] In fact, unpredictable and excessive changes and even permanent corneal distortion have resulted from the cold turkey method.[17, 59] In one reported case, a patient who lost one of her PMMA lenses was examined 3 days later with the following results:[13]

OS: Baseline Spectacle Rx: $-4.25 - 1.50 \times 180$ 20/20
Keratometry: 43.00 @ 180; 44.75 @ 090
OS: 3 days after lens loss: $-8.50 - 1.00 \times 170$ 20/25
Keratometry: 45.50DS with mire distortion
OS: 6 days after lens loss: $-14.25 - 1.00 \times 170$ 20/50
Keratometry: 44.50 @ 150; 50.25 @ 060 with mire distortion
OS: 6 months later (after successful refitting into RGPs)
Spectacle Rx: $-12.00 - 2.00 \times 150$ 20/25
Keratometry: 45.75 @ 180; 47.25 @ 090 with slight mire distortion

Because spectacle lens wear was unsatisfactory, she never discontinued wear of a rigid lens in her right eye, and her refraction, which was similar to the baseline value for the left eye, experienced much less of an increase in myopic refractive error after refitting into an RGP material. According to Rengstorff,[125] the amount of corneal distortion and refractive changes these patients experience is caused by sudden exposure to high oxygen levels resulting from abrupt cessation of PMMA lens wear. The amount of distortion is related to the number of years of PMMA lens wear, with the greatest changes occurring the first few days after lens removal.

In the absence of corneal distortion, it has been found that the refractive error stabilizes more quickly if immediate cessation of wear is the method of choice.[20] Stabilization usually occurs on the average in about 2 weeks, although there is much individual variation. Rengstorff[116, 117, 128] found a specific pattern of progressive corneal flattening, as measured by keratometry, in both the vertical and horizontal meridians for 1 and 3 days, respectively, followed by corneal steepening to the 48th day of the observation period. (Fig 4–3).[73, 116, 117, 128] The magnitude of corneal curvature changes was less for patients who wore their lenses less than all waking hours, particularly when some time was allowed to elapse between contact lens removal and sleep.

Refractive changes for long-term PMMA lens wearers who suddenly discontinued contact lens wear appeared to be correlated with corneal curvature changes. Corneal curvature changes were accompanied by a steady decrease in myopia during the first 3 days (average decrease = 1.32D), followed by a return toward baseline during the next several weeks. The extent and duration of these changes correlated with the number of years the lenses had been worn. Although in general there has been agreement that in most cases the refractive error changes will be accompanied by the corresponding corneal curvature changes, there have been cases in which this has not been true.[118] A possible cause for this difference in some cases pertains to keratometer use. The keratometer measures only anterior corneal surface power and does not account for the correct index of refraction of the cornea, thickness of the cornea, steepening of the posterior corneal curvature, or changes in axial length; all of these factors may influence refractive error.

Astigmatic changes, with the rule, usually increases in the first few days after PMMA lens removal and then reverts toward baseline.[20, 114, 126] The amount of astigmatic change, however, can be large, unpredictable, and permanent.[59]

The refractive error, measured immediately on PMMA lens removal or after corneal stabilization, is often unchanged from the prefitting refractive error.[30] However, because excessive refractive and corneal curvature changes are possible between these times, especially if corneal distortion is present, satisfactory vision through spectacles is often impossible. Therefore, the cold turkey technique is not the recommended method of managing a long-term PMMA wearer.

Deadaptation.—As originally suggested by Arner,[7, 8] a gradual reduction in wearing time may permit corneas to deadapt or adjust their metabolic system to non–contact lens wear. Typically this procedure consists of reducing wearing time by 1 to 2 hours/day until the patient has discontinued contact lens use. Refraction and corneal curva-

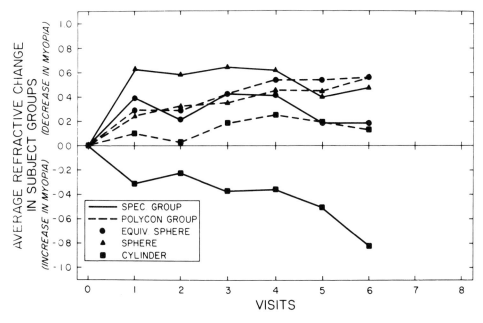

FIG 4–3.
Average change in refractive state for each of two groups of patients discontinuing long-term wear of PMMA lenses. One group wore spectacles, the other Polycon lenses, until stability of the components of refraction was achieved. (From Bennett ES, Tomlinson A: *AM J Optom Physiol Opt* 1983; 60:139–145. Used by permission.)

ture values are monitored until stabilization has occurred; at that time the patient is refitted into a an RGP lens material. Overall this is an acceptable method of management. It has been found that gradually reducing wearing time minimizes the incidence of both visual acuity loss and corneal distortion during the rehabilitation process.[122, 129, 130] In addition, a reduced risk of large astigmatic change is present. The primary disadvantage of this method is patient dissatisfaction. Many patients are unable to adequately function during the period required for the corneas to recover and stabilize for reasons related to work or lifestyle.[16] When temporary spectacles are prescribed, the visual acuity obtained at different times may not be adequate for the patient's needs. In addition, as with the cold turkey method, corneal sensitivity will recur, necessitating a readaptation process with the RGP lenses.

Immediate Refitting With Rigid Gas-Permeable Materials.—This management approach has been strongly recommended in recent years and has definite advantages over the other two methods.[13, 20, 46, 56, 130] There is little or no patient inconvenience, and corneal rehabilitation and refractive error stabilization can occur during RGP lens wear.

Bennett and Tomlinson[20] compared corneal curvature and refractive stabilization of immediate refitting with RGP lenses (Polycon I) vs. immediate cessation of wear (i.e., cold turkey) with two groups of non–corneal warpage syndrome PMMA wearers. Results from this study showed that initial corneal flattening changes, associated with a decrease in myopia, occurred with both groups, and astigmatic changes were significant in the spectacle-wearing group but not in the immediate refit group (Fig 4–4). It was concluded that immediate refitting with RGP lenses

did not generally inhibit any corneal rehabilitative changes occurring after PMMA removal, because vision was significantly better and more stable in this group. In another study in which the corneal curvature changes with 60 previous PMMA wearers immediately refit into Boston II were compared with 72 new patients fitted with the same material, it was found that no significant deviation from baseline occurred in the horizontal or vertical meridians in either group.[36]

These reports also indicated that few lens changes were necessary during the rehabilitation process. It is apparent that the former PMMA-wearing patient who is immediately refitted into a RGP lens material may still experience fairly large corneal curvature changes without an accompanying change in the refractive power and while maintaining a good lens-cornea fitting relationship.[73, 94] This occurs because the tear lens has nearly the same index of refraction as the cornea and thereby masks the effects of corneal changes. Likewise, if the fluorescein pattern does not change, it is most likely the result of a compensating paracentral–midperipheral corneal curvature change, which would result in an unchanged sagittal depth. Note that the keratometer evaluates the curvature of only approximately the central 3 mm of the cornea.

If corneal warpage syndrome is present, however, a longer recovery period will be necessary, but stabilization with loss of corneal distortion does typically result. In one study involving 76 corneal warpage syndrome patients (74 with PMMA, 2 with hydrogel), all were refitted into an RGP material (Boston I); of these patients, 57 were refitted without loss of wearing time.[99] There was a loss of corneal warpage in 66 patients, improvement in 4 patients, and no change in 6 patients. The resolution of corneal warpage

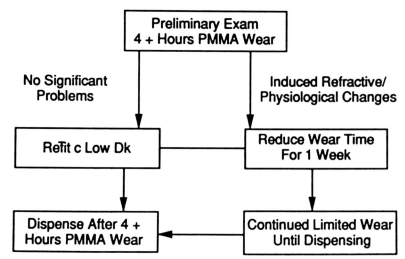

REFIT - PMMA OVERWEAR

FIG 4–4.
Management nomogram for long-term PMMA wearers. (From Grohe RM, Bennett ES: Problem-solving, in Bennett ES, Weissman BA [eds]: *Clinical Contact Lens Practice.* Philadelphia, JB Lippincott Co, 1991, pp 1–15. Used by permission.)

was achieved in one half of these patients within 3 months.

Refitting Procedure.—Once the decision to proceed has been made, the patient can be refit the same day as the initial evaluation, especially if corneal distortion is absent or minimal.[13, 16] The corneal curvature and refractive findings obtained within 15 minutes after PMMA lens removal should be used as baseline values for determining the diagnostic fitting lens parameters. If moderate or severe corneal distortion is present, making keratometry readings of little value, it is advisable to decrease any further adverse

effects from long-term wear of PMMA lenses. The patient's wearing time should be reduced to the minimum number of hours that can be tolerated and a return visit scheduled in 1 week for the fitting (Fig 4–5). Often these patients do not have up-to-date or useful spectacles, but they can usually function adequately during normal working hours with a reduction in contact lens wearing time to 8 to 12 hours/day. If the patient adheres to this schedule, dramatic improvement is often observed at the 1-week visit. Both the initial visit and the 1-week visit should be at approximately the same time of day, preferably after a minimum of 4 hours of lens wear to evaluate the effects of

FIG 4–5.
The vision contrast test system contrast sensitivity chart.

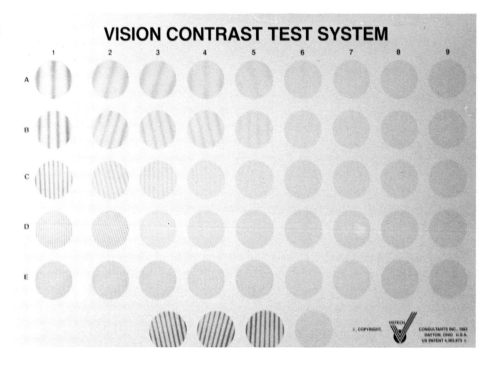

edema and to ensure comparability of corneal and refractive measurements.

Although success has been achieved by simply duplicating the PMMA lens parameters in the new RGP lens material,[137] I prefer to diagnostically fit RGP lenses because (1) diagnostic fitting typically results in fewer lens exchanges than so-called empirical fitting,[19] and (2) RGP lens materials often benefit from a different lens design than was traditionally used with PMMA lenses.[14] Newer materials are usually prescribed in larger overall or optical zone diameters, flatter base curves, greater center thicknesses, and steeper peripheral curve radii.

When an RGP material is selected to refit previous PMMA wearers, it is essential to remember that PMMA lens wearers are changing from a durable, forgiving lens material to one that is less durable and less forgiving.[65] As the oxygen permeability increases, the softness of the material increases as well, leading to greater likelihood of problems such as surface scratches and warpage.[63] Previous PMMA wearers usually have acquired poor care habits of cleaning the lenses between the index finger and thumb, storing the lenses dry, and using unusual methods of cleaning, including dishwashing detergent and lighter fluid. Therefore, thorough reeducation is required to prevent warpage, scratches, and poor surface wettability of RGP lenses based on these poor habits alone. Therefore, it is optimum to refit PMMA patients immediately into a low Dk (i.e., 25–50). The lower Dk material should exhibit greater stability and hardness. In addition, it is possible that less dramatic refractive and corneal curvature changes could occur during the rehabilitation process with low Dk than with the more flexible and higher oxygen-transmissible rigid lens materials. Once corneal stabilization has resulted, the patient can be refitted into a higher Dk material if corneal edema is still present.

Once the refitting process has been completed, these patients should be carefully monitored, especially if corneal distortion is present. Patients should be evaluated within 1 week of dispensing, then at 2 weeks, 1 month, 3 months, and then every 6 months.

Patients with PMMA lenses usually have an out-of-date spectacle prescription if, in fact, one is present. Therefore, the importance of a current spectacle prescription for wear on awakening and in the evening must be emphasized. Spectacles can be prescribed, on average, 3 weeks after initiating wear of the RGP lenses.[20, 110] If corneal warpage syndrome is present, this time period may be longer.

Continued Use of PMMA Lenses

Although the number of lenses is steadily decreasing, PMMA lenses are still fitted today. Typically this is a result of either one or a combination of the following:

1. Material stability. The durability and flexure resistance of PMMA is advantageous in cases such as high astigmatism, keratoconus, orthokeratology, and presbyopia.
2. RGP failures. Often this is the result of subjective dryness or frequent lens replacement resulting from warpage.
3. Clinician preference. The PMMA lenses will be fitted when clinicians are accustomed to fitting them and are less motivated to try other, newer rigid lens materials.

However, continued use of PMMA should be avoided. The results of long-term PMMA lens wear, including induced refractive changes, corneal edema and distortion, and loss of tolerance are well documented. In addition, clinicians may be liable if they fit (or refit) an outdated material or abandon follow-up care on present PMMA wearers and complications later occur.[57]

Polymethylmethacrylate Lens Wear as an Etiological Factor in Keratoconus

Much controversy has been generated on whether long-term PMMA lens wear is a causative mechanism in keratoconus in some patients. It is important to initially differentiate keratoconus from corneal warpage syndrome. Patients with keratoconus exhibit gradual progression of central corneal steepening, corneal thinning (ectasia), and Vogt's straie.[15] These changes are irreversible. Patients with corneal warpage syndrome have some keratometric mire distortion and astigmatic changes, but these changes tend to revert to normal either after removal of contact lenses or after refitting with an RGP lens material.

There have been several reports of keratoconus developing in PMMA contact lens wearers who were previously asymptomatic.[29, 39, 45, 60, 61, 76, 104, 109, 139] It has been postulated that the long-term wear of rigid contact lenses may result in the onset of keratoconus in certain individuals, particularly those with a history of atopic disease, poorly fitted lenses, or low ocular rigidity. It has been suggested that early measurement of ocular rigidity might identify a high-risk patient group,[62, 76] although the relevance of low ocular rigidity as a predisposing factor has been questioned.[109] In addition, it has been theorized that keratoconus can be triggered by corneal changes accompanying PMMA-induced biochemical and physiological alterations,[59] long-term PMMA wear resulting in an interference with corneal metabolism, corneal fatigue, and finally keratoconus. Contact lens–induced keratoconus is claimed to be most often unilateral, not bilateral,[61] and it rarely progresses to the point where a keratoplasty is required.[104]

The published reports attempting to associate PMMA lens wear with keratoconus, although informative, have largely been anecdotal. Gasset et al.[45] examined 162 patients with keratoconus and discovered that 26.5% had worn PMMA lenses before keratoconus developed. Conversely, in a group of 1,248 controls who were fitted with soft lenses and observed over 1 to 6 years of lens wear, only 1 was observed with keratoconus. Because Gasset compared a retrospective group of cases (with keratoconus) with a prospective group of controls (hydrogel lens patients), however, this study has been criticized for poor methodology.[138, 153] Brightbill and Stainer[29] examined 120 keratoconus patients and found a positive history of keratoconus in 17.5%. However, no control group was available.

The possibility of keratoconus development in PMMA lens wearers being a coincidence has not been ruled out. In fact, it has been observed that the incidence of keratoconus would be expected to be higher in a contact lens–wearing population than in the general public because the contact lens population is at an age when keratoconus is initiated, and keratoconus patients usually become myopic before the keratoconus is manifested and may be corrected with contact lenses.[92]

These arguments are countered by reports that the age of onset of contact lens–associated keratoconus cases is typically much later than the usual teenage onset of naturally occurring keratoconus.[109] A summary of reports linking keratoconus and contact lens wear is provided in Table 4–1.

In summary, this is a difficult, perhaps impossible, issue to settle. Rigid contact lenses may play a role in some cases of keratoconus; this is likely a result of some (unknown) predisposition for this condition elicited by PMMA contact lens wear. However, as argued by Zadnik,[153] because rigid contact lens application is a treatment option for keratoconus and early keratoconus can be difficult to diagnose, a causative relationship between the two may be impossible to ascertain.

Rigid Gas Permeable–Induced Changes

Wearing an RGP contact lens can alter the refractive error and corneal curvature of the eye. As a result of the molding force of the lens (notably the base curve radius) against the eye, even in lieu of edema-related changes, increases

TABLE 4–1.

Published Reports on Astigmatism and Keratoconus After Contact Lens Wear*†

Authors	No. of Cases	Duration of CL Wear (yr)	Refraction After CL Wear	Comments
Hartstein[60]	4	3, 4, 7, 7	The more affected of 3 pairs of eyes had a net increase in cylinder of −3.75, −4.25, and −4.50. The less affected increased by −1, −2, and −1.75.	3/4 patients had unilateral keratoconus; 1 bilateral.
Ing[76]	131	Mean 4.4 (range 1–12)	4/131 had greater than 2D astigmatism.	An additional 5 eyes are mentioned with keratoconus after years of hard CL wear. Low ocular rigidity was cited as predisposing factor.
Gasset et al.[45]	34	Mean 7 (range 0.25–22)	?	These cases had worn CLs before keratoconus was diagnosed, but the authors suggested correlation not cause.
Steahly[139]	2	31, 35	Increase in cylinder of −6D, OU.	Bilateral keratoconus in 1 case and unilateral in other case.
Levenson[91]	50	3–21	Change: 1-6.25D including 5 with keratoconus. Most patients changed 1-3D, usually with the rule.	Refitted all patients with RGP lenses, usually with good resolution; only 2 failed.
Nauheim and Perry[104]	1	13	?	Patient persisted with CLs for 6 more yr and required corneal graft OS.
Eggink et al.[39]	47	4–20	?	803 keratoconus patients wearing CLs were surveyed; of them, 47 (5.9%) had developed keratoconus (42 PMMA, 4 HEMA, 1 PMMA and CAB) 4–20 yr after beginning CL wear.
Phillips[109]	8	6–10	In almost every case, refractive cylinder increased a minimum of 3D.	6 PMMA cases (1 switched to soft, 1 to RGP before diagnosis) and 2 soft lens cases.

*Adapted from Phillips CI: *Acta Ophthalmol* 1991; 69:661–668.
†CL = contact lens; OU = each eye; RGP = rigid gas-permeable; OS = left eye; PMMA = polymethylmethacrylate; HEMA = hydroxyethylmethacrylate; CAB = cellulose acetate butyrate.

or decreases in refractive error and astigmatism are not uncommon.[43] Studies performed with the 12-ring Corneascope (Kera Corporation), which has the benefit of evaluating a much larger corneal area than the keratometer, have concluded that when rigid lenses align properly to the corneal periphery and exhibit adequate clearance, all 12 rings are clear and not distorted.[74] However, steep rigid lenses, even with a high Dk value, that tend to impinge on the midperipheral region of the cornea can cause distortion in this region. In addition, as noted earlier, when a rigid lens decenters, the tendency is to cause flattening and corneal warpage in the regions of bearing.[150]

Early RGP extended wear clinical studies demonstrated a trend toward significant corneal flattening during the first few months of lens wear with as much as 1D of change in the vertical meridian, followed by steepening toward the baseline.[63, 112, 134, 135] However, recent studies with higher Dk materials have demonstrated much more moderate keratometric and refractive changes, often not exceeding 0.25D.[111, 128] It appears that the reduction in edema may make the cornea less susceptible to the mechanical force of the lens, and less corneal and refractive change results. According to Schnider et al.,[134] changes that result in sphericalization of the cornea with less than one line of visual acuity change through the baseline spectacle prescription are probably acceptable. Any large change (unless flexure-related) in refractive error, astigmatism, or reduction in best-corrected spectacle visual acuity should warrant a change to a higher Dk material or change in lens design, typically to achieve more lens movement and greater peripheral edge clearance.

Sphericalization of mild-to-moderate astigmatic corneas fitted with spherical lenses is typically the result of corneal molding by the back surface of the contact lens.[63, 112] It is also apparent that quite frequently, as a result of lid forces during sleep and uneven pressure distribution occurring with rigid extended wear lenses, subtle changes in corneal shape can occur.[9, 72] Badowski[9] compared the effects on vision, corneal topography, and refractive error of fitting the Boston Equalens for extended wear 1D flatter than the "K" reading (eight eyes), 1D steeper than K (six eyes) and "on the K" reading (six eyes). Interestingly, although not statistically significant, the trend with keratometry was toward progressive flattening in both meridians in all groups. Likewise, the evaluation of peripheral corneal topography did not reveal a significant change between fitting methods, although the periphery again showed flattening from baseline. As previously reported with PMMA lens wearers, cases of inferior corneal steepening were induced by the flat-fitting lenses. In terms of refractive error, the steep group showed considerable variation and was slightly more myopic at the end of this 4-month study. The other two groups both showed a trend toward decreasing myopia that could affect spectacle wear. A slight decrease in refractive cylinder was also reported. It was concluded that the alignment- and flat-fitting lenses resulted in the greatest changes in corneal shape; specifically, the alignment-fitting lenses induced the most change, and the most irregular changes were induced by the flat-fitting lenses.

The role of lens adherence in rigid extended wear is also important. Adherence of the lens to the cornea during sleep has been reported in as many as 50% of rigid extended wear patients.[111, 112, 143] It has been claimed that a steep-fitting relationship could cause adherence as a result of centration forces provided by the tear layer.[18] Likewise, a lens design that results in peripheral sealoff (i.e., peripheral curve is too steep, resulting in an absence of fluorescein in this region) could encourage adherence.[51] Remediation can include changing to a more flexural resistant material and using a design with a flat peripheral curve system. If this fails, reducing the patient to daily wear often succeeds.[18, 134]

Hydrogel-Induced Changes

Mode of Lens

It is uncommon to find a large change in the corneal curvature of a soft lens wearer,[11, 12, 93] although both corneal steepening[52, 58, 68] and flattening[52] have been reported. As a result of the flexible nature of hydrogel lenses, there is less opportunity for significant localized areas of pressure to develop. Therefore, regular and irregular corneal distortion and molding are less marked with these lens materials.[143] Likewise, although epithelial edema may be present, because it is typically uniform across the cornea, the corneal curvature does not change significantly.[68, 69, 93] For this reason, soft lens patients rarely experience spectacle blur.

As with rigid lenses, hydrogel lens adherence to the cornea can cause changes in both refraction and corneal curvature, albeit of less magnitude. One cause of adherence is hydrogel lens dehydration, which can result in a steeper-fitting relationship and edema via the reduced oxygen transmission.[2, 90] Another hydrogel-induced complication, often occurring with extended wear, is *myopic creep,* a form of progressive myopia.[81] It appears to result from low-level, chronic epithelial edema and subtle changes in corneal contour and can be permanent if not diagnosed early and managed properly.[97] Management should consist of either reducing the patient's wearing time or switching to a higher oxygen-transmissible lens material.

Comparison With Rigid Lenses

Iacona[74, 75] performed an interesting comparative study. A total of 50 patients, 25 with hydrogel lenses and 25 with

RGP lenses, all successful wearers for a minimum of 6 months, were enrolled into the study. All 50 patients exhibited some corneal distortion with the 12-ring Corneascope and were all refitted into RGP lenses using the Corneascope values as a basis for obtaining the best fit. Approximately 80% were fit between 0.50D and 0.75D flatter than K. Almost all of the soft lens patients exhibited a large variation in the roundness of the central three rings and a lack of uniform curvature of the outermost three rings. The most common region of distortion was inferior. After 1 week of RGP lens wear, the central rings cleared up completely, whereas the outermost (peripheral) rings improved only slightly. There was also some paracentral (fourth to sixth rings) flattening, accompanied by a decrease in both with-the-rule astigmatism and minus sphere. When distortion remained, it was inferior in location. The RGP patients also exhibited corneal distortion in the central and outermost three rings, which improved after 1 week in the new lenses. However, as opposed to the inferior location of hydrogel lens–induced corneal distortion, rigid lenses tended to maintain some amount of distortion in the horizontal midperipheral (seventh to ninth rings) even after refitting, an apparent result of corneal desiccation in those regions. These patients also exhibited corneal flattening in most regions after being refitted into the new rigid lenses.

The use of computerized corneal mapping has been used to compare corneal topographical changes induced by both rigid and hydrogel lens materials.[79] Using the Corneal Modeling System in a case report on one patient, Kame et al.[79] found that both a hydrogel lens material (Acuvue, Jacksonville, FL) and a low Dk RGP lens material (Polycon) in a spherical design resulted in superior peripheral corneal flattening and inferior peripheral corneal steepening. The use of a posterior aspheric design in a higher Dk material, however, resulted in a more symmetrical change in corneal shape.

Effect of Contact Lenses on the Quality of Vision

The subjective complaint of many contact lens wearers that their vision is inferior to that with spectacles has led to attempts to define the nature of this difference. Most of the studies have focused on the quality of vision with hydrogel lenses, although some attention has been directed to vision with hard lenses. Several techniques have been employed in these investigations; these fall into three general categories of optotypes, variable contrast acuity charts, and contrast sensitivity devices.

Methods of Measurement

Snellen Chart Visual Acuity.—Several causes have been suggested for reduced vision with the different types of contact lenses. Hydrogel lens wearers can experience this problem as a result of uncorrected refractive cylinder (or poor rotational stability with toric lenses), the aforementioned myopic creep phenomenon, strain induced with lathe-cut lenses during the manufacturing process,[93] and soft lens–induced flexure. The latter appears to be limited to plus power lenses.[149] El-Nashar and Larke[40] found after calculating the wave front aberration from photokeratoscopy measurements of the cornea and a soft lens in situ, under low illumination (large pupil–diameter conditions), visual function is likely to be impaired. Reduced vision in RGP lens wearers is usually the result of either lens-induced flexure,[66] warpage,[63, 64] or poor surface wettability.[50]

Two studies have directly compared letter chart visual acuity in extended wear patients with hydrogel and rigid lenses.[44, 148] In both studies the visual acuity was found to be better with RGP lenses than with hydrogel lenses.

Variable-Contrast Acuity Charts.—The use of low- and high-contrast Bailey-Lovie (Log MAR) charts have the advantages over conventional Snellen acuity charts of being able to compare visual ability under high- and low-contrast conditions. They are quick and reliable and provide equal letter spacing between rows and letters, a fixed number of letters per line, and a constant logarithmic size progression.[9, 70]

Contrast Sensitivity Function Testing.—The traditional, and still most commonly used method of measuring visual ability is the use of the Snellen visual acuity chart. A patient having 20/20 visual acuity is generally considered to have excellent vision, and the presence of any vague complaints are sometimes ignored by the attending clinician. These complaints may not only be real but can be confirmed clinically by evaluating contrast sensitivity function (CSF).

The evaluation of a patient's contrast sensitivity involves measuring the ability to distinguish light and dark bands (sine-wave gratings) (Fig 4–6).[47] There are two variables to consider when one is performing CSF testing: (1) contrast and (2) spatial frequency.[25] The sine-wave grating, which appears as alternate light and dark bars (with ill-defined borders), is used as a target. The contrast difference between the light and dark bars is varied. If the visual system is very sensitive to the stimuli, little difference in contrast between the light and dark bars is necessary for the target to be observed. Conversely, if the visual system is not sensitive to the stimuli, a large difference in contrast is necessary. The second variable is spatial frequency or the width of the bars on the target. The human visual system is most sensitive to gratings of three to five cycles/degree, with one cycle equal to one light and one dark band pair. At the optimum size, very little contrast is required between the dark and light bars for the pattern to

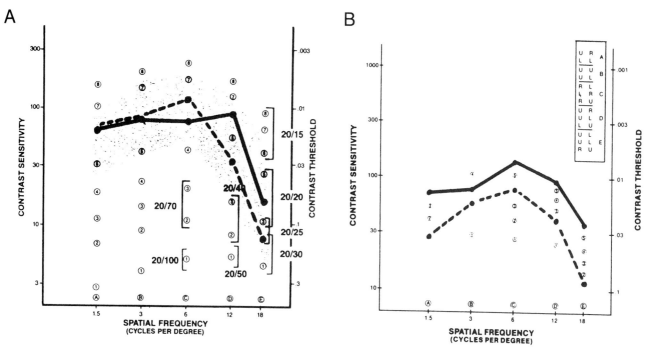

FIG 4–6.
A, contrast sensitivity measured through spectacles *(solid line)* and spherical soft contact lens with mild residual astigmatism. **B,** contrast sensitivity measured through two different brands of spherical soft contact lenses on an eye with 0.75D of astigmatism. Visual acuity was 20/20 through either contact lens. (From Bosse JC: *Contact Lens J* 1989; 18:75–78. Used by permission.)

be recognized. As the bars become thinner, or higher in spatial frequency, the pattern is increasingly more difficult to differentiate. Likewise, as the bars become thicker, or lower in spatial frequency, once again the pattern becomes more difficult to observe and greater contrast is required. Measuring many spatial frequencies at varied contrasts will derive the complete CSF curve.[25]

Snellen visual acuity measures the minimum resolvable object under high-contrast conditions. Therefore, it cannot be compared directly to CSF,[47] although 20/20 acuity is roughly equal to 30 cycles/degree on the CSF test. With Snellen visual acuity, the clinician is unable to measure middle to low spatial frequencies or how the patient sees under moderate- to low-contrast situations (i.e., under more normal, or real life, conditions). Using the Snellen visual acuity test to evaluate a patient's vision has been compared with testing one's hearing by using only one tone.[25]

Simplified clinical tests for evaluating CSF have been developed. These include a wall chart, a projector slide version, and a computerized method that evaluates both contrast sensitivity and the effects of central and peripheral glare sources.[25, 144]

Effects of Contact Lens Wear
Hydrogel Lenses.—Numerous clinical research studies have compared the CSF obtained between different contact

lens materials. Early reports suggested superior vision with spectacle correction. Applegate and Massof[5] measured six spectacle-wearing ametropes.[5] Baseline measurements were performed and then measured again after three patients were fitted with PMMA lenses and three patients were fitted with hydrogel contact lenses. They concluded that a large decrement in CSF resulted with hydrogel (Bausch & Lomb [B & L] Soflens) lens wear vs. spectacles. Uncorrected residual (astigmatic) refractive error was implicated for the decrease in CSF. Other initial studies provided similar results.[98, 152] The decrease in CSF at all spatial frequencies occurring after 2 weeks in a study by Mitra and Lamberts[98] with the B & L Soflens was attributed to several possible causes, including, uncorrected refractive error, optical aberrations from the contact lens, and corneal edema.

Later studies have confirmed the effects of corneal edema and residual astigmatism on CSF. Hess and Garner[67] found that mild edema affects only high spatial frequencies, whereas larger amounts of edema affect all spatial frequencies. Uncorrected refractive astigmatism, even in small amounts, will result in a decrease in CSF, especially at higher spatial frequencies.[55] Gundel et al.[55] investigated the effect of mild residual astigmatism (X = 0.75D) on CSF. They concluded that all but the highest spatial frequency tested was affected by residual astigmatism and that this decrease was not solely from the hydrogel lenses and not only from the absence of cylinder correction (a spherical equivalent in spectacle form did not lead to as much loss in CSF) (Fig 4–7). Hydrogel lens–induced flexure was implicated as a possible cause of reduced CSF. Contrast sensitivity function testing was deemed much more beneficial than Snellen visual acuity in differentiating significant visual impairment with contact lenses.

More recently, better controlled experiments with more rigorous statistical analyses of results have led to the current consensus view that hydrogel contact lenses do not significantly reduce contrast sensitivity.[49, 107, 145, 146] The visual impairment suggested in the early studies was negated by tighter controls, eliminating the effects of residual astigmatism, contact lens adaptation, chronic corneal edema, and deposited contact lenses.[25] Teitelbaum et al.[145] controlled for adaptation and astigmatism and used only brand new lenses. They concluded that there was no significant difference in CSF in hydrogel lens wear compared with spectacle lens wear. In addition, no significant difference in CSF was found between three polymers of differing water content. Likewise, other clinical studies using nonastigmatic hydrogel lens wearers have found no significant difference in CSF between spectacle and hydrogel lens wear.[107, 146] In addition, no significant difference was found for lens fit, thickness, and water content.[107]

Rigid Lenses.—Few clinical studies have evaluated the effects of rigid contact lenses. In one study, the effect on CSF of rigid extended wear was determined.[154] Baseline readings were obtained from PMMA, hydrogel, and spectacle lens wearers. These patients were then refitted into a rigid extended wear lens material (Boston IV, Polymer Technology Corporation, Wilmington, MA). After 1 year of contact lens wear, the CSF had improved in all three groups. Another study compared the effects on CSF and glare (the latter using a two-channel tachistoscope developed by Applegate)[4, 6] of a tricurve vs. a progressive aspheric design, both in a fluorosilicone/acrylate lens material.[144] The aspheric design performed as well as the spherical design. This was considered a positive result because it can be suggested that a possible fault of aspheric designs is that the manufacturing process (specifically the polishing of the many curves) can result in optical aberrations and a compromise in the quality of vision.

Two clinical studies have evaluated the effects of rigid diffractive lens designs on CSF.[38, 78] The diffractive optics design which, although providing a multi-focal correction, using the simultaneous vision concept, nevertheless provides an equal, but reduced, amount of light for distance and near vision images. Two studies suggest that this design may compromise CSF.[34, 38, 78] Eggink et al.[38] found that the CSF was significantly lower with the diffractive design than with a conventional RGP lens design. Jones et al.[78] reported a large decrement with a rigid diffractive lens when compared with single-vision spectacle lenses.

Recently a short-duration stimulus, CSF test has been developed to measure temporal fluctuations in vision after the blink in contact lens wearers.[146] Loss of sensitivity has been shown to occur for short periods (generally up to 50 msec) after the blink, which is caused by shifts in the retinal image as a result of lens movement. Losses have been found in both hydrogel and RGP lens wearers, but because visual reduction is related to the degree of lens movement, the magnitude of change is greater with RGP lenses. These findings indicate the need for good lens design in the fitting of all lenses and particularly hard lenses, where good centration and controlled movement (consistent with good physiology) are essential.

DELIBERATE REFRACTIVE ERROR AND CORNEAL CURVATURE CHANGES

Orthokeratology

Definition

Orthokeratology has been defined as a deliberate attempt to modify the corneal curvature to produce a reduction or elimination of a refractive anomaly by programmed application of contact lenses.[89] It is typically a 1- to 2-year program, with a cost ranging from $1,000 to $2,000.

Suitable for orthokeratology are low-myopic or astigmatic patients and individuals with high motivation, availability for frequent follow-up visits, and a degree of affluence. Patients are often motivated to undergo orthokeratology to meet an occupational vision requirement. This includes airline pilots, military personnel, fire fighters, police officers, and bus drivers.

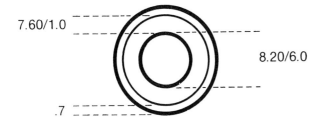

7.60/1.0

8.20/6.0

.7

7.6 P.S.B.C.
6.0 Diameter of P.B.C.
1.0 Diameter of P.S.B.C. (Tear reservoir)
.7 Aspheric edge lift-design

FIG 4–7.
Diagram of the Ortho-K 60 lens, Contex, Inc. (From Wlodyga RJ, Bryla C: *Contact Lens Spectrum* 1989; 4(8):58–65. Used by permission.)

Fitting Philosophies

Original fitting philosophies recommended the "radical flattening" approach.[77, 106] Fits were so flat that the lacrimal layer corrected the amount of existing myopia. However, because the amount of central bearing would be excessive in these cases, increasing the risk of corneal distortion, clinicians initiated "best fit" approaches to orthokeratology.

A well-known fitting philosophy for use in orthokeratology was introduced by Grant and May.[48] For myopic patients, they selected a base curve radius only 0.25D to 0.75D flatter than K. Visits are scheduled every 6 to 8 weeks, and lens changes are made in 0.50D flatter base curve radius increments as the corneal curvature flattens until a low minus or plano refractive error is obtained. Hyperopes are fitted 0.25D steeper than K, and the time interval for lens change is longer than with myopes (i.e., 2–4 months vs. 6–8 weeks). Once a near-plano prescription has been obtained, the rigid contact lenses are worn on a retainer basis for 6 months, and then wearing time is gradually decreased; eventually the contact lenses are discarded.

The Tabb fitting method claims good success despite actually recommending a steeper than K fitting philosophy.[35] Patients with less than 1D of corneal astigmatism are fitted 0.25D steeper than K; greater than 1D, astigmatic patients are fitted 0.50D to 0.75D steeper than K. The overall diameter and base curve radius remain unchanged, whereas the optical zone is reduced incrementally such that the resultant tear reservoir is gradually increased. A positive correlation has been found for refractive and visual acuity changes.

A more recent fitting philosophy has been introduced by Wlodyga and Bryla[151] using the Ortho-K lens (Contex). In addition to taking central keratometry readings, they asked patients to view nasally at the + sign on the B & L keratometer ring. If the observed temporal, horizontal readings were flatter than the central value, the chances of

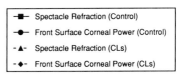

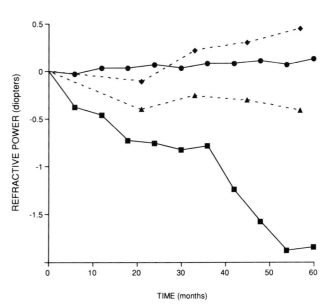

FIG 4–8.
Cumulative frequency curves showing rates of change per year in myopia in the control group and contact lens group. (From Stone J: *Br J Physiol Opt* 1977; 32:89–114. Used by permission.)

adequate corneal flattening centrally were considered excellent. The Ortho-K lens material has a Dk value of 88; the specific lens design is given in Figure 4–8. Four sets of Ortho-K 60 lenses are ordered for each patient. Set 1 is 1D flatter than K, or 50% of the difference between the flat central K reading and the flat temporal K value. The second set is ordered 1D flatter than set 1, and so on with sets 3 and 4. The best case results were obtained with patients who were first-time contact lens wearers and with those individuals having average to steep, corneal curvature readings. A summary of orthokeratology fitting philosophies is provided in Table 4–2.

Efficacy

Several clinical studies have evaluated the success and long-term effectiveness of orthokeratology. Kerns[82–89] evaluated 36 eyes fitted 0.12D to 0.37D flatter than K in the orthokeratology group and 26 eyes wearing conventional alignment-fitting contact lenses and 6 eyes wearing spectacles. These patients were evaluated over 1,000 days of wear, followed by 60 days of lens discontinuation. Kerns concluded that even though some patients were capable of achieving quite excessive changes, others exhib-

TABLE 4–2.

Some Philosophies of Orthokeratology Fitting

Authors	Base Curve Relationship/Lens Design
Jessen[77]	Flattening factor equals amount of myopia to create a plano-powered contact lens
Nolan[106]	Same as Jessen[77]; controlled wearing time for effect
Grant and May[48]	Fit on flat K reading; changed center thickness
Kerns[84]	0.12D–0.37D flatter than flat K reading
Binder et al.[24]	0.75D–2.50D flatter than flat K reading
Coon[35]	Lenses fit 0.25D–0.75D steeper than flat K reading
Brand et al.[28]	0.30D flatter than flat K reading

ited much smaller, if any, changes with orthokeratology. On discontinuation of lens wear, both corneal curvature and visual acuity tended to regress toward the prefitting values, although neither returned to the original state.

Binder et al.[24] reported on 23 orthokeratology patients fitted 0.75D to 2.50D flatter than K. These patients were compared with 16 patients wearing rigid lenses fitted on K; all patients were observed for 40 months. Three levels of change were reported. Five patients exhibited little change; the uncorrected visual acuity never improved greater than three lines from the baseline visual acuity. Another group of six patients showed partial/variable responses, characterized by initial unresponsiveness, accompanied by an improvement in unaided visual acuity and ultimately a deterioration in vision and regression in refractive values. Nine patients achieved good responses, defined as 20/20 unaided visual acuity sometime during the study, usually early in the process, and maintenance of that level of vision throughout the study. They concluded that even though orthokeratology produces unpredictable results, it is able to achieve an average of 1.50D reduction of myopia. Although it appears to be safe on a short-term basis, it can result in moderate spectacle blur, increased with-the-rule astigmatism, and a quality of unaided vision that is less than the same level of best corrected vision. Furthermore, retainer lenses were required to maintain the improvements in visual acuity. Total lens removal resulted in a return toward the prefitting values.

The most comprehensive and controlled investigation on the safety and efficacy of orthokeratology is the Berkeley study.[26-28] The treatment group consisted of 40 patients fitted approximately 0.30D flatter than 40 rigid lens-wearing control patients. It was found that rigid contact lenses, worn in a controlled manner, can reduce myopia 1D. The study concluded that this value can be clinically significant in low myopes. The induced change was not permanent; when contact lens wear was reduced to 4 hours/day, 45% of the refractive error change returned. A complete return to baseline, however, did not occur. It was also found that the visual acuity was variable during the periods of non–contact lens wear. The study concluded that orthokeratology is an unscientific method because no consistent mathematical relationship is present. However, orthokeratology was not determined to be unsafe, although more monitoring of these patients for maintenance of a good lens-cornea fitting relationship was recommended.

Corneal Curvature and Refractive Changes

A comprehensive overview on corneal curvature and refractive changes with orthokeratology has been reported by Kerns.[89] He discusses change under the headings of base curve to corneal fitting relationship, lens position, temporal effects, and sphericalization of the cornea.

Base Curve–Corneal Relationship Versus Corneal Curvature.—The horizontal corneal curvature tends to change regardless of the base curve to cornea fitting relationship. There is a poor correlation with the amount of flatness of base curve radius and degree of induced corneal flattening. The corneal curvature responses are much more variable when the base curve radius-cornea relationship exceeds 0.50D flat. An analysis of the results suggest that the curvature could flatten, steepen, or remain unchanged with each base curve–corneal relationship.

The vertical corneal curvature tends to flatten with base curve–cornea relationships of on K to 0.50D flatter than K. A base curve–cornea relationship exceeding 0.50D results in an average steepening effect, therefore, inducing corneal toricity. As with the horizontal meridian, change could occur in any direction; the average change is 0.12D steep. For both horizontal and vertical meridians it was concluded that the flatter the fit, the greater the variability of responses and the greater the probability of increasing corneal toricity.

Contact Lens Position.—Typically, as the corneal topography became more spherical, lens positioning was affected. Hence, change in lens position was influenced by changes in corneal topography. Because mechanical pressure forces are constantly on the horizontal meridian, on blinking the eyelid, interaction compounds the pressure effect. In addition, the contact lens rocks on the horizontal meridian, resulting in varying pressure along the vertical meridian of the cornea. It is this concept that is proposed to account for the variability of change in the vertical corneal curvature meridian.

Temporal Effects.—During the first 200 days or so, uniform corneal curvature changes were noted, regardless of the lens-cornea fitting relationship. It was proposed that the limit of the effects of orthokeratology seem directly related to corneal topography and probably ocular rigidity. This is supported by several studies in which most corneal changes had ceased after about 300 to 400 days.[84, 85, 87] Changes observed after this time were forced, erratic, and thus less predictable.

Sphericalization.—Because sphericalization typically produces a flatter central curvature and a steeper peripheral corneal curvature, a more spherical cornea results. Furthermore, when the cornea becomes more spherical, there is no longer an area available for displacement other than in the posterior direction. This may account for fewer corneal curvature changes occurring as the cornea becomes spherical and may represent a practical limit to the effects of orthokeratology.

Adverse Effects

Adverse effects pertaining to corneal curvature, refraction, and vision induced in the practice of orthokeratology can be summarized as follows:

1. Induced corneal astigmatism is produced by the pressure applied when a lens with excessively flat base curve radii is used or is produced from the effects of long-term lens decentration.
2. Peripheral corneal distortion can result from using a "too flat, too soon" fitting approach, especially with patients having flatter than average peripheral corneas.
3. Decreased quality of vision is typically described as hazy or "watery" vision; this is most often caused by corneal and astigmatic changes.
4. Visual problems at near are reported as an increased difficulty at near as orthokeratology process proceeds. This may be a result of a hyperactivity of the accommodative system.
5. Regression toward the prefit level is often manifest as a regression of corneal curvature, refraction, and vision toward the baseline values.

Myopia Progression in Young People

There have been a large number of early published reports that contact lens wear may slow the regression of myopia in young people.[101–106] Certainly the benefits of slowing this progression would be numerous, including a decreased reliance on spectacles and possibly a decrease in retinal pathological conditions.[140] However, others have tended to present the opposite view, citing, among other reasons, that contact lens wear is typically initiated when myopia has already stabilized.[11] Only through controlled clinical studies could this controversy be resolved.

Polymethylmethacrylate Lens Wear

The first major clinical study that addresses this issue was performed by Stone[140–142] in the 1970s with PMMA lenses. The experimental group consisted of 80 patients with a mean age of 12.8 years and a range equal to 8.42 to 16.58 years. The control group consisted of 40 spectacle wearers with a mean age of 12.19 years and a range equal to 6.58 to 16.08 years. Keratometry and a cycloplegic refraction were performed at 6-month intervals.

After 5 years the results showed significantly less increase in myopia in the contact lens wearers compared with the spectacle-wearing controls. The mean rate of change in the contact lens wearers was 0.17D more myopia per year; for the control group the increase was 0.38D per year. Only about one half of the refractive change could be accounted for by corneal flattening; therefore, it was concluded that contact lenses have other effects in addition to changing corneal curvature that may correct the development of myopia. These effects could include either slowing down the rate of increase in axial length or reducing the power of the crystalline lens.

Rigid Gas-Permeable Lens Wear

Recent reports have described a similar clinical study to that of Stone in which an RGP lens material was fitted.[53, 54, 108] One hundred myopic children between the ages of 8 and 13 years were fitted with a 39 Dk silicone-acrylate lens material (Paraperm O2 +, Paragon Optical, Mesa, AZ) This group was matched in age and refractive error with a control group of 20 spectacle lens wearers.

After 3 years of contact lens wear, the mean increase for the 56 subjects remaining in the study was 0.48D (0.16D/year) compared with 1.53D (0.51D/year) for the spectacle-wearing group. The mean change in corneal curvature values was a decrease or corneal flattening of 0.37D in the contact lens–wearing group. Because this amount was less than one half of the effect of contact lenses in controlling myopia progression, it was proposed that although the keratometer provides a valid measurement of corneal refracting power for a normal cornea, it fails to provide a valid measurement for a cornea that has been flattened by a contact lens. Specifically, the keratometer does not measure the axial portion of the cornea, which may, in fact, flatten at a greater rate than the paracentral region.[41] Therefore, the actual amount of apical flattening could be greater than the actual measured values with a keratometer. Future use of a computerized corneal modeling instrument or similar device should provide an answer. Definitive conclusions from this study were compromised by the absence of keratometry readings for the control group and the fact that no axial length measurements were performed. Nevertheless, this study tends to support Stone's hypothesis that rigid contact lenses may have an effect on the axial elongation of the eye.

Hydrogel Lens Wear

A recent study by Andreo[3] compared the rate of myopia progression with one group of 28 hydrogel lens wearers with 28 spectacle-wearing controls. The age range in these groups was 14 to 19 years. No difference in the rate of progression of refractive error occurred in this study. Andreo concluded that there was no effect of hydrogel contact lens wear on the progression of myopia.

SUMMARY

It is quite apparent that all contact lens materials have an effect on refractive error and corneal topography. Rigid lens materials, especially PMMA, tend to have the greatest effect as a result of edema, corneal molding, and changes in corneal astigmatism. Hydrogel lenses can also induce changes as a result of corneal edema and lens adherence. The benefits of RGP lens materials in minimizing edema-related corneal complications have been well documented in this text; however, the importance of obtaining an optimum lens-cornea fitting relationship to minimize the possibility of corneal distortion by a decentered or adhered lens cannot be overemphasized. Finally, contact lens–induced refractive error and corneal curvature changes can occur with all patients, and it is imperative that procedures be performed at every progress evaluation visit to determine any changes taking place.

REFERENCES

1. Anderson RH: Apparent arrest of myopia by contacts. *Contacto* 1968; 12:3–4.
2. Andrasko G: The amount and time course of soft contact lens dehydration. *J Am Optom Assoc* 1982; 53:207.
3. Andreo LK: Long-term effects of hydrophilic contact lenses on myopia. *Ann Ophthalmol* 1990; 22:224–227.
4. Applegate RA, Jones DH: Disability glare and hydrogel lens wear revisited. *Am J Optom Physiol Opt* 1989; 66:756–759.
5. Applegate RA, Massof RC: Changes in the contrast sensitivity function induced by contact lens wear. *Am J Optom Physiol Opt* 1975; 52:840–846.
6. Applegate RA, Wolf M: Disability glare increased by hydrogel lens wear. *Am J Optom Physiol Opt* 1987; 64:309–312.
7. Arner RS: Prescribing new contact lenses or spectacles for the existing contact lens wearer. *J Am Optom Assoc* 1970; 41:253–256.
8. Arner RS: Corneal deadaptation: The case against abrupt cessation of contact lens wear. *J Am Optom Assoc* 1977; 48:339–341.
9. Badowski L: Refractive error and corneal topographical changes with daily and extended wear of rigid gas permeable contact lenses. Master's thesis, Ohio State University College of Optometry, Columbus, Ohio, 1991.
10. Bailey NJ: New contact lens development. Possible factors in the control of myopia with contact lenses. *Contacto* 1958; 2:114–117.
11. Bailey NJ, Carney LG: Corneal changes from hydrophilic contact lenses. *Am J Optom Arch Am Acad Optom* 1973; 50:299–304.
12. Baldone JA: Corneal curvature changes secondary to the wearing of hydrophilic gel contact lenses. *Contact Intraoc Lens Med J* 1975; 1:175–176.
13. Bennett ES: Immediate refitting of gas permeable lenses. *J Am Optom Assoc* 1983; 54:239–242.
14. Bennett ES: Silicone/acrylate lens design. *Int Contact Lens Clin* 1985; 12:45–53.
15. Bennett ES: Keratoconus, in Bennett ES, Grohe RM (eds): *Rigid Gas-Permeable Contact Lenses*. New York, Professional Press, 1986, pp 297–344.
16. Bennett ES: Treatment options for PMMA-induced problems, in Bennett ES, Grohe RM (eds): *Rigid Gas-Permeable Contact Lenses*. New York, Professional Press, 1986, pp 275–295.
17. Bennett ES, Gilbreath MK: Handling PMMA-induced corneal distortion: A case study. *Optom Monthly* 1983; 74:529–533.
18. Bennett ES, Grohe RM: How to solve stock lens syndrome. *Rev Optom* 1987; 124(12):51–52.
19. Bennett ES, Henry VA, Davis LJ, et al: Comparing empirical and diagnostic fitting of daily wear fluoro-silicone/acrylate contact lenses. *Contact Lens Forum* 1989; 14:38–44.
20. Bennett ES, Tomlinson A: A controlled comparison of two techniques of refitting long-term PMMA contact lens wearers. *Am J Optom Physiol Opt* 1983; 60:139–145.
21. Bennett ES, Tomlinson A, Mirowitz MC, et al: Comparison of overnight swelling and lens performance in RGP extended wear. *CLAO J* 1988; 14:94–100.
22. Berman MR: Central corneal curvature and wearing time during contact lens adaptation. *Optom Weekly* 1972; 63(6):27–30.
23. Bier N: Myopia controlled by contact lenses. *Optician* 1958; 135:427.
24. Binder PS, May CH, Grant SC: An evaluation of orthokeratology. *Am Acad Ophthalmol* 1980; 87:729–744.
25. Bosse JC: Use of contrast sensitivity testing for contact lens fitting and management. *Contact Lens J* 1990; 18:75–78.
26. Brand RJ, Polse KA, Schwalbe JS: The Berkeley orthokeratology study, part I: General conduct of the study. *Am J Optom Physiol Opt* 1983; 60:175–186.
27. Brand RJ, Polse KA, Schwalbe JS, et al: The Berkeley orthokeratology study, part II: Efficacy and duration. *Am J Optom Physiol Opt* 1983; 60:187–198.
28. Brand RJ, Polse KA, Schwalbe JS, et al: The Berkeley orthokeratology study, part III: Safety. *Am J Optom Physiol Opt* 1983; 60:321–328.
29. Brightbill FS, Stainer GA: Previous hard contact wear in keratoconus. *Contact Introc Lens Med J* 1979; 5:43–47.
30. Brungardt TF, Potter CE: Measuring refractive error change in the contact lens wearer. *Am J Optom* 1971; 48:497–503.
31. Carney LG: Corneal topography changes during contact lens wear. *Contact Lens J* 1974; 3:5–16.
32. Carney LG: The basis for corneal shape change during contact lens wear. *Am J Optom* 1975; 52:445–454.

33. Carney LG: Refractive error and visual acuity changes during contact lens wear. *Contact Lens J* 1975; 5:28–34.

34. Cohen AL, Cohen HR: Bifocal optics: Diffractive bifocal designs vs. simultaneous vision. *Contact Lens Spectrum* 1989; 4:49–51.

35. Coon LJ: Orthokeratology: part II. Evaluating the Tabb method. *J Am Optom Assoc* 1984; 55:409–418.

36. DeRubeis MJ, Shily BG: The effects of wearing the Boston II gas permeable contact lens on central corneal curvature. *Am J Optom* 1985; 62:497–500.

37. Dickinson F: The value of microlenses in progressive myopia. *Optician* 1957; 133:263–264.

38. Eggink FAGJ, Pinkers AJLG: Visual acuity and contrast sensitivity with Diffrax contact lenses. *Contact Lens J* 1990; 18:37–39.

39. Eggink FAGJ, Pinkers AJLG, et al: Keratoconus, a retrospective study. *Contact Lens J* 1988; 16:204–206.

40. El-Nashar NF, Larke JR: Wave front aberration in the hydrogel lens wearing eye. *Am J Optom Physiol Opt* 1986; 63:409–412.

41. Erickson P, Thorn F: Does refractive error change twice as fast as corneal power in orthokeratology? *Am J Optom Physiol Opt* 1977; 54:581–597.

42. Finnemore VM, Korb JE: Corneal edema with polymethylmethacrylate versus gas permeable rigid polymer contact lenses of identical design. *J Am Optom Assoc* 1980; 51:271–274.

43. Fonn D: Progress evaluation procedures, in Bennett ES, Weissman BA (eds): *Clinical Contact Lens Practice*. Philadelphia, JB Lippincott Co, 1991, pp 1–10.

44. Fonn D, Holden BA: RGP versus hydrogel lenses for extended wear. *Am J Optom Physiol Opt* 1988; 65:545–551.

45. Gasset AR, Houde WL, Garcia-Bengochea M: Hard contact lens wear as an environmental risk in keratoconus. *Am J Ophthalmol* 1978; 85:339.

46. Ghormley NR: Update on Polycon: It's hard to beat. *Contact Lens Forum* 1980; 5(10):33–41.

47. Goldberg SM: The effect of contact lens wear on contrast sensitivity. *J Missouri Optom Assoc* January 1984, pp 122–127.

48. Grant SC, May CH: Orthokeratology control of refractive errors through contact lenses. *J Am Optom Assoc* 1971; 42:1277–1283.

49. Grey CP: Changes in contrast sensitivity during the first six months of soft lens wear. *Am J Optom Physiol Opt* 1987; 64:768–774.

50. Grohe RM, Caroline PJ: RGP non-wetting lens syndrome. *Contact Lens Spectrum* 1989; 4(3):32–44.

51. Grohe RM, Lebow HA. Vascularized limbal keratitis. *Int Contact Lens Clin* 1989; 16:197–209.

52. Grosvenor T: Changes in corneal curvature and subjective refraction in soft contact lens wearers. *Am J Optom Physiol Opt* 1975; 52:405.

53. Grosvenor T, Perrigin DM, Perrigin J, et al: Houston myopia control study: A randomized clinical trial: part 2. Final report by the patient care team. *Am J Optom Physiol Opt* 1987; 64:482–498.

54. Grosvenor T, Perrigin J, Perrigin D, et al: Use of silicone acrylate contact lenses for the control of myopia: Results after two years of lens wear. *Optom Vis Sci* 1989; 66:41–47.

55. Gundel RE, Kirshen SA, DiVergilio D: Changes in contrast sensitivity induced by spherical hydrogel lenses on low astigmats. *J Am Optom Assoc* 1988; 59:636–640.

56. Harris MG: Refitting contact lenses, in Miller D, White PF (eds): *Complications of Contact Lenses*. Boston, Little, Brown & Co, 1981, pp 95–104.

57. Harris MG: Legal issues in contact lens practice, in Bennett ES, Weissman BA (eds): *Clinical Contact Lens Practice*. Philadelphia, JB Lippincott Co, 1991, pp 1–31.

58. Harris MG, Sarver MD, Polse KA: Corneal curvature and refractive error changes associated with wearing hydrogel contact lenses. *Am J Optom Physiol Opt* 1975; 52:313.

59. Hartstein J: Corneal warping due to contact lenses: A report of 12 cases. *Am J Ophthalmol* 1965; 60:1103–1104.

60. Hartstein J: Keratoconus that developed in patients wearing corneal contact lenses. *Arch Ophthalmol* 1968; 80:345.

61. Hartstein J: Keratoconus and contact lenses. *JAMA* 1969; 208:539.

62. Hartstein J, Becker B: Research into the pathogenesis of keratoconus. *Arch Ophthalmol* 1970; 84:728–729.

63. Henry VA, Bennett ES, Forrest JF: Clinical investigation of the Paraperm EW rigid gas permeable contact lens. *Am J Optom Physiol Opt* 1987; 64:313–320.

64. Henry VA, Bennett ES, Sevigny J: Rigid extended wear problem solving. *Int Contact Lens Clin* 1990; 17:121–133.

65. Henry VA, Campbell RC, Connelly S, et al: How to refit contact lens patients. *Contact Lens Forum* 1991; 16(2):19–27.

66. Herman JP: Flexure of rigid contact lenses on toric corneas as a function of base curve fitting relationship. *J Am Optom Assoc* 1983; 54:209–213.

67. Hess RF, Garner LF: The effect of corneal edema on visual function. *Invest Ophthalmol Vis Sci* 1977; 16:5–13.

68. Hill JF: A comparison of refractive and keratometric changes during adaptation to flexible and non-flexible contact lenses. *J Am Optom Assoc* 1975; 46:290–294.

69. Hill JF: Variation in refractive error and corneal curvature after wearing hydrophilic contact lenses. *J Am Optom Assoc* 1975; 46:1136–1138.

70. Ho A, Bilton SM: Low contrast charts effectively differentiate between types of blur. *Am J Optom Physiol* 1986; 63:202–208.

71. Holden B: Suffocating the cornea with PMMA. *Contact Lens Spectrum* 1989; 4(5):69–70.

72. Holden BA, Swarbrick HA: Extended wear: Physiologic considerations, in Bennett ES, Weissman BA (eds): *Clinical Contact Lens Practice*. Philadelphia, JB Lippincott Co, pp 1–15, 1991.

73. Hom MM: Thoughts on contact lens refractive changes. *Contact Lens Forum* 1986; 11(11):16–20.

74. Iacona GD: Corneal contour changes with contact lenses: part I. *Contact Lens Spectrum* 1989; 4(4):54–55.

75. Iacona GD: Corneal contour changes with contact lenses: part II. *Contact Lens Spectrum* 1989; 4(5):34–38.

76. Ing MR: The development of corneal astigmatism in contact lens wear as an environmental risk in keratoconus. *Ann Ophthalmol* 1976; 8:309–314.

77. Jessen GN: Contact lenses as a therapeutic device. *Arch Acad Optom* 1964; 41:429–435.

78. Jones D, Yawitz M, Bennett ES, et al: A clinical investigation of the Diffrax™ bifocal contact lens. Poster presented at the Annual Meeting of the American Academy of Optometry, New Orleans, December 1989.

79. Kame RT, Caroline PJ, Hayashida JK, et al: Computerized mapping of corneal contour changes with various contact lenses. *Contact Lens Spectrum* 1989; 4(6):35–40.

80. Kame RT, Hayashida JK: Lens evaluation procedures and problem solving, in Bennett ES, Weissman BA (eds): *Clinical Contact Lens Practice*. Philadelphia, JB Lippincott Co, 1991, pp 1–10.

81. Kame R, Herskowitz R: The corneal consequences of hypoxia, in Bennett ES, Grohe RM: *Rigid Gas Permeable Contact Lenses*. New York, Professional Press, 1986, pp 21–30.

82. Kerns RL: Research in orthokeratology: part II. Experimental design, protocol and method. *J Am Optom Assoc* 1971; 42:1277–1283.

83. Kerns RL: Research in orthokeratology: part I. Introduction and background. *J Am Optom Assoc* 1976; 47:1047–1050.

84. Kerns RL: Research in orthokeratology: part III. Results and observations. *J Am Optom Assoc* 1976; 47:1505–1515.

85. Kerns RL: Research in orthokeratology: part IV. Results and observations. *J Am Optom Assoc* 1977; 48:227–238.

86. Kerns RL: Research in orthokeratology: part V. Results and observations—recovery aspects. *J Am Optom Assoc* 1977; 48:345–359.

87. Kerns RL: Research in orthokeratology: part VI. Statistical and a clinical analysis. *J Am Optom Assoc* 1977; 48:1134–1147.

88. Kerns RL: Research in orthokeratology: part VII. Examination of techniques, procedures and control. *J Am Optom Assoc* 1977; 48:1541–1553.

89. Kerns RL: Research on orthokeratology: part VIII. Results, conclusions and discussion of techniques. *J Am Optom Assoc* 1978; 49:308–314.

90. Kohler JE, Flanagan GW: Clinical dehydration of extended-wear lenses. *Int Contact Lens Clin* 1985; 12:152–157.

91. Levenson DS: Changes in corneal curvature with long-term PMMA contact lens wear. *CLAO J* 1983; 9:121–125.

92. Mandell RB: Keratoconus, in Mandell RB: *Contact Lens Practice*, ed 4. Springfield, Ill, Charles C Thomas Publisher, 1988, pp 824–849.

93. Mandell RB: Symptomatology and aftercare, in Mandell RB: *Contact Lens Practice,* ed 4. Springfield, Ill, Charles C Thomas Publisher, 1988, pp 598–643.

94. Mandell RB: Symptomatology and refitting, in Mandell RB: *Contact Lens Practice,* ed 4. Springfield, Ill, Charles C Thomas, Publisher, 1988, pp 388–439.

95. Masnick K: A preliminary investigation into the effects of corneal lenses on central corneal thickness and curvature. *Aust J Optom* 1971; 54:87–98.

96. Miller JP: Contact lens-induced corneal curvature and thickness changes. *Arch Ophthalmol* 1968; 80:420–432.

97. Miller JP, Coon LJ, Meier RF: Extended wear of Hydrocurve II 55 soft contact lenses. *J Am Optom Assoc* 1980; 51:225–233.

98. Mitra S, Lamberts DW: Contrast sensitivity in soft lens wearers. *Contact Intraoc Lens Med J* 1981; 7:315–322.

99. Morgan JF: For keratoconus diagnosis: "Qualitative" ophthalmometry. *Ophthalmol Times* 1982; 7(4):33–35.

100. Morrison RJ: Contact lenses and the progression of myopia. *Optom Weekly* 1956; 47:1487–1488.

101. Morrison RJ. Contact lenses and the progression of myopia. *J Am Optom Assoc* 1957; 28:711–713.

102. Morrison RJ: Observations on contact lenses and the progression of myopia. *Contacto* 1958; 2:20–25.

103. Morrison RJ: The use of contact lenses in adolescent myopic patients. *Am J Optom Arch Am Acad Optom* 1960; 37:165–168.

104. Nauheim JS, Perry HD: A clinicopathologic study of contact lens related keratoconus. *Am J Ophthalmol* 1985; 100:543–546.

105. Nolan JA: Progress of myopia and contact lenses. *Contacto* 1964; 8(1):125–126.

106. Nolan JA: Orthokeratology. *J Am Optom Assoc* 1971; 42:355–360.

107. Nowozyckyj A, Carney LG, Efron N: Effect of hydrogel lens wear on contrast sensitivity. *Am J Optom Physiol Opt* 1988; 65:263–271.

108. Perrigin J, Perrigin D, Quintero S, et al: Silicone-acrylate contact lenses for myopia control: 3-year results. *Optom Vis Sci* 1990; 67:764–769.

109. Phillips CI: Contact lenses and corneal deformation: Cause, correlate or co-incidence? *Acta Ophthalmol* 1991; 69:661–668.

110. Polse KA, Rivera RK: Corneal rehabilitation following hypoxic stress, in Bennett ES, Weissman BA (eds): *Clinical Contact Lens Practice*. Philadelphia, JB Lippincott Co, 1991, pp 1–6.

111. Polse KA, Rivera RK, Bonanno J: Ocular effects of hard gas permeable lens extended wear. *Am J Optom Physiol Opt* 1988; 65:358–364.

112. Polse KA, Sarver MD, Kenyon E, et al: Gas-permeable hard contact lens extended wear: Ocular and visual responses to a 6-month period of wear. *CLAO J* 1987; 13:31–38.

113. Pratt-Johnson JA, Warner DM: Contact lenses and corneal curvature changes. *Am J Ophthalmol* 1965; 60:852–855.

114. Rengstorff RH: Corneal curvature and astigmatic changes subsequent to contact lens wear. *J Am Optom Assoc* 1965; 36:996–1000.

115. Rengstorff RH: The Fort Dix report: Longitudinal study of

the effects of contact lenses. *Am J Optom Arch Am Acad Optom* 1965; 42:153–163.

116. Rengstorff RH: Variations in myopia measurements: An after-effect observed with habitual wearers of contact lenses. *Am J Optom* 1967; 44:149–161.

117. Rengstorff RH: An investigation of overnight changes in corneal curvature. *J Am Optom Assoc* 1968; 39:262–265.

118. Rengstorff RH: Relationship between myopia and corneal curvature changes after wearing contact lenses. *Am J Optom* 1969; 46:357–362.

119. Rengstorff RH: Studies of corneal curvature changes after wearing contact lenses. *J Am Optom Assoc* 1969; 40:298–299.

120. Rengstorff RH: Variation in corneal curvature measurements: An after-effect observed with habitual wearers of contact lenses. *Am J Optom Arch Am Acad Optom* 1969; 46:45–51.

121. Rengstorff RH: Diurnal variations in myopia measurements after wearing contact lenses. *Am J Optom* 1970; 47:812–815.

122. Rengstorff RH: Corneal curvature: Patterns of change after wearing contact lenses. *J Am Optom Assoc* 1971; 42:264.

123. Rengstorff RH: Diurnal variations in corneal curvature after wearing of contact lenses. *Am J Optom* 1971; 48:239–244.

124. Rengstorff RH: Diurnal constancy of corneal curvature. *Am J Optom* 1972; 49:1002–1005.

125. Rengstorff RH: Prevention and treatment of corneal damage after wearing contact lenses. *J Am Optom Assoc* 1975; 46:277–278.

126. Rengstorff RH: Astigmatism after contact lens wear. *Am J Optom Physiol Opt* 1977; 54:787–791.

127. Rengstorff RH: Circadian rhythm: Corneal curvature and refractive changes after wearing contact lenses. *J Am Optom Assoc* 1978; 49:443–444.

128. Rengstorff RH: Changes in corneal curvature associated with contact lens wear. *J Am Optom Assoc* 1979; 50:375–376.

129. Rengstorff RH: Refitting long-term wearers of hard contact lenses. *Rev Optom* 1979; 116:75–76.

130. Rengstorff RH: Strategies for refitting PMMA lens wearers. *Rev Optom* 1981; 118:49–50.

131. Rengstorff RH: Refractive changes after wearing contact lenses, in Stone J, Phillips AJ: *Contact Lenses*, ed 2. Stoneham, Mass, Butterworth, 1984, pp 527–534.

132. Saks SJ: Fluctuation in refractive state in adapting and long-term contact lens wearers. *J Am Optom Assoc* 1966; 37:229–238.

133. Schapero M: Tissue changes associated with contact lenses. *Am J Optom Arch Am Acad Optom* 1966; 43:477–485.

134. Schnider CM, Bennett ES, Grohe RM: Rigid extended wear, in Bennett ES, Weissman BA (eds): *Clinical Contact Lens Practice*. Philadelphia, JB Lippincott Co, 1991, pp 1–14.

135. Sevigny J: Clinical comparison of the Boston IV contact lens under extended wear versus the Boston II lens under daily wear. *Int Eye Care* 1986; 2:260–264.

136. Silbert M: Comments on myopia control by contact lenses. *Optom Weekly* 1962; 53:961–963.

137. Snyder AC, Gordon A: Refitting long-term asymptomatic PMMA wearers into gas permeable lenses. *J Am Optom Assoc* 1985; 56:192–197.

138. Sommer A: Keratoconus in contact lens wear [letter to the editor]. *Am J Ophthalmol* 1978; 86:442.

139. Steahly LP: Keratoconus following contact lens wear. *Ann Ophthalmol* 1978; 10:1177.

140. Stone J: Contact lens wear and the young myope. *Br J Physiol Opt* 1973; 28:90–124.

141. Stone J: Possible influence of contact lenses on myopia. *Br J Physiol Opt* 1976; 31:89–114.

142. Stone J: The possible influence of contact lenses on myopia. *Br J Physiol Opt* 1977; 32:89–114.

143. Swarbrick HA, Holden BA: Rigid gas permeable lens binding: Significance and contributing factors. *Am J Optom Physiol Opt* 1987; 64:815–823.

144. Tardibuono L, Nelson J, Bennett ES, et al: A comparison of spherical versus aspheric fluoro-silicone/acrylate lens design based on contrast sensitivity function, disability glare and overall performance. Poster presented at the Annual Meeting of the American Academy of Optometry, Denver, December 1987.

145. Teitelbaum BA, Kelly SA, Gemoules G: Contrast sensitivity through spectacles and hydrogel lenses of different polymers. *Int Contact Lens Clin* 1985; 12:162–166.

146. Tomlinson A, Mann G: An analysis of visual performance with soft contact lens and spectacle correction. *Ophthal Physiol Opt* 1985; 5:53–57.

147. Tomlinson A, Ridder WH: Effects of lens movement on vision with RGP contact lenses. *J Br Contact Lens Assoc* (In press.)

148. Weiss L: Clinical study of extended wear lenses: Hydrogel versus gas permeable. *Contact Lens Forum* 1987; 12(9):41–46.

149. Weissman BA: Loss of power with flexure of hydrogel plus lenses. *Am J Optom* 1986; 63:166.

150. Wilson SE, Lin DTC, Klyce SD, et al: Rigid contact lens decentration: A risk factor for corneal warpage. *CLAO J* 1990; 16:177–182.

151. Wlodyga RJ, Bryla C: Corneal molding: The easy way. *Contact Lens Spectrum* 1989; 4(8):58–65.

152. Woo G, Hess R: Contrast sensitivity function and soft contact lenses. *Int Contact Lens Clin* 1977; 6:171–176.

153. Zadnik KS: Keratoconus, in Bennett ES, Weissman BA (eds): *Clinical Contact Lens Practice*. Philadelphia, JB Lippincott Co, 1991, pp 1–10.

154. Ziel CJ, Gussler JR, Van Meter WS, et al: Contrast sensitivity in extended wear of the Boston IV lens. *CLAO J* 1990; 16:276–278.

Corneal Anesthesia Following Contact Lens Wear

Michel Millodot, O.D., Ph.D.

The cornea of the eye is probably the most sensitive tissue in the body. A small speck of dust, which would remain unnoticed on the tip of the finger, for example, can cause a lot of discomfort. Such extraordinary response is linked to the alarm signal of the cornea, which warns that the tissue is at risk and its ultimate "raison d' être" (i.e., transparency) may be jeopardized. This high sensitivity is linked to the palpebral reflex mechanism that closes the eyelids and protects the eye against potential trauma.

However, contact lenses represent one of the modern disturbances to an exquisite metabolic system. The way in which contact lenses affect corneal metabolism are well known, and many of them are described in other chapters of this book. One aspect of the consequences of corneal metabolic disturbances is a variation in corneal sensitivity. In all forms of contact lens wear, corneal sensitivity is reduced to some extent, depending on the type of material, the fit of the lenses, and the length of wear.

Nevertheless, this loss of sensation of the cornea and the eyelids accompanying contact lens wear has some initial value inasmuch as contact lens wear, especially the rigid type, becomes more comfortable with time. Of course, the sensation does not disappear entirely, and in a large percentage of cases it remains sufficiently acute to preclude complete adaptation at least as far as comfort is concerned.[39] On the other hand, the loss of corneal sensation is not altogether a bonus, because the cornea is deprived of its unique alarm signal, with the possibility of serious consequences.

MEASUREMENT OF CORNEAL SENSITIVITY

Although corneal sensitivity is sometimes assessed with a piece of cotton wool, it is impossible with this technique to obtain a quantitative evaluation. The first measurements of von Frey in 1894 were made with horse hairs of different lengths attached with wax to the tip of a glass rod. These hairs had different tip configurations, thus evoking touch and pain sensation, and calibration left a lot to be desired. Boberg-Ans[5] devised a clinical instrument with a single nylon filament that produced various forces when applied to the cornea by varying its length and was more appropriate for assessing the touch sensation of the cornea. A commercial form of this instrument was devised by Cochet and Bonnet.[10] It is the most widely used clinical instrument today (Fig 5–1) because of its simplicity, low cost, and relatively good performance. It can produce pressures ranging from 2 to 90 mg/0.005 mm^2 for model I and from 11 to 200 mg/0.0113 mm^2 for model II (the standard model). The area of cornea tested is small, covering at most a dozen epithelial cells.

Over the years other instruments have been built, some of them more advanced and others more accurate than the Cochet-Bonnet aesthesiometer. These instruments are cited in a review of the corneal sensitivity.[43] None of these has gained wide popularity among clinicians. This may be accounted for by the fact that in corneal aesthesi-

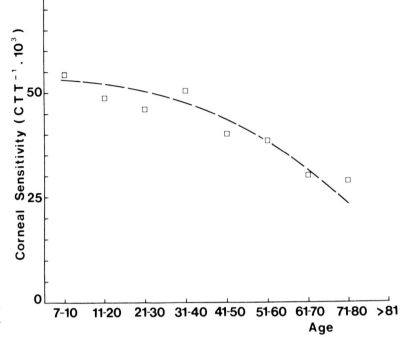

FIG 5–3.
Corneal touch threshold as a function of age.
(From Millodot M: *Invest Ophthalmol* 1977; 16:241.
Used by permission.)

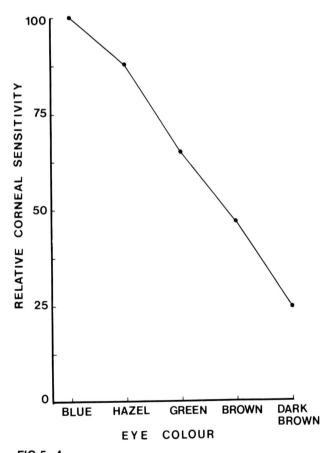

FIG 5–4.
Relative corneal sensitivity as a function of eye color. (From Millodot M: *Nature* 1975; 255:151. Used by permission.)

contraceptive pill is used) and in the last few weeks of pregnancy, sensitivity in women was found to be greatly reduced.[50, 57, 75] Surprisingly, the decrease in corneal sensitivity before menstruation was not observed by Riss et al.,[74] but they found a change at the end of pregnancy.[75]

Ambient temperature also affects corneal sensitivity. Kolstad[32] observed a ninefold reduction as the outside temperature varied between 22° C and −14° C. This may explain the relative comfort of contact lens wearers outside when it is cold.

Also of interest to the contact lens practitioner is that in diabetic[68, 70, 78] eyes and keratoconic eyes,[64] corneal sensitivity is greatly reduced. Thus, contact lens wear is likely to be more comfortable. However, it must also be kept in mind that the fragility of the corneal epithelium is greater in these eyes, and contact lens wear must be monitored and limited to shorter periods of time than in normal eyes.[64, 70]

SHORT-TERM EFFECT OF CONTACT LENS WEAR

Hard Contact Lens

Earlier investigations of the effect of contact lens wear on corneal sensitivity dealt with hard (polymethylmethacrylate [PMMA]) lenses and for short wearing periods (months to 3 years of wear). The first such report appears to be that of Boberg-Ans[5] using his own aesthesiometer. He found a slight reduction in corneal sensitivity after about 2 hours of wear, progressing to a loss of nearly three times that throughout the day. This was followed by numerous other investigations using, in most cases, the Cochet-Bonnet aesthesiometer. Unfortunately, not all of these studies controlled all of the variables or gave all of the information needed.[10, 12, 14, 18, 19, 21, 23, 24, 35, 37, 46, 48, 56, 66, 67, 73, 76, 77, 80]

The unequivocal conclusions from almost all these studies is that corneal sensitivity decreases with hard (PMMA) contact lens wear. One investigator, Millodot,[48] obtained data in subjects who had worn their lenses for at least 3 months asymptomatically. Readings were taken before the lenses were inserted in the morning and then after 4, 8, and 12 hours of continuous uninterrupted wear. These data are shown in Figure 5–5 and labeled hard lenses. This figure shows that the average sensitivity diminishes appreciably after 3 hours of wear and progressively falls by about one half after 12 hours' wear. It is also worth noting that there is a physiological diurnal variation in corneal sensitivity,[41] as shown by the curve labeled physiological variation. Therefore, the average percentage loss is even slightly greater if that is taken into account.

However, corneal sensitivity does not diminish in all subjects. Some subjects exhibit little or no change in sensitivity. This interindividual subject variation is accounted for by biological differences and also by the fit of the lenses and has been noted by many authors[12, 19, 23, 66, 80] The quality of the fit of the lenses was believed to be mainly responsible for the interindividual variations.[5, 10, 14, 18, 66, 76] A well-designed and well-fitted lens will enable optimum tear exchange and consequently minimum interference with corneal metabolism.

Recovery

Several authors have specifically carried out measurements after removal of the lenses.[5, 18, 21, 31, 46, 73, 80] Recovery of sensitivity always occurred. However, the length of time for recovery varies between 20 minutes and 1 week. This variation depends again on biological differences to some extent but to a larger extent on the fit and length of time that the patient has been wearing the lenses. If patients have worn hard lenses for more than 10 years, it takes a great deal longer than 1 week to regain the original threshold level. Figure 5–6 shows the mean data of Millodot[46] on 11 subjects who had worn their lenses for 14 months (median). However, recovery is not complete in ½ hour because CTT should have dropped to a level below the original baseline (before contact lens wear) if one considers the diurnal variation in corneal sensitivity. If we take into account diurnal variations, several hours are required to reach complete recovery.

Soft Lenses

The first study of the effect of soft (hydroxyethylmethacrylate [HEMA]) lenses on corneal sensitivity was carried out by Knoll and Williams,[30] followed by the work of Larke and Sabell.[35] Both investigations concluded that soft lenses gave rise to no statistically significant loss of sensitivity. However, in both instances they were unaware of the existence of a diurnal variation in corneal sensitivity,[41] which should be taken into account. Millodot[44, 48] measured CTT before and after 4, 8, and 12 hours of continuous, uninterrupted wear of HEMA lenses by 15 subjects. A small but significant increase in CTT was observed after 8 hours of wear, becoming more significant after 12 hours. If the diurnal variation is also taken into account, the difference becomes very significant after 8 hours. The data are shown in Figure 5–5, labeled soft lenses. Similar results were found by Draeger et al.,[18] Guillon,[22] and Beuerman and Rozsa.[4] Wide interindividual differences, which may be the result of biological differences and the fit of the lenses, are also noted.

Recovery from loss of corneal sensitivity induced by soft lenses is usually more rapid than with hard lenses but also depends on the nature and duration of wear. Data on

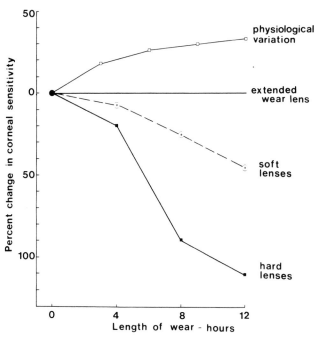

FIG 5–5.
The effect of various types of contact lenses on corneal sensitivity. The physiological variation indicates the diurnal change in CTT in noncontact wearers. (From Millodot M: *Acta Ophthalmol* 1976; 54:721. Used by permission.)

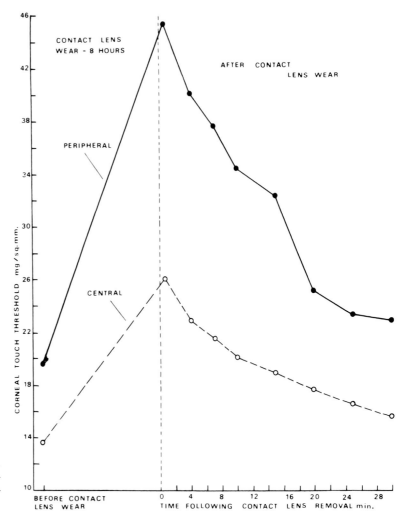

FIG 5–6.
Recovery of CTT after hard contact lens wear. Data were obtained in the center and periphery of the cornea. (From Millodot M: *Acta Ophthalmol* 1975; 53:579. Used by permission.)

recovery have been obtained by Millodot[44] and Draeger et al.[18]

High water content soft lenses produce practically no change in corneal sensitivity over 12 hours, although different lenses and different fits may cause slightly different results.[34, 48, 55] Such data obtained by Millodot[48] are also illustrated in Figure 5–5, labeled extended wear.

LONG-TERM WEAR

Hard Lenses

Several authors have reported on the effect of wear of contact lenses on corneal sensitivity after periods of some months and years of wear. Most of these studies are cross-sectional, but some are longitudinal.

Cochet and Bonnet[10] report some longitudinal measurements made after 4 hours' wear in 22 myopes over 6

months. They found that CTT increased rapidly, being highest after 1 month's wear, and then decreased progressively in the next few months to regain almost normal threshold levels at 6 months. At about the same time, Hamano[24] reported on a cross-sectional investigation involving four groups of contact lens patients who had worn lenses for different periods of time: 1, 2 to 3, 4 to 8, and more than 12 months. The greatest change in CTT compared with the control group was found after 1 month's wear and CTT diminished afterward, although it did not return to normal level. Hamano[24] did not specify after how many hours of wear measurements were taken. Ko and Tomiyama[31] also found that subjects who had worn lenses for more than 3 years exhibited marked decrease in corneal sensitivity (by two or three times) immediately after removing their lenses. Gould and Inglima[23] observed little change after 10 weeks' wear and 1 year, but, again, no reference was made to the number of hours the patient had worn the lenses on the day of measurement. This is important because measurements made in the morning before the lenses are inserted would indeed show no change (because there is usually complete recovery) in the first few years of wear. Sabell[76] mentioned that he found CTT to increase two or three times after adaptation and that in some rare cases of long-term contact lens use, CTT had increased tenfold. Kemmetmueller[29] mentioned that contact lens patients have their corneal sensitivity rapidly and completely restored, although he does not present any data to support his view. Morganroth and Richman[67] measured two groups, one in which lenses had been worn for no more than 3 months and the other for 5 to 9 years. Both of these groups showed CTT higher than a third control group. The group wearing lenses for the longest time had a CTT twice as high as the group wearing lenses for a short time.

In a longitudinal investigation lasting 20 weeks, Larke and Sabell[35] observed a progressive and significant reduction in corneal sensitivity. Millodot[48] measured the same group of nine subjects 2 years in a row and found a small but not significant difference; some subjects exhibited an improvement, whereas others showed a degradation of sensitivity. Draeger et al.[18] measured CTT in several groups of subjects having worn hard lenses for up to 36 months and found a remarkable increase in CTT (more than ten times) up to 2 years, diminishing slightly thereafter. However, with the wear of rigid gas-permeable (RGP) lenses, Lydon[37] obtained a small loss of corneal sensitivity that did not appear to progress over 6 months, whereas PMMA lenses induced a substantial and progressive loss of sensitivity over the same period of time.

What would happen, though, if lenses were worn for more than, say, 5 years? Morganroth and Richman[67] already noted a twofold increase in CTT in a group with 5 to 9 years of wear compared with another group of patients with less than 3 months of wear. Millodot[52] carried out a systematic cross-sectional investigation of patients wearing their PMMA lenses for up to 22 years. His data obtained in the morning before inserting the lenses showed that up to 2 to 3 years of wear, recovery was more or less complete overnight. However, after 5 years of wear, there was a significant increase in CTT, indicating that recovery was not complete even 12 hours after removal. Corneal touch threshold was found to increase progressively with the number of years of lens wear. The mean data are given in Figure 5–7.

Recovery

In view of the dramatic loss of corneal sensitivity accompanying the long-term wear of hard (PMMA) lenses, it was important to discover whether removal of the lenses leads to recovery or whether this loss was irreversible. Some of the subjects who participated in the Millodot[52, 53] studies were persuaded to temporarily cease

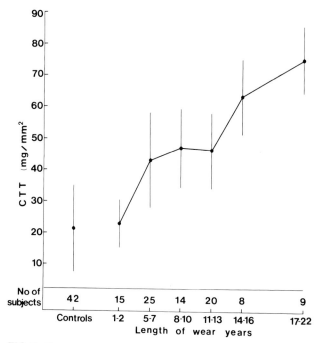

FIG 5–7.
Corneal touch threshold as a function of length of wear of hard contact lenses. Controls indicate non–contact lens wearers. (From Millodot M: *Contacto* 1978; 22:9. Used by permission.)

lens wear. In all, seven people who had worn lenses for 10 to 21 years obliged. It took between 1 and 4 months to regain normal corneal sensitivity (Fig 5–8). It also appeared that the longer the initial wear, the longer it took to recover, all other factors (e.g., fit) being the same. Hence, long-term wear of hard lenses may induce a greater risk because corneal sensation is chronically depressed.

Therefore, lenses with high oxygen transmissibility (GP or soft) should be the choice for long-term daily use to prevent loss of corneal sensitivity. However, empirical evidence of the effect of very long-term use of these lenses still remains to be presented.

Soft Lenses

A glimpse of what may happen, in the long term, to corneal sensitivity with wear of soft lenses (HEMA or high water lenses) may be provided by looking at two longitudinal studies with high water extended wear lenses. Larke and Hirji[34] followed patients who were wearing Sauflon 85 lenses, and Millodot[55] monitored people who were wearing X-Ten lenses for either 1 week at a time or for 3 months before removal. These studies were carried out for periods up to 13 weeks (Fig 5–9). In both instances corneal sensitivity diminished progressively with the number of weeks of wear, reaching about 50% increase in CTT by the end of the 13th week with the X-Ten lens (Dk = 45).

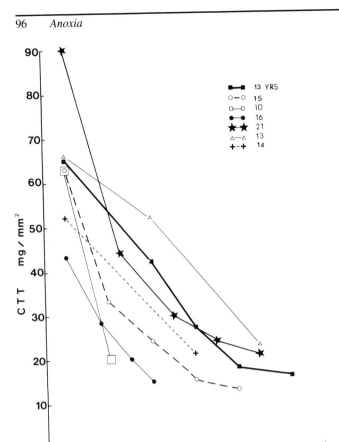

FIG 5–8.
Recovery of corneal sensitivity in seven patients who had worn hard (polymethylmethacrylate [PMMA]) contact lenses for many years. (From Millodot M: *Contacto* 1978; 22:10. Used by permission.)

FIG 5–9.
Change in CTT with two types of high water content soft lenses worn either continuously (Sauflon 85 and X-Ten continuous) or 1 week at a time (X-Ten weekly), or with a solution of saline water morning and night each day (Sauflon solution users). (From Millodot M: *Int Contact Lens Clin* 1984; 11:16. Used by permission.)

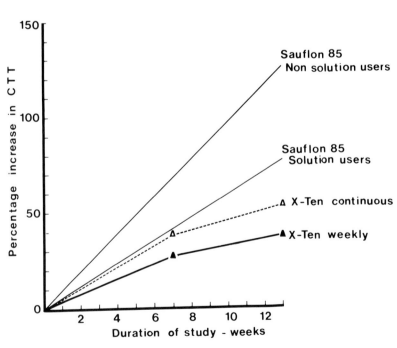

Thus, it may be inferred that even with lenses of high oxygen transmissibility, some loss of corneal sensitivity eventually occurs.

MECHANISM OF CORNEAL SENSITIVITY LOSS

The dramatic decline and recovery of corneal sensitivity accompanying short- and long-term asymptomatic contact lens wear is perplexing. Sufficient evidence exists to show that it is not a direct consequence of edema. Indeed, daily wear of lenses for short and long term can give rise to little or no edema but large losses of corneal sensitivity.[26, 37, 53, 55, 73] This loss could be attributed to sensory adaptation to mechanical stimulation. The most obvious support for this view stems from the fact that contact lenses that produce less mechanical stimulation, for example, hard compared with soft lenses, give rise to smaller decreases in corneal sensitivity. Therefore, at face value the effect of mechanical stimulation could contribute to the reduction in corneal sensitivity when one is wearing contact lenses. However, this suggestion is irreconcilable with the following two observations. First, when the eyes are closed, corneal sensitivity declines dramatically and progressively (Fig 5–10) as a result of the lower oxygen pressure at the corneal surface and not as a result of mechanical stimulation.[61] Second, exposing the cornea to reduced partial pressure of atmospheric oxygen clearly yields a progressive loss of corneal sensitivity starting 2 or 3 hours

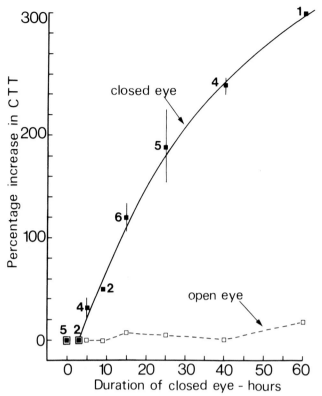

FIG 5–10.
Corneal touch threshold as a function of eyelid closure. The open eye served as a control. (From Millodot M, O'Leary D: *Exp Eye Res* 1979; 29:419. Used by permission.)

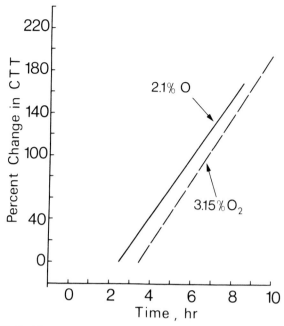

FIG 5–11.
Change in CTT as a function of time with exposure to partial oxygen mixtures of 2.1% and 3.15%. (From Millodot M: *Int Ophthalmol Clin* 1981; 21:52. Used by permission.)

after exposure (Fig 5–11). Yet the cornea is free of any mechanical stimulation.[62]

Fitting identically designed GP and PMMA lenses to different groups of people and fitting one type of lens to one eye and the other lens to the other eye of the same subject led Douthwaite and Connelly[15] to observe that PMMA lenses produce a greater loss of corneal sensitivity than GP lenses. Over 3 months, CTT was not only higher but progressively increased with PMMA lenses, whereas it remained practically the same (or even tended to diminish) with GP lenses. In fact, the data obtained for several types of GP lenses tended to show that the greater the Dk, the smaller the loss of corneal sensitivity.[13] In a similar study, Lydon[37] compared the effect of three types of rigid contact lenses and arrived at the same conclusion that epithelial oxygen availability was directly related to changes in corneal sensitivity.

Bergenske and Polse[3] noted that patients who are refitted with RGP lenses after having worn PMMA lenses often regain lens awareness. They substantiated this clinical observation by finding that corneal sensitivity had returned to almost normal levels (in most subjects of a group of seven) 6 months after refitting.

All the results just described confirm the hypothesis

presented by Millodot and O'Leary[62] that corneal sensitivity is dependent on the epithelial oxygen tension (Po_2) level. For any level below the normal or near-normal corneal oxygen pressure, corneal sensitivity does not remain constant; it decreases slowly and progressively. There is a direct relationship between the time necessary to produce a given loss of corneal sensitivity (e.g., one half the initial value) and epithelial oxygen pressure (Fig 5–12). Therefore, contact lenses with the greatest transmissibility, all other factors being equal, should least affect corneal integrity. For example, daily wear not exceeding 16 hours would require an epithelial Po_2 of at least 55 mm Hg (or epithelial oxygen pressure of about 8%) to avoid a significant loss of corneal sensitivity. Such Po_2 is easily obtained with material having a permeability of at least 10 and a thickness of no more than 0.1 mm (or any other combination of Dk and L that arrives at the same oxygen transmissibility). However, if tear interchange occurs with each blink, the values could be smaller. For extended wear or for many years of daily wear, oxygen transmissibility needs to be higher and the lens fitted somewhat loose to facilitate tear exchange. On the basis of corneal edema, Holden et al.[27] have found that a Po_2 of 74 mm Hg (or 10.1%) was required to maintain normal corneal physiology (see Chapter 1). This value indicates that adopting a loss of corneal sensitivity equal to one half is probably too high. A lower criterion of corneal sensitivity loss (e.g., one fourth the initial value) may be more appropriate and in good accord with these results of Holden et al.[27]

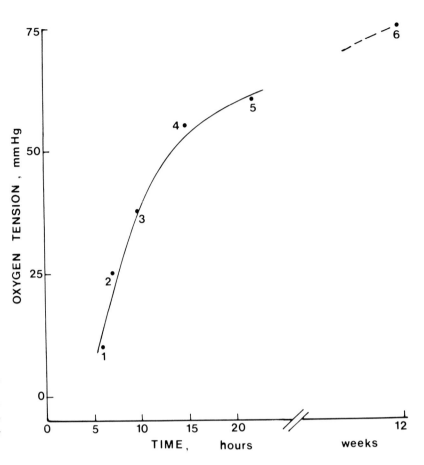

FIG 5–12.
Oxygen tension at the corneal surface and time to produce a reduction of one half in corneal sensitivity with *1*, 2.1 oxygen mixture[62]; *2*, 3.15% oxygen mixture[62]; *3*, hard (PMMA) contact lenses[62]; *4*, eyelid closure[61]; *5*, a point based on some assumptions concerning soft lenses, namely, soft lenses (HEMA 38%) would produce a loss of one half in sensitivity when the data of Millodot[48] is extrapolated. Oxygen transmissibility of such lenses and of that thickness (about 0.18 mm) should lead to an epithelial oxygen tension far lower than the value suggested here, and therefore it is hypothesized that appreciable tear exchange wtih each blink might take place. *6*, extended wear lenses (Sauflon 85).[34] Lenses with greater oxygen transmissibility would take longer to induce a reduction by one half in corneal sensitivity.

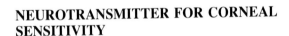

NEUROTRANSMITTER FOR CORNEAL SENSITIVITY

The search for a neurotransmitter to modulate corneal sensitivity is still open, but evidence is steadily accumulating in favor of acetylcholine. The corneal epithelium is known to possess a high concentration of this substance.[7, 20, 25] Hellauer[25] already suggested that the epithelial cholinergic system was involved in corneal sensitivity because he found that, by and large, the higher a species' corneal acetylcholine content, the greater the sensitivity. Other evidence included the fact that the concentration of acetylcholine and corneal sensitivity are greater in the center than in the periphery of the cornea,[65] and acetylcholine concentration is lower in older animals.[25] Nevertheless, the evidence is not unequivocal, and attempts at blocking or enhancing corneal sensitivity with cholinergic drugs have not been one sided. For example, atropine (a drug that prevents the action of acetylcholine) was found to depress corneal sensitivity in some studies[69, 85] but did not affect it in studies by d'Amato[1] and Tanelian et al.[81] Similarly, von Oer[69] found that eserine (which neutralizes acetylcholinesterase, leaving the action of acetylcholine to continue) enhances sensitivity slightly, whereas d'Amato[1] found that eserine decreased it.

In a controlled study, O'Leary et al.[71] demonstrated that atropine significantly depresses corneal sensitivity and that eserine and pilocarpine significantly increase it. Tanelian et al.[81] found that acetylcholine applied to the corneal epithelium increased action potential frequency. These last two investigations provide strong evidence supporting the hypothesis that epithelial acetylcholine is a neurotransmitter to the corneal nerves. Moreover, indirect evidence was provided several years earlier in an experiment in which the eyelids were closed for various periods of time and corneal sensitivity was found to decrease progressively.[61] This was analogous to the observations of Mindel et al.,[65] who noted that lid closure in rabbits led to a suppression of epithelial acetylcholine.

Other substances such as potassium[38] and substance P[82, 84] have been considered as possible neurotransmitters, but so far little or no evidence has substantiated these suggestions.[8, 84] Nevertheless, the ultimate test of acetylcholine as a corneal neurotransmitter will rest on direct evidence obtained by actually measuring this substance in the epithelium under various experimental conditions simultaneously with corneal sensitivity. The mechanism by which stimulation of the corneal epithelium is transduced into a nerve impulse may have to be reconsidered because there does not seem to be any cholinergic receptor in the epithelium of the rabbit.[72] Recently, however, Cavanagh and Colley[9] detected some cholinergic receptors in rabbit corneal epithelium. It remains to be shown whether such receptors exist in the human cornea.

CONCLUSIONS

The utility of testing corneal sensitivity in contact lens practice is becoming apparent. Formerly many authors[2, 10, 18, 24, 33, 67, 77] thought that it would serve as a screening device for predicting contact lens intolerance, hypertensive people being unable to endure the lenses. Unfortunately, it was found that clinical correlation of corneal sensitivity to success appeared poor because patient's motivation is probably more important in adapting to contact lenses. Perhaps more important is the sensitivity of the eyelids, because corneal sensitiveness is not a consideration per se with hydrogel contact lenses.

On the other hand, it is useful to detect cases of hypoesthesia before fitting. These people must be advised to heed the slightest discomfort, because failure to do so could lead to serious corneal complications. Moore and McCollum[66] reported the case of a patient with a corneal ulcer who was unaware of it while wearing hard lenses with total comfort.

After fitting, the benefit of testing corneal sensitivity using the prefit CTT as a baseline is to assess the state of corneal metabolism accompanying the wear of contact lenses. It is a precocious and sensitive indicator of corneal disturbances. For that reason it can help in establishing the optimum fit of a lens[10, 66, 76] and whether the lens is being worn properly or overworn. Some diminution of corneal sensitivity will occur in any case with contact lens wear, but the lower the epithelial oxygen pressure, the greater the sensitivity loss. However, it is important to ensure that the amount of hypoesthesia does not exceed a given amount (e.g., one half or less its initial value). Otherwise, as corneal sensitivity continues to decline, the cornea loses a unique alarm signal warning it of serious problems.

The value of corneal sensitivity testing is lessened only by the care that must be taken in measuring CTT. If appropriate precautions are taken, the information derived can be invaluable to contact lens practitioner in evaluating the fit of the lens and the physiological effect of the lens material. Such a suggestion has been made by several authors.[3, 10, 15, 37, 54] In fact, Douthwaite and Connelly[15] and Lydon[37] believed that aesthesiometry was the most sensitive test compared with refraction, keratometry, and pachometry for monitoring the status of the cornea fitted with various types of rigid contact lenses.

REFERENCES

1. d'Amato A: Richerche di estesiometria corneale in condizioni normali, patalogische e dopo instillazione e iniezione sottoconjiuntivale di colliri. *Gior Ital Oftal* 1956; 9:223–234.
2. Berens C, Girard L, Foree K: Corneal contact lenses. *Trans Am Ophthalmol Soc* 1952; 50:55–75.
3. Bergenske PD, Polse KA: The effect of rigid gas permeable lenses on corneal sensitivity. *J Am Optom Assoc* 1987; 58:212–215.
4. Beuerman RW, Rozsa AJ: Threshold and signal detection measurements of the effect of soft contact lenses on corneal sensitivity. *Curr Eye Res* 1985; 4:742–744.
5. Boberg-Ans J: Experience in clinical examination of corneal sensitivity. *Br J Ophthalmol* 1955; 39:709–726.
6. Bonnet R, Millodot M: Corneal aesthesiometry: Its measurement in the dark. *Am J Optom* 1966; 43:238–243.
7. Brucke von H, Hellauer HF, Umrath K: Azetylcholin und aneuringehat der hornhaut und seine beziehungen zur nerven versorgung. *Ophthalmalogica* 1949; 117:19–35.
8. Bynke G, Hakanson R, Sundler F: Is substance P necessary for corneal nociception? *Eur J Pharmacol* 1984; 101:253–258.
9. Cavanagh HD, Colley AM: Beta-adrenergic and muscarinic binding in corneal epithelium. *Invest Ophthalmol* 1981; 37(ARVO suppl).
10. Cochet P, Bonnet R: L'esthésie cornéenne. *Clin Ophthalmol* 1960; 4:3–27.
11. Collins M, Seeto R, Campbell L, et al: Blinking and corneal sensitivity. *Acta Ophthalmol* 1989; 67:525–531.
12. Dixon JM: Ocular changes due to contact lenses. *Am J Ophthalmol* 1964; 58:424–442.
13. Douthwaite WA: Personal communication, 1986.
14. Douthwaite WA, Atkinson HL: The effect of hard (PMMA) contact lens wear on the corneal curvature and sensitivity. *J Br Contact Lens Assoc* 1985; 8:21–25.
15. Douthwaite WA, Connelly AT: The effect of hard and gas permeable contact lenses on refractive error, corneal curvature, thickness and sensitivity. *J Br Contact Lens Assoc* 1986; 9:14–20.
16. Douthwaite WA, Kaye NA: Is corneal sensitivity related to corneal thickness? *Ophthalmic Opt* 1980; 20:753–758.
17. Draeger J: Klinische Ergebnisse der Aesthesiometrie der Hornhaut. *Ber Dtsch Ophthalmol Ges* 1979; 76:389–395.
18. Draeger J, Heid W, Luders M: L'esthésiometrie chez les porteurs de lentilles de contact. *Contactologia* 1980; 2:83–93.
19. Edmund J: The cosmetic indication for using contact lenses. *Acta Ophthalmol* 1967; 45:760–768.
20. Fitzgerald GG, Cooper JR: Acetylcholine as possible sen-

sory mediator in rabbit corneal epithelium. *Biochem Pharmacol* 1971; 20:2741–2748.

21. Gligo D, Vojnikovic B, Volkoric A, et al: The effect of hard contact lenses on corneal sensitivity, ocular pressure and coefficient of outflow, in PDT Roper (ed): *The Cornea in Health and Disease.* New York, Academic Press, 1981.

22. Guillon M: Long term effects of soft contact lenses. A preliminary report. *J Br Contact Lens Assoc* 1981; 4:50–58.

23. Gould HL, Inglima R: Corneal contact lens solutions. *Eye Ear Nose Throat Monthly* 1964; 43:39–49.

24. Hamano H: Topical and systemic influences of wearing contact lenses. *Contacto* 1960; 4:41–48.

25. Hellauer HF: Sensibilitat und acetylcholingehalt der hornhaut verschieder tiere und des menschen. *Z Verg Physiol* 1950; 32:303–310.

26. Hirji N: Some aspects of the design and ocular response to synthetic hydrogel contact lenses intended for continuous usage. *Doctoral dissertation*, Birmingham, England, University of Aston, 1978.

27. Holden BA, Sweeney DF, Sanderson G: The minimum precorneal oxygen tension to avoid corneal edema. *Invest Ophthalmol* 1984; 25:476–480.

28. Jalavisto E, Orma E, Tawast M: Aging and relation between stimulus intensity and duration in corneal sensitivity. *Acta Physiol Scand* 1951; 23:224–233.

29. Kemmetmueller H: Corneal sensitivity and contact lens fitting. *J Jpn Contact Lens Soc* 1969; 20:7–12.

30. Knoll HA, Williams J: Effects of hydrophilic contact lenses on corneal sensitivity. *Am J Optom* 1970; 47:561–563.

31. Ko LS, Tomiyama SK: The influence of contact lens application on the corneal sensitivity. *Trans Ophthalmol Soc Republic China* 1963; 2:1–9.

32. Kolstad A: Corneal sensitivity by low temperatures. *Acta Ophthalmol* 1970; 48:789–793.

33. Kraar RS, Cummings CM: Lacrimation, corneal sensitivity and corneal abrasive resistance in contact lens wearability. *Optom Weekly* 1965; 56:25–32.

34. Larke JR, Hirji NK: Some clinically observed phenomena in extended contact lens wear. *Br J Ophthalmol* 1979; 63:475–477.

35. Larke JR, Sabell AG: A comparative study of the ocular response to two forms of contact lens. *Optician* 1971; 162(4187):8–12.

36. Lowther GE, Hill RM: Sensibility threshold of the lower lid margin in the course and adaptation to contact lenses. *Am J Optom* 1968; 45:587–594.

37. Lydon DPM: Effects of rigid contact lens materials on the cornea and tear film of the human eye. Submitted doctoral dissertation, Sydney, Australia, University of New South Wales, 1986.

38. Maurice DM: The cornea and sclera, in Davson H (ed): *The Eye.* New York, Academic Press, 1984, vol 1B.

39. Millodot M: One year after: Analysis of a group of contact lens wearers. *Optician* 1967; 154(3982):79–82.

40. Millodot M: Studies on the sensitivity of the cornea. *Optician* 1969; 157(4067):267–271.

41. Millodot M: Diurnal variation of corneal sensitivity. *Br J Ophthalmol* 1972; 56:844–847.

42. Millodot M: Objective measurement of corneal sensitivity. *Acta Ophthalmol (Copenh)* 1973; 51:325–334.

43. Millodot M: A review of research on the sensitivity of the cornea. *Ophthal Physiol Opt* 1984; 4:305–318.

44. Millodot M: Effect of soft lenses on corneal sensitivity. *Acta Ophthalmol (Copenh)* 1974; 52:603–608.

45. Millodot M: Do blue eyed people have more sensitive corneas than brown eyed people? *Nature* 1975; 255:151–152.

46. Millodot M: Effect of hard contact lenses on corneal sensitivity and thickness. *Acta Ophthalmol* 1975; 53:576–584.

47. Millodot M: Corneal sensitivity in people with the same and with different iris colour. *Invest Ophthalmol* 1976; 15:861–862.

48. Millodot M: Effect of the length of wear of contact lenses on corneal sensitivity. *Acta Ophthalmol* 1976; 54:721–730.

49. Millodot M: Influence of age on the sensitivity of the cornea. *Invest Ophthalmol* 1977; 16:240–242.

50. Millodot M: The influence of pregnancy on the sensitivity of the cornea. *Br J Ophthalmol* 1977; 61:646–649.

51. Millodot M: Corneal sensitivity in albinos. *J Pediatr Ophthalmol* 1978; 15:300–302.

52. Millodot M: Effect of long term wear of hard contact lenses on corneal sensitivity. *Arch Ophthalmol* 1978; 96:1225–1227.

53. Millodot M: Long term wear of hard contact lenses and corneal integrity. *Contacto* 1978; 22:7–12.

54. Millodot M: Corneal sensitivity. *Int Ophthalmol Clin* 1981; 21(2):47–54.

55. Millodot M: Clinical evaluation of an extended wear lens. *Int Contact Lens Clin* 1984; 11:16–23.

56. Millodot M, Henson D, O'Leary DJ: Measurement of corneal sensitivity and thickness with PMMA and gas permeable contact lenses. *Am J Optom* 1979; 56:628–632.

57. Millodot M, Lamont A: Influence of menstruation on corneal sensitivity. *Br J Ophthalmol* 1974; 58:49–51.

58. Millodot M, Larson W: Effect of bending of the nylon thread of the Cochet-Bonnet aesthesiometer upon recorded pressure. *Contact Lens* 1967; 1(3):5–28.

59. Millodot M, Larson W: New measurements of corneal sensitivity: A preliminary report. *Am J Optom* 1969; 46:261–265.

60. Millodot M, Lim CH, Ruskell GL: A comparison of corneal sensitivity and nerve density in albino and pigmented rabbits. *Ophthalmic Res* 1978; 10:7–12.

61. Millodot M, O'Leary DJ: Loss of corneal sensitivity with lid closure in humans. *Exp Eye Res* 1979; 29:417–421.

62. Millodot M, O'Leary DJ: Effect of oxygen deprivation on corneal sensitivity. *Acta Ophthalmol (Copenh)* 1980; 58:434–439.

63. Millodot M, O'Leary DJ: Corneal fragility and its relationship to sensitivity. *Acta Ophthalmol (Copenh)* 1981; 59:820–826.

64. Millodot M, Owens H: Sensitivity and fragility in keratoconus. *Acta Ophthalmol (Copenh)* 1983; 61:908–917.

65. Mindel JS, Szilagyi PIA, Zadunaisky JA, et al: The effects of blepharorrhaphy induced depression of corneal cholinergic activity. *Exp Eye Res* 1979; 29:463–468.

66. Moore CD, McCollum TH: Corneal sensitivity and contact

lenses, in Girard LJ (ed): *Corneal and Scleral Contact Lenses.* St Louis, CV Mosby Co, 1967, pp 408–412.

67. Morganroth J, Richman L: Changes in the corneal reflex in patients wearing contact lenses. *J Pediatr Ophthalmol* 1969; 6:207–208.

68. Neilsen HV: Corneal sensitivity and vibratory perception in diabetes mellitus. *Acta Ophthalmol* 1978; 56:406–412.

69. Oer von S: Uber die beziehung des acetycholins des hornhautepithels zur erregungsubertragung von diesem auf die sensiblen nervenden. *Pflugers Arch Gesamte Physiol* 1961; 273:325–334.

70. O'Leary DJ, Millodot M: Abnormal epithelial fragility in diabetes and contact lens wear. *Acta Ophthalmol* 1981; 59:827–833.

71. O'Leary DJ, Nazarian J, Millodot M: Which neurotransmitters modulate corneal sensitivity? *Clin Exp Optom* 1986; 69:108–111.

72. Olsen JS, Neufeld AH: The rabbit cornea lacks cholinergic receptors. *Invest Ophthalmol* 1979; 18:1216–1225.

73. Polse KA: Etiology of corneal sensitivity accompanying contact lens wear. *Invest Ophthalmol* 1978; 17:1202–1206.

74. Riss B, Binder S, Riss P, et al: Corneal sensitivity during the menstrual cycle. *Br J Ophthalmol* 1982; 66:123–126.

75. Riss B, Riss P: Corneal sensitivity in pregnancy. *Ophthalmologica* 1981; 183:57–62.

76. Sabell AG: Ocular changes in contact lens wearers. *Ophthalmic Opt* 1968; 8:1051–1057.

77. Schirmer KE: Corneal sensitivity and contact lenses. *Br J Ophthalmol* 1963; 47:493–495.

78. Schwartz DE: Corneal sensitivity in diabetics. *Arch Ophthalmol* 1974; 91:174–178.

79. Strughold H: The sensitivity of cornea and conjunctiva of the human eye and the use of contact lenses. *Am J Optom* 1953; 30:625–630.

80. Tanelian DL, Beuerman RW: Recovery of corneal sensation following hard contact lens wear and the implication for adaptation. *Invest Ophthalmol* 1980; 19:1391–1394.

81. Tanelian DL, Beuerman RW, Young M: Stimulation of rabbit corneal nerves by acetylcholine and nicotine [abstract]. *Soc Neurosci* 1982; 8:858.

82. Tervo T, Tervo K, Eranko L, et al: Substance P immunoreaction and Acetylcholinesterase activity in the cornea and gasserian ganglion. *Ophthalmic Res* 1983; 15:280–288.

83. Tota G, Le Marca F: Correlazioni tra sensibilita corneale e colore dell iride. *Atti Fond Contri Ist Ottica* 1982; 37:59–69.

84. Tullo AB, Keen P, Blyth WA, et al: Corneal sensitivity and substance P in experimental herpes simplex keratitis in mice. *Invest Ophthalmol* 1983; 24:596–598.

85. Umrath K, Mussbichler H: Die blockierung der erregringsubertragung von sekundaren sinneszellen auf die herabsetzung der hornhautemfindlichkeit durch atropin. *Z Vitamin-Hormaon Fermentforsch* 1951; 4:182–190.

PART II

Abrasion

Keratitis

Cristina M. Schnider, O.D.

The term keratitis is a nonspecific one that refers to a wide range of disturbances of the cornea affecting one or more of its layers. Using the classification set forth by Waring and Rodrigues,[63] we can artificially divide the cornea into four zones when discussing pathological processes: (1) the epithelium; (2) the subepithelial zone, which consists of the epithelial basement membrane, Bowman's layer, and anterior stroma; (3) the stroma; and (4) the endothelium and Descemet's membrane. These authors also describe six types of pathological responses, which include defects (partial or complete loss of corneal tissue), fibrosis and vascularization, edema and cysts, deposits, inflammatory and immune responses, and proliferation. Although the term keratitis can be used in association with any of these responses, this chapter focuses specifically on superficial nonulcerative keratitis induced by contact lens wear.

The cornea serves as the primary refracting surface of the eye and acts as a barrier to penetration of offending agents as well. Its integrity is therefore critical to the health of the eye and is also essential for the maintenance of optical imagery so vital to human function. The addition of a contact lens offers many opportunities for disruption of the corneal surface through mechanical, chemical, and physiological means. By far, epithelial defects represent the most common contact lens–induced complication of the cornea. In the contact lens–wearing eye, the epithelium is continually exposed to the mechanical forces involved in lens movement, chemicals and preservatives in the care system products, environmental desiccation, oxygen deprivation, and immunological stimuli from lens deposits. The chief manifestation of most of these types of trauma is superficial punctate keratitis (SPK), a term coined more than 100 years ago by Fuchs[17] to describe small dotlike epithelial changes he saw in association with epidemic conjunctivitis. Today the term is commonly used to describe the appearance seen when sodium fluorescein dye is instilled in the eye and fills in gaps in the epithelial surface created when epithelial cells are damaged or missing. In some cases, these superficial changes are also accompanied by edema, inflammation in the subepithelial layer, and, more rarely, fibrosis and vascularization, which can affect several layers.

Because the cornea is a highly organized avascular tissue, it has a limited set of responses to a wide variety of stimuli. Therefore, most contact lens–related complications with SPK as a clinical feature closely mimic conditions seen in the non–contact lens wearing eye as well. This chapter provides descriptions of the clinical appearance and physiological bases for the changes induced and the course and management of various disorders related to contact lens wear that manifest themselves in some form of epithelial punctate keratitis.

Diffuse superficial punctate epithelial changes, sometimes also accompanied by involvement of the subepithelial region, are common in response to contact lens wear, primarily as a result of complications involving contact lens solutions. The lens polymers themselves are nontoxic and biologically inert, but they require additional aqueous solutions for cleaning, disinfection, and storage. Although the vehicle for most solutions is physiological saline, the antimicrobial preservatives, buffers, chelators, emulsifiers, and viscosity agents also present may induce toxic or allergic reactions. Toxic and hypersensitivity reactions to contact lens solutions are discussed in the context of the ocular inflammatory response in Chapter 10.

TOXIC REACTIONS

Irritation and tissue damage caused by toxicity occur because of a chemical's inherent biological characteristics.[38] These effects are dose related, so concentration and exposure time influence the magnitude of the effect. Antimicrobial agents used in contact lens solutions act by one of several mechanisms to render the microbe essentially nonviable, including cell wall disruption or cell membrane lysis and inhibition of protein synthesis. They can exert the same effects on appropriate human cells, however, and a balance must be reached between the safety and efficacy of the various agents. In fact, the *U.S. Pharmacopeical Convention*[59] for preservatives states, "Any antimicrobial agent may exhibit the protective properties of a preservative. However, all useful antimicrobial agents are toxic substances. For maximum protection of the consumer, the concentration of the preservative shown to be effective in the final packaged product should be considerably below the concentration of the preservative that may be toxic to human beings." In vitro studies have shown that many preservatives used in contact lens solutions can damage epithelial tissues when used in sufficiently high concentrations, and some will even cause changes when used in the concentrations commonly found in available care products. However, differences in behavior exist when the same solutions are studied in the human eye.

Thimerosal, a mercurial compound long used as a preservative in the pharmaceutical industry because of its relatively good antimicrobial activity and low toxicity, was shown in early scanning electron microscopy (SEM) studies to cause loosening of the corneal epithelium in isolated rabbit corneas using concentrations as low as 4 ppm, but such effects were not demonstrable with the in vivo rabbit model.[44] Later studies using rabbit corneal epithelium cultures also demonstrated significant toxic effects with concentrations lower than those used in commercially available products.[50] However, evidence throughout the years linking thimerosal with mainly hypersensitivity reactions (rather than toxic) suggests that the buffering and dilution provided by the tear film can be effective in limiting the effects of some potentially toxic substances on the cornea.

Chlorbutanol, another preservative used in the early development of contact lens care products, also produced in vitro epithelial toxicity not found in the in vivo model. However, unlike thimerosal, this chemical has the ability to accumulate in soft lens materials and hence may reach a concentration sufficient to cause toxicity with time in some cases.[6] Chlorhexidine gluconate (CHG), benzalkonium chloride (BAK), and alkyltriethanol ammonium chloride (ATAC) are cationic molecules used as preservatives and are also capable of binding to many lens materials, particularly in the presence of protein deposits.[30, 49] They therefore can accumulate to toxic levels over time and have been implicated in adverse reactions involving the corneal epithelium.[40, 42] Gasset[19] has demonstrated cytotoxicity of BAK, a common preservative in rigid lens solutions, even at routinely used concentrations. It is a quaternary cationic surfactant that has been shown to contribute to epithelial disruption and tear film destabilization in laboratory studies[25] but has been shown to be safe and effective in clinical studies by other authors.[4] Conflicting reports have also been published concerning the ability of BAK to bind to rigid gas-permeable (RGP) lens materials,[46, 65] further fueling the controversy surrounding this antimicrobial agent.

Most commonly, chemicals with toxic potential are intended to be rinsed off after the appropriate cleaning or disinfection procedure and thus should have little or no opportunity to contact the ocular surface. Such is the case with hydrogen peroxide, which has been demonstrated to be toxic to corneal tissue when present in sufficiently high concentrations and can cause ocular discomfort unless neutralized or diluted to a concentration less than 100 ppm.[27, 41] In cases of improper neutralization, significant amounts of peroxide are delivered to the epithelial surface and can result in significant corneal insult (Fig 6–1). In addition, particularly with hydrophilic lenses, residues can be physically or chemically adherent to a lens when it is placed on the eye, and the addition of soilants and mechanical defects in the lens, which occur with age, can exacerbate such problems.

A number of the newer available contact lens solution preservatives are purported to have lower levels of toxicity than the more traditional agents. These include polyaminopropylbiguanide (PAPB, Dymed), polyquaternium-1 (Polyquad), benzyl alcohol,[15] and chlorine.[51] Polyquad and PAPB have very large molecular weights and therefore are said to resist lens uptake and binding, even with ionically charged and high water content polymers. They have been shown to be effective microbiologically even at low concentrations, and toxicity studies have shown them to be less toxic than their predecessors in both in vitro[22] and in vivo studies.[11, 33] One author,[2] however, has reported toxic effects on rabbit epithelia with the Boston Advance (formerly Avant) conditioning solution. This is an RGP wetting and soaking solution preserved with PAPB, but it also contains additional viscosity and wetting agents not present in the formulation for hydrogel lenses. The solution was shown on SEM studies to cause cell sloughing, alterations in microvilli, and an increase in intracellular vacuoles. In addition, there have been unpublished reports of superficial punctate staining and associated symptoms in users of this particular conditioning solution. The manufacturer (Polymer Technology Corporation, Wilmington, MA) attributes these effects to inconsistencies in large

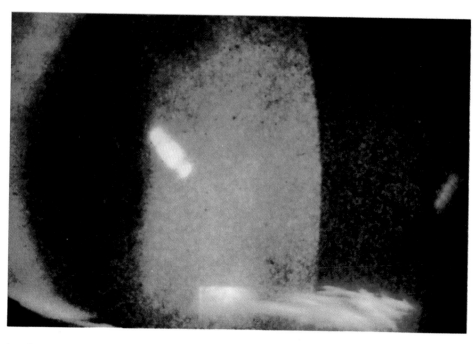

FIG 6–1.
Epithelial disruption after accidental instillation of 3% hydrogen peroxide into the eye with a contact lens that was not neutralized after disinfection.

batch processing and is proceeding with steps to rectify the problem, which they claim is unrelated to the PAPB preservative.

The principal corneal sign of solution toxicity is a diffuse superficial punctate keratitis, often accompanied by ocular injection and symptoms of ocular stinging or burning at the time of lens insertion. It can be mild to severe, depending on the concentration and duration of exposure, and usually occurs within the first hours or days of lens wear. Toxic reactions can occur more readily in compromised eyes when the normal defenses are diminished or inactivated. Figures 6–2 through 6–4 are such examples in which a severe toxic reaction to a BAK-preserved solution occurred after use of a topical anesthetic for applanation tonometry. It is hypothesized that the anesthetic softened the epithelium, allowing a higher than normal concentration of the preservative to remain in contact with the cornea, thus causing the severe epithelial disruption noted. Fonn et al.[16] and Soni et al.[52] have each reported mild to severe toxic reactions to chlorhexidine resulting from the use of a new tablet disinfection system for soft contact lenses (OptimEyes, Igel, U.K.). Chlorhexidine is a biguanide, like PAPB, but its smaller size and charge allow it to bind to hydrogels, thus facilitating the conditions for a toxic reaction. Other reports of chemically induced keratitis can be found in the literature, and they implicate primarily BAK and peroxide as the offending agents. Sterling and Hecht[55] reported on two cases of apparent BAK toxicity that resulted only after use of a BAK-preserved RGP lens solution. Both patients exhibited acuity reductions and bilateral SPK, with accompanying symptoms of redness and irritation after lens insertion. Each resolved within 48 hours of discontinuing use of the BAK solution, but signs and symptoms returned when one patient re-

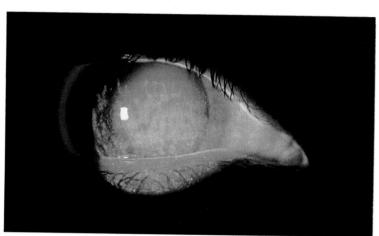

FIG 6–2.
Severe epithelial disruption of the right eye of a 41-year-old woman resulting from use of a BAK-preserved solution after Goldmann tonometry and use of a topical anesthetic.

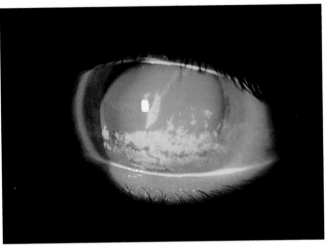

FIG 6–3.
Corneal disruption on the left eye of the patient in Figure 6–2. Note the obvious change in appearance that corresponds to the location of the lid after a partial blink.

sumed use of the BAK preservative. More severe reactions have been noted after unintentional instillation of hydrogen peroxide into the eye or after inadequate neutralization.[14] Peroxide is an oxidative agent, but its mechanism of action as an antimicrobial and cytotoxic agent may be linked to the generation of hydroxyl free radicals.[14] These molecules can aggressively attack organic substances and cause cellular disruption by rupturing cell membranes of both pathogen and mammalian cells.[26] The tear film and cornea do possess some protective mechanisms that can dilute and neutralize small amounts of residual peroxide harmlessly, but the presence of larger amounts could lead to epithelial damage. Another interesting toxic phenomenon has been observed with the use of peroxide disinfection of tonometer tips.[45] A severe central punctate keratitis was observed after applanation tonometry in a 50-year-old man who had undergone penetrating keratoplasty 6 years previously. The lesion appeared as a circular epithelial opacity corresponding in size to the tonometer tip, with adjacent small stromal bubbles. The bubbles disappeared after 6 hours, and the epithelial defect cleared 2 days later. The authors suggested that the peroxide, which had been allowed to evaporate overnight on the probe, was the cause of the severe disruption. In animal studies, they found that fresh 3% hydrogen peroxide applied to corneas using the tonometer tips would not cause epithelial staining, but defects similar to that observed in their patient could be produced when the peroxide was allowed to evaporate on the tonometer tips. The mechanism of the effect remains unclear; however, it does appear that significant chemical changes occur during evaporation of peroxide. This could have implications for contact lens storage as well, particularly with rigid lenses stored in small quantities of peroxide.

Mild cases of solution toxicity can be expected to recover quickly on removal of the offending agent and even with continued lens wear in some cases, but more severe

FIG 6–4.
Retroillumination photograph of the left eye of the patient in Figures 6–2 and 6–3, showing the marked irregularities of the cornea after the preservative reaction.

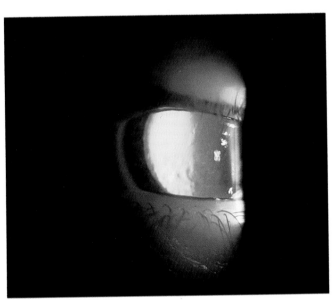

cases require cessation of lens wear and sometimes replacement of the lens. In cases of documented or suspected deviation from the prescribed care regimen, such as inadequate rinsing or neutralization of the disinfectant, simple reinstruction should be adequate to prevent recurrence of the keratitis. However, many cases of toxicity involving solutions require selection of an alternate system for disinfection and storage. To definitively diagnose a solution toxicity, simply discontinue its use or replace the suspected agent with a nonpreserved solution for several days. If the keratitis clears, alternate solutions can be substituted until an acceptable one is identified. Most peroxide regimens available in the United States now consist of essentially preservative-free products (assuming the peroxide is adequately neutralized) and offer viable alternatives to chemically preserved solutions that cause toxic reactions in some patients. However, several different neutralization systems are used to neutralize the peroxide to varying degrees and over different time spans, so toxic reactions secondary to peroxide exposure may still occur in some individuals with some systems.

As mentioned previously, various degrees of SPK have been reported in association with contact lens solutions. Although many of these occurrences are labeled as toxic reactions, the presence of itching should alert the practitioner to the possibility of an allergic response.

ALLERGIC AND HYPERSENSITIVITY REACTIONS

Allergic or hypersensitivity reactions represent a more common response to contact lens solutions and contaminants and are manifested in many forms. Hypersensitivity or allergic reactions that are immediate (anaphylactic) are mediated by IgE, as in the case of hayfever or drug allergies. These reactions manifest themselves as itching, vasodilation, conjunctival edema, tearing, and photophobia but rarely involve the cornea.[33] Delayed hypersensitivity is a cell-mediated, T cell–dependent reaction that occurs after prolonged contact with a chemical. It is believed that the chemicals act as haptens, which require combination with a tissue protein to initiate an allergic response.[7] Thimerosal, a compound of organic mercury and thiosalycilic acid, is the chemical most commonly implicated in delayed hypersensitivity reactions, with other reports involving chlorhexidine as well. Thimerosal has been shown to cause contact dermatitis,[38] which is a confirmed form of a delayed hypersensitivity reaction. Hallmarks of allergic ocular reactions are burning, itching, photophobia, and conjunctival hyperemia, often accompanied by corneal staining, infiltrates, and even vascularization and dendri-

form lesions. Such reactions are caused by the release of inflammatory factors such as histamine, serotonin, or eosinophils. The delayed hypersensitivity reactions represent a diagnostic and therapeutic challenge to the contact lens clinician, because they can masquerade as a variety of conditions resembling both contact lens–related and non–contact lens related complications. We will begin by discussing the superficial responses, such as SPK, and progress through more severe reactions, such as pseudodendrites and nummular keratitis, and, finally, consider conditions affecting the limbal area.

SUPERFICIAL PUNCTATE KERATITIS

Thygeson's Superficial Punctate Keratitis

Superficial punctate keratitis is not a diagnosis in itself, except when one is referring to the specific entity of Thygeson's SPK.[43] This disease is a chronic, noncontagious disorder of the epithelium associated with characteristic punctate epithelial changes. It was first described by Thygeson[57] in 1950, with findings of bilateral, asymmetrical lesions confined to the corneal epithelium. The lesions were described as round or oval, discrete gray-white intraepithelial dots about 0.2 mm in diameter, with a predilection for the central cornea. The lesions wax and wane over the course of the disease. During the active stage, they are dense and slightly elevated, with a central area that stains with fluorescein, and can then resolve fully or partially during stages of remission. The lesions can last hours to weeks and may recur over 3 to 16 years before resolving completely. Both sexes are affected, and symptoms can include burning, lacrimation, and blurred vision. Its etiology has not been established, although evidence exists to indicate a viral etiology.[34] Corticosteroid treatment has been suggested for suppressive therapy, but the lesions frequently return after cessation of medication. Soft lenses have also been shown to provide symptomatic relief, with resolution of lesions within days of application, but recurrence is possible after lens removal.[20]

Several other non–contact lens related conditions can produce a keratitis similar in appearance to Thygeson's, including staphylococcal, viral, and chlamydial infections, such as adenovirus, molluscum contagiosum, inclusion conjunctivitis, and trachoma. In addition, keratitis sicca and exposure can produce obvious punctate lesions of the epithelium.

Lens Dehydration

A common contact lens–related complication causing punctate lesions of the central cornea occurs with dehydra-

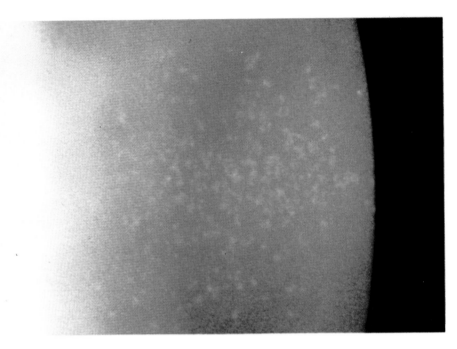

FIG 6–5.
Punctate epithelial lesions associated with dehydration of a thin, high water content hydrogel lens worn 4 hours.

tion of hydrogel lenses (Fig 6–5). Tiny grayish white epithelial erosions can usually be observed centrally with white light and will stain when fluorescein is instilled as well. This staining is more commonly seen with thin, high water content (>50%) hydrogel lenses[24, 36] and is thought to be caused by the movement of water from the cornea into the lens replacing water lost to dehydration. The phenomenon is directly related to lens thickness and water content and, though less common, can also be observed with thin low water content hydrogel lenses, particularly in arid environments or in patients with poor blink habits.

The lesions will disappear within hours of lens removal and will not recur without lens wear. However, the staining will recur in the same central location if lenses of the same type are worn again. Symptoms, if present at all, are usually mild, and the use of ocular lubricants is of little value because of the need for chronic use to maintain hydration. A change to a thicker lens in the same material will often suffice, but occasionally a change to a thicker, lower water content material may be necessary to eradicate the staining. A more complete discussion of corneal drying with contact lens wear can be found in Chapter 9.

FIG 6–6.
Lesions caused by the eruption of microcysts through the anterior epithelial layers.

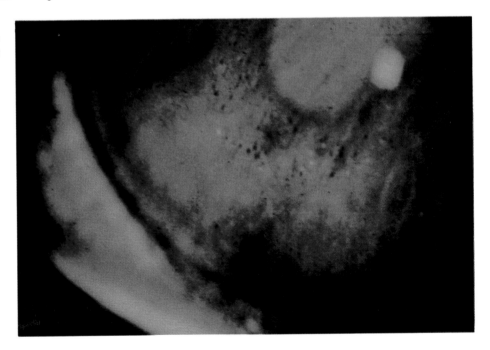

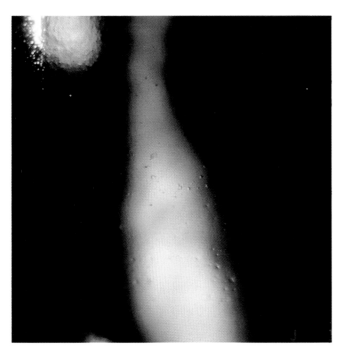

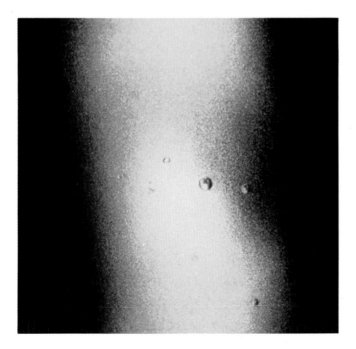

Hypoxia

Central punctate lesions of the cornea in the presence of contact lens wear can also occur secondary to hypoxia, particularly in the case of microcystic corneal edema. In this case the superficial lesions are often deeper than those observed with dehydration and may even appear as tiny pits in which fluorescein pools (Fig 6–6). These lesions are generally surrounded by tiny refractile bodies that display reversed illumination when viewed in marginal ret-

FIG 6–7.
Epithelial microcysts showing reversed illumination.

roillumination, indicating that their refractive index is higher than that of surrounding tissues (Fig 6–7). These bodies are epithelial microcysts, which are thought to be pockets of dead cellular matter that form adjacent to intraepithelial sheets at the basement membrane.[66] They then migrate to the surface of the epithelium and create epithelial punctate lesions when they erupt through the surface. They are often observed with epithelial vacuoles, small bubbles that display nonreversed illumination (Fig 6–8). Epithelial microcysts are commonly observed with ex-

FIG 6–8.
Epithelial vacuoles: bubblelike objects showing nonreversed illumination.

tended wear soft lenses[13, 23] and are indicative of a recent or ongoing period of chronic hypoxia. The significance of vacuoles is not known.

Microcysts are also associated with Cogan's microcystic or epithelial basement membrane dystrophy, however, and may be early signs of the site of a recurrent erosion. Therefore, if they are noted in a contact lens patient not known to be wearing lenses on an extended wear basis, careful scrutiny of the cornea should take place, along with a thorough history, to rule out the presence of the dystrophy. Contact lens wear of any kind is discouraged in the presence of an epithelial dystrophy, given the increased chances of recurrent erosion, which can be further exacerbated by mechanical irritation, desiccation, and hypoxia during contact lens wear. When microcysts are caused solely by hypoxia, an increase in oxygen transmission is required, which can be accomplished by changing lens materials, lens thickness, or wearing schedule. Microcysts will resolve over a period of months after cessation of lens wear, although they may actually increase in numbers during the first few weeks after lens removal. A more detailed discussion of complications relating to hypoxia can be found in Chapter 2.

DENDRIFORM LESIONS

Pseudodendrite

Before the introduction of preservative-free peroxide regimens and second- and third-generation preservatives, more

severe adverse reactions were occasionally observed. Rather than the diffuse punctate staining observed in mild to moderate cases, the lesion exhibited a dendritic appearance (Fig 6–9) similar to the corneal epithelial ulcer seen in ocular herpes simplex keratitis. This lesion was termed a pseudodendrite and appeared as a slightly raised, gray, irregular epithelial plaque[35], with no end bulbs, which stained variably with fluorescein and rose bengal. Udell et al.[58] reported on nine patients with this condition and found that all nine patients had been exposed to thimerosal and that most had also been exposed to CHG. The patients also displayed a mild papillary-follicular conjunctivitis, and all were wearing daily wear soft contact lenses. It is unclear whether this is a primarily toxic reaction or a delayed hypersensitivity reaction. The absence of infiltrates or symptoms of itching seem to indicate a toxic etiology, but the presence of a papillofollicular response and the later onset of the condition could also indicate a delayed hypersensitivity reaction. The key differential diagnostic features between dendriform keratitis caused by contact lens wear and herpes simplex and herpes zoster, the two other conditions most frequently associated with dendriform lesions, are listed in Table 6–1.

Herpes Simplex Virus Infections

The staggering incidence of nonocular herpes simplex virus (HSV) infections (between 70% and 90% of the adult population[62]) means that the chances of a contact lens wearer suffering from an attack are significant, further complicating the diagnosis. Classically, HSV infections

FIG 6–9.
Pseudodendrite produced in response to severe corneal reaction to thimerosal-preserved solution in a soft contact lens wearer. (Courtesy of Rochester Eye Associates.)

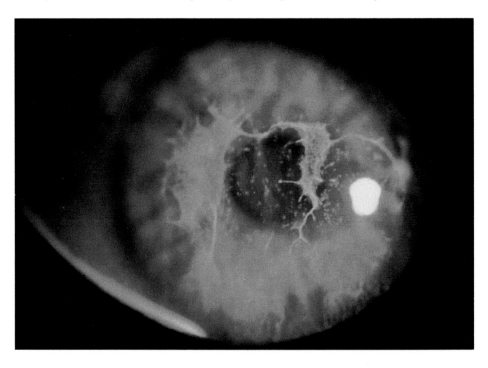

TABLE 6–1.

Differential Diagnosis of Dendriform Epithelial Lesions

	Solution Toxicity	Herpes Simplex	Herpes Zoster
Appearance	Annular, sinuous	Delicate, lacy	Medusa-like
Terminal bulbs	None	Frequent	Rare
Fluorescein stain	Patchy, apical	Bright	Irregular
Depth of lesion	Plaque	Excavated	Elevated
Usual occurrence	Often bilateral	Unilateral	Unilateral

produce true dendritic lesions (Fig 6–10 and 6–11), which are said to be uniquely associated with focal hypoesthesia.[54] Primary HSV infections typically respond well to antiviral agents, whereas a contact lens–induced lesion may actually worsen with therapy, particularly if the antiviral agent is preserved with thimerosal. Herpes simplex virus infections are sometimes associated with a follicular conjunctivitis and lid or cutaneous vesicles and usually occur unilaterally. Herpes zoster can also mimic these conditions, by producing pseudodendrites, often in response to trauma or exposure. These lesions are usually self-limiting, however, and often heal with no intervention or sequellae (see Chapter 7).

NUMMULAR KERATITIS

Another common variant of solution-related keratitis involves an inflammatory response of the subepithelial region and has been termed nummular, or infiltrative, kera-titis. The term nummular means coin shaped and refers to the appearance of the opacities seen in the superficial and deeper layers of the corneal stroma (Fig 6–12).[10] Although more common in the British literature than in American journals, the term nummular keratitis is preferred over the term infiltrative keratitis, which often implies a noninfective ulcerative keratitis. The mechanisms of corneal infiltration secondary to contact lens wear are discussed in detail in Chapter 10.

Contact Lens–Related Hypersensitivity Reaction

Corneal infiltrates represent one of the most common adverse reactions in contact lens wearers and can be seen in both daily and extended wear patients, as well as in non-lens wearers.[29] They have been reported in association with tight-fitting lenses,[21, 37] allergic or toxic reactions to solution preservatives,[39] chlamydial (trachoma inclusion conjunctivitis) infection,[39] and adenoviral infections.[32] Because any or all of these entities may occur in the contact lens–wearing patient, diagnosis by exclusion is indicated.

Reports of corneal infiltrates with contact lens wear

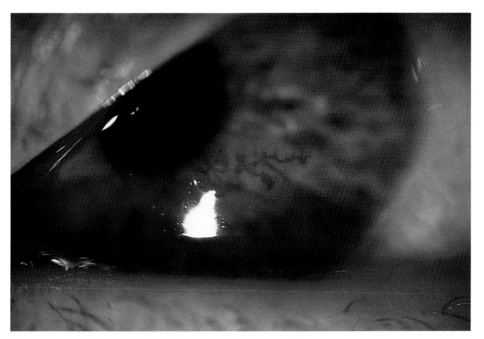

FIG 6–10.
True dendrite observed in a patient with herpes simplex virus keratitis, viewed after instillation of rose bengal. (Courtesy of M. Williams.)

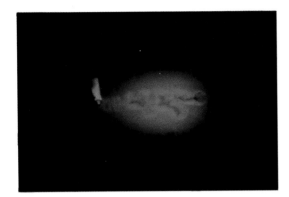

FIG 6–11.
True dendrite with fluorescein and rose bengal staining.
(Courtesy of M. Williams.)

were first seen in the early 1970s, soon after the introduction of hydrogel lenses in a large-scale fashion. In the early reports, the contact lens material itself was blamed for the reaction,[3] but later reports pointed to the contact lens solutions as the cause.[5]

Mondino and Groden[39] used intradermal and occlusive patch tests with thimerosal-containing solutions to demonstrate delayed hypersensitivity to thimerosal in three patients who developed anterior stromal infiltrates, accompanied by red, itchy eyes, after switching from heat disinfection system to a chemical system. They ruled out bacterial, viral, and chlamydial infections with cultures and staining. They also noted that the symptoms did not return with heat disinfection but did return on challenge with chemically disinfected lenses. Others[5, 64] have reported on

similar series of patients wearing hydrogel contact lenses, and Dart[10] has also observed a similar reaction in a rigid lens wearer who was using a thimerosal-preserved cleaning and wetting solution.

Discomfort and hyperemia are characteristic features of nummular keratitis, with the observation of coin-shaped opacities in the subepithelial layers being its hallmark sign. Patients typically experience a rapid decrease in lens tolerance. Lesions that occur secondary to thimerosal use will resolve slowly after removal of the preservative from the regimen and will resolve more quickly in the presence of corticosteroids, without showing the recurrence characteristic of lesions caused by epidemic keratoconjunctivitis (EKC) after corticosteroid therapy. The lesions appear semiopaque to opaque in direct illumination and are also easily visible in retroillumination (Fig 6–13). Gordon and Kracher[21] found in their series of 51 patients (54 eyes) that 93% of infiltrates were located in the corneal periphery, within 3 mm of the limbus. They detected a lucid interval between the limbus and the infiltrate and found that 67% of these infiltrates occurred between 10 and 2 o'clock in the superior cornea. They also found that a single well-demarcated inferior infiltrate (Fig 6–14) was also common. Most infiltrates were found in the subepithelial region. The infiltrates occurred after 3 weeks to 5 years of lens wear, and 41% occurred during the first year of an extended wear regimen. They postulated that a tight-fitting lens was the primary causative factor because thimerosal was not as widely used as a contact lens preservative in this group and because all 51 patients were able to resume wear without a recurrence of the keratitis

FIG 6–12.
Scattered central subepithelial infiltrates, characteristic of nummular keratitis. (Courtesy of M. DePaolis.)

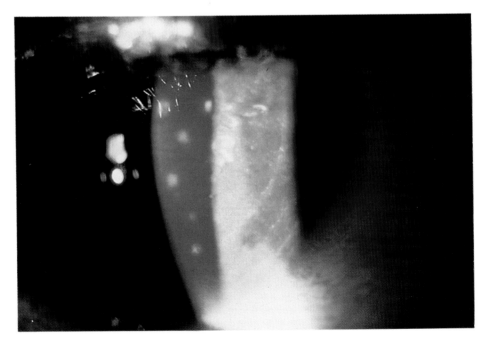

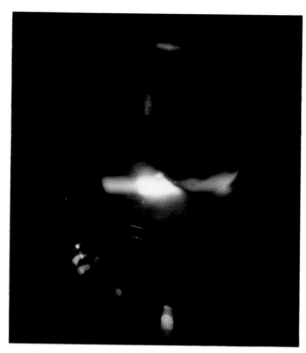

FIG 6–13.
Three subepithelial infiltrates viewed in indirect illumination.
(Courtesy of M. Williams.)

after refitting with a looser lens. They cited corneal hypoxia and trapped debris as a factor, with subsequent release of intrastromal inflammatory kinins that mediate the reaction.

The peripheral location of infiltrates supports the idea that leukocytes can enter the cornea from the limbal ves-

sels, as suggested by Chusid and Davis.[8] Wallace[60] suggests that Langerhans cells present in the corneal epithelium are involved in antigen processing, with T-cell recognition and cellular infiltration to follow. Numerous stimuli can act as facilitators in this reaction, chiefly by increasing the blood flow to the limbal region but possibly also by causing slight alterations in the corneal epithelium. These can include hypoxia, tight lenses, solution hypersensitivity reactions, and bacteria.

Marginal corneal infiltrates can be caused by conditions relating to the contact lenses themselves, such as deposits, drying, or mechanical irritation, but can also occur secondary to an underlying microbial allergy.[60] In the case of contact lens involvement, corticosteroids, generally accompanied by prophylactic antibiotic therapy, have been advocated. However, the underlying cause of the irritation or disruption must be identified and removed before the patient resumes wear. Corneal infiltrates seen with a largely intact overlying epithelium are often caused by exotoxins produced by bacteria such as *Staphylococcus aureus*. These reactions represent allergic responses and, as such, are often accompanied by significant conjunctival edema, hyperemia, and symptoms of itching. The infiltrative region will lie close to the limbus in such cases, and the discharge will be watery (Fig 6–15). In cases such as these, it is important to treat the underlying bacterial lid disease, which is the source of the toxins, before or concurrently with any corticosteroid or antibiotic therapy. By way of contrast, Figure 6–16 shows a central bacterial ulcer with the characteristic features of severe conjunctival hyperemia, accompanied by matted lashes and a purulent

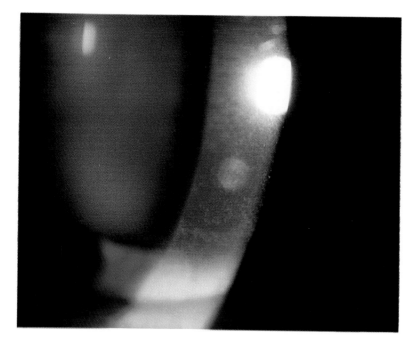

FIG 6–14.
Large, circular infiltrate in the inferior cornea.

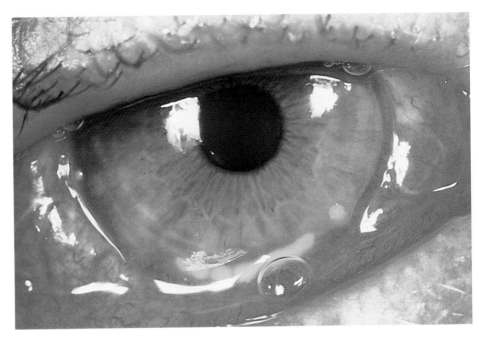

FIG 6–15.
Chemotic conjunctiva with peripheral corneal infiltrate typical of allergic reactions to bacterial exotoxins. (Courtesy of Rochester Contact Lens Associates.)

discharge. A discussion of ulcerative processes affecting the cornea can be found in Chapter 12.

Epidemic Keratoconjunctivitis

A key differential diagnosis for central corneal infiltrates is EKC. Follicular conjunctivitis, often accompanied by petechial hemorrhages, is the earliest and most common sign of adenoviral infection[32] (although follicular responses are also common in allergic conditions). Preauricular lymphadenopathy is said to be a hallmark of EKC, but the degree of hypertrophy and tenderness is quite variable from individual to individual. The palpebral follicular response may progress to create a pseudomembrane. The chief corneal signs do not occur for 3 to 4 days after the initial symptoms and can include a fine, diffuse punctate epithelial keratitis. This is then followed by a coalescence of the finer lesions into areas of focal keratitis resembling those of Thygeson's SPK approximately 1 week after the initial symptoms. The third stage of corneal involvement is the subepithelial infiltration that appears beneath the focal epithelial spots. The infiltrates can continue for weeks to years and may remain permanently in some patients. The management of the EKC condition is largely symptomatic. Lubricants or cold compresses may be helpful, but topical corticosteroids are not typically employed because they

FIG 6–16.
Deep hyperemia of conjunctiva and matted lashes with central bacterial ulcer. (Courtesy of Rochester Contact Lens Associates.)

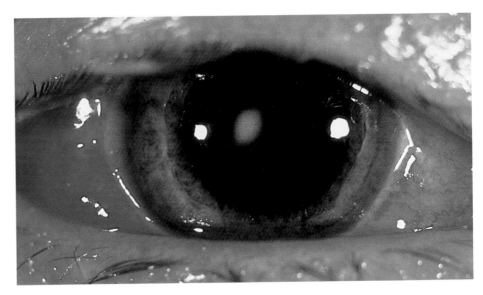

can actually prolong the course of the infection. Hyperosmotic agents may be helpful in cases of accompanying edema.

MARGINAL KERATITIS

Superior Limbic Keratoconjunctivitis

Marginal keratitis secondary to contact lens wear can also involve vascularization and proliferation of tissue, typically in response to long-term corneal insult, whether as a result of mechanical, chemical, or immunological stimuli. Another condition observed in soft contact lens wearers that is thought to be related to solution hypersensitivity is contact lens–induced superior limbic keratoconjunctivitis, or CLKC. It is so named because it shares many of the diagnostic features of Theodore's superficial limbic keratoconjunctivitis (SLKC). Theodore[56] first described SLKC in 1963 as a painful, usually bilateral inflammation of the superior limbus and bulbar conjunctiva with papillary hypertrophy of the superior tarsal conjunctiva. The inflammatory nature of CLKC is discussed in Chapter 10. Accompanying symptoms can also include burning, a foreign body sensation, photophobia, and blepharospasm. A key corneal sign is SPK, with filamentary keratitis occurring in between 35% and 50% of cases.[1] Vision is not often affected, because the corneal disruption is usually limited to the superior cornea. Although all ages can be affected, the condition occurs most commonly in older women (80% of cases) who suffer from hyperthyroid conditions. Histological studies show epithelial keratinization, acanthosis, nuclear degeneration, and intracellular glycogen granules.[1, 12] The treatment may consist of a bandage soft contact lens, as well as ocular lubricants, cauterization with silver nitrate, or surgical resection of the superior conjunctival region. More recent reports have also suggested cromolyn sodium, a mast cell stabilizer, as appropriate therapy.[9]

Contact Lens–Related Superior Limbic Keratoconjunctivitis

The contact lens condition (CLKC) was first described in the 1970s after the introduction of widespread use of hydrophilic contact lenses. Like Theodore's SLKC, the condition in contact lens wearers affects the superior bulbar conjunctiva, beginning with poor wetting of the conjunctiva, followed by injection and inflammation of the surrounding tissue.[48] The epithelium displays variable staining in the superior portion, often in a swirled pattern,[61]

and the superior epithelium can become dull and hazy. However, these patients are typically younger than the SLKC patients and do not have the thyroid condition. In addition, filamentary keratitis is rarely seen in this group of patients.

The CLKC condition begins after 2 months to 3 years of lens wear, whereupon the patients may begin to complain of burning, itching, red eyes with increased photophobia and secretions.[1] Lid eversion will often reveal papillary hypertrophy, with petechiae and inflammation of the superior tarsus. The superior bulbar conjunctiva may become loose, boggy, and keratonized, with injection noted prominently in a vertical band pointing to the insertion of the superior rectus (Fig 6–17; see also Figs 10–16 to 10–18).[48] Punctate staining of the superior one to two thirds of the cornea can usually be observed, and it most frequently occurs bilaterally. The epithelium near the limbus may appear dull and eventually, a U- or V-shaped micropannus and a subepithelial haze or opacities begin to encroach on the cornea and can eventually affect vision. In rare cases, hyperplasia is observed in a spokelike pattern radiating from the superior limbus. Histologically, a mild to moderate neutrophilic response is present, mild prekeratinized epithelial cells can be observed, and goblet cell density may be decreased.

Many theories have been advanced as to the cause of CLKC, the most promising one related to thimerosal hypersensitivity. Sendele et al.[47] studied a series of 40 patients who suffered from ocular redness, irritation, and decreased lens tolerance to determine a possible etiology. On slit-lamp examination, 15 patients showed superior bulbar infiltration that was bilateral and symmetrical, with perilimbal vascular injection and micropannus. Irregular thickening and redundancy of the superior bulbar conjunctiva, limbus, and cornea were noted and confirmed the diagnosis of CLKC. Acting on the suspicion that solution preservatives might be involved, they selected 15 subjects, who were challenged in one eye with thimerosal, with the contralateral eye receiving either ethylenediamine tetraacetic acid (EDTA) or BAK. An additional ten subjects who were asymptomatic but using the same chemical contact lens disinfection regimens were studied, as well as ten asymptomatic contact lens wearers not using chemicals systems. Five test subjects also underwent biopsy testing.

For their study, they first discontinued all lens wear and gave artificial tears and ointments for symptomatic relief. After resolution of symptoms, the subjects were challenged with the thimerosal and control solutions every hour. Of the 15 test patients, 5 tested positively for a thimerosal allergy, whereas none of the asymptomatic patients on chemical regimens responded to the challenge, nor did any of the test patients react to BAK or EDTA.

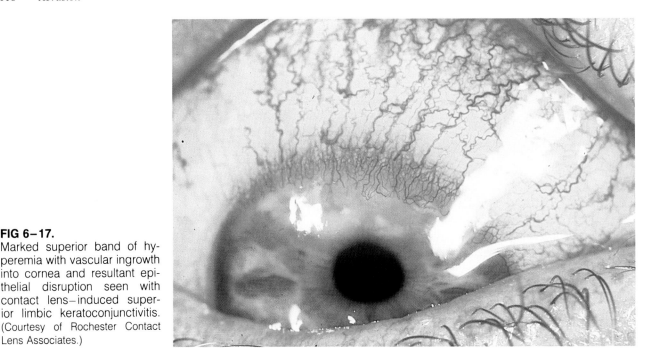

FIG 6–17.
Marked superior band of hyperemia with vascular ingrowth into cornea and resultant epithelial disruption seen with contact lens–induced superior limbic keratoconjunctivitis. (Courtesy of Rochester Contact Lens Associates.)

However, despite the relatively low allergic response rate to thimerosal in the symptomatic group, several factors point to thimerosal allergies as a related feature: All 15 CLKC subjects were using a thimerosal preserved–contact lens solution and had bilateral signs and symptoms that resolved after they stopped using the preserved contact lens solutions, and the syndrome recurred if thimerosal was reintroduced to the care regimen but not if thimerosal-free solutions were used.

Fuerst et al.[18] also reported on 13 cases of CLKC and noted that the signs and symptoms can persist for up to 15 months after cessation of lens wear. In their series, patch testing failed to show consistent hypersensitivity reactions, and some patients experienced a recurrence of the condition even after switching to nonthimerosal-preserved systems. Other reports also dispute thimerosal as a primary cause. Of four CLKC patients studied by Stenson,[53] three experienced resolution of signs after lens removal and were able to resume a limited wearing schedule with thinner lenses. The last patient took 2 years to heal without lens wear. The key symptoms reported in Stenson's study were discomfort, dryness, burning, itching, and blurred vision, which was exacerbated by lens wear. Conjunctival and corneal scrapings revealed a neutrophilic response with prekeratinized epithelial cells, similar to findings by other authors. She, however, was unable to identify any common lens factors. The patients had worn their lenses from 5 months to 3 years, two patients had lenses that were 18 months old, and excess movement was noted in two of the patients. Abel et al.[1] point out that if CLKC were solely a hypersensitivity reaction to solutions, it should not be confined to just the superior region of the cornea. This may point to a hypoxic component, as suggested by Ajamian, because the region under the lid would be relatively deprived of oxygen during lens wear.[61] In their report on eight cases, Abel's group[1] also suggests that thimerosal may not be the only factor. All patients were required to discontinue wear of their lenses until the condition was clear, which took between 5 days and 10 months for their group. Patients were given ocular lubricants for relief of symptoms, and one more severe case required corticosteroids to quiet the response. They noted a sequence of events in the regression of the CLKC. The edema and injection of the conjunctiva resolved first, followed by clearing of the epitheliopathy, and finally the papillary changes after several months. They also found that several of the patients would experience a recurrence of symptoms if thimerosal were used again but only if the original lenses were worn. When new lenses were substituted with the thimerosal regimen, there was not an immediate return of the symptoms, as had been the case with the old lenses. The authors suggest a mechanical effect of excess lens movement, possibly combined with the deposits on the contact lenses, because most cases displayed movement in excess of 1.5 mm. They recommended changing both lens material and design parameters for the post-CKLC patient. Because of the high association of solution hypersensitivity, it is also recommended that the patient be switched to a preservative-free care regimen and that new lenses be issued to remove any source of chemical or immunological contamination before resuming lens wear.

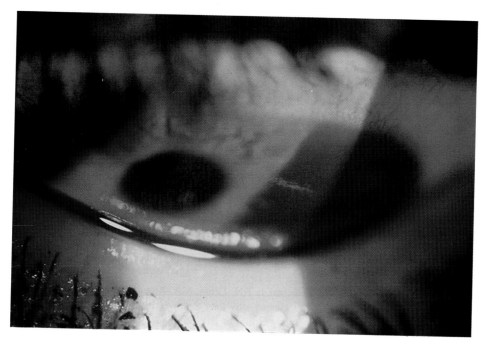

FIG 6–18.
Lacy white line of epithelial splitting seen with white light.

Superior Epithelial Arcuate Lesions

One other entity, which has been infrequently described in the literature but is a rather common occurrence in practice, is superior epithelial arcuate lesions, also known as epithelial splitting. A report by Kline and DeLuca[31] in 1977 described light superior staining that developed into a more concentrated punctate appearance with time, and which eventually evolved into bunching and whitish pitting of the superior epithelium. These lesions were found within 3 mm of the superior limbus and occurred frequently in patients wearing large-diameter, thin, high wa-

ter content lenses with lens movement up to 1.5 mm. Patients were largely asymptomatic in the early stages but complained of burning, itching, and redness as the condition progressed. Staining, which persisted up to 15 hours after lens removal, was observed. Josephson[28] reported a similar phenomenon that he observed with lathe-cut hydrogels. These lesions initially appear as diffuse, scattered punctate dots, aligned in a linear or arcuate fashion in the superior cornea, under the upper lid. As coalescence progresses, the lesions can be viewed in white light and appear as a lacy line or arc (Fig 6–18). When viewed with fluorescein, they will fluoresce brightly, with penetration

FIG 6–19.
Staining with fluorescein seepage from superior epithelial arcuate lesions.

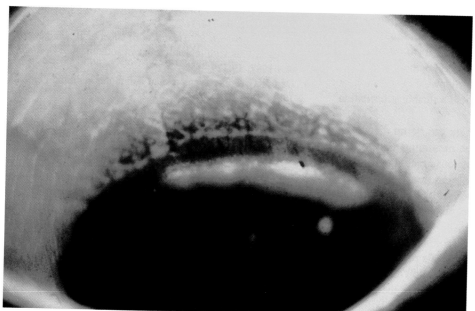

TABLE 7–1.

Various Forms of Diagnostic Fluorescein

Type	Form	Preservative
Sodium fluorescein (9 mg)	Strips	Chlorobutanol
Sodium fluorescein (20 mg)	Liquid dropperettes	Thimerosal
Fluoresoft* (0.35%)	Liquid dropperettes	Nonpreserved

*Holles Laboratories, Cohasset, Mass.

to prevent their contamination with the dye. Or, clinicians can use the high moleculer weight fluorescein known as Fluoresoft (0.35% concentrations, Holles Laboratories, Cohasset, Mass.), which in solution does not bind to a hydrogel matrix or surface. It is so simple and so useful, yet many clinicians do not routinely stain soft lens–wearing patients unless dramatic symptoms are reported. Ideally, staining of the cornea is best visualized without any lens on the cornea. It is more marked if the dye is instilled within a short time after lens removal and may be more evident if the lens has been worn for a long time before removal. Table 7–1 summarizes the various types of fluorescein available.

METHODS OF STAINING AND OBSERVATION

In the application of dyes to the cornea, rose bengal is useful in staining dead, dying, or degenerative tissues such as insulted corneal epithelium, conjunctiva, and mucus strands (Fig 7–2,A).[67] Sodium fluorescein, on the other hand, is invaluable in staining areas of the cornea where the epithelial cells are absent. True staining of an epithelial defect can often be differentiated from negative staining or indentation staining by use of a sterile irrigating solution after the dye has been initially instilled and observed. Negative staining represents an area of tissue where the dye will not flow smoothly. Indentation staining represents an area of pooling rather than true tissue absorption of the dye. Enhancement of abrasion staining can be achieved by using the technique of sequential staining.[37] This entails several applications of dye at specific time intervals to promote absorption into the compromised tissue, thus producing a highlighted effect.

Other ways in which enhancement of staining can be achieved is by using filters to improve contrast with certain stains.[11, 21] White light observation with a slit lamp may define certain abrasions with or without dye instillation, but cobalt blue, Tiffen, or specific Wratten filters used in conjunction with dyes such as fluorescein are much more definitive of lesions (Fig 7–2,B and C). Most slit-lamp biomicroscopes use a white light source with corresponding cobalt blue or red-free filters. Additional filters that can be handheld or fitted to most slit-lamp biomicroscopes include yellow barrier filters such as Wratten no. 12 and 15, Tiffen no. 2, or the Volk Universal Yellow filter shown in Figure 7–3. These barrier filters are placed in front of the objective lens system of the microscope and the eye surface to be viewed. Blue enhancing filters such as a Wratten no. 45 or 49 are applied over the light source of the slit lamp. Although these filters can be either handheld or taped to most instrument housings, a simple retainer ring

A

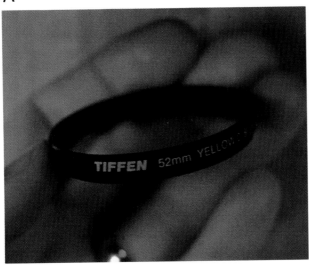

B

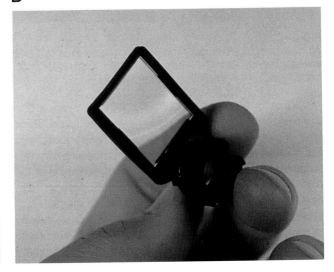

FIG 7–3.
A, handheld Tiffen yellow no. 2 photographic filter to be held over objective area of slit lamp. (Courtesy of R. Grohe.) **B,** Volk Universal yellow filter attachment to slit-lamp post. (Courtesy of R. Grohe.)

to hold the barrier filter can be made by the clinician to allow convenient attachment and removal to the biomicroscope. It can be as simple as using a round plastic bottle with an inside diameter that matches the outside diameter of the objective lens; an 8-oz saline solution bottle fits many biomicroscopes. The bottle is cut off on the bottom ½ in. from the end. A 1¾ in. hole is then cut out of this bottom piece, which then becomes the retainer for the filter and fits snugly to the microscope.[39]

The concept of grading the intensity of the abrasion staining is very useful for documentation and helpful in determining the degree of resolution on follow-up examination (Fig 7–4). Photodocumentation through still photographs or videotape procedures is an asset if the clarity and resolution of the abrasion is apparent.

Slit-lamp biomicroscopy is an essential tool for the contact lens diagnostician. The art, skill, and experience of the clinician dictates the utility of the results when staining patterns are observed. Evaluations of abrasion stain involve the use of various illumination modalities for the slit lamp. Direct focal, and indirect illumination, retroillumination, sclerotic scatter on specular reflection with optic sections, broad beam, or pinpoint illumination, independently or in combination, can make observation and evaluation of specific abrasions easier.[18, 43] In addition, the degree of magnification and the quality of the optics of the biomicroscope, as well as the visual acuity, skill, thoroughness, and patience of the clinician, will dictate how precisely the abrasion is seen and assessed. It is important that clinicians are aware that rapid and accurate identifica-

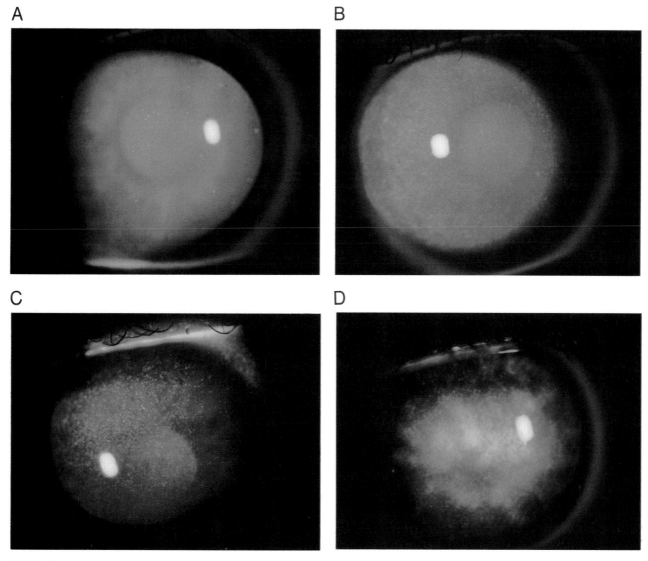

FIG 7–4.
A, grade 1+ chemical staining. **B,** grade 2+ chemical staining. **C,** grade 3+ chemical staining. **D,** grade 4+ chemical staining. (Courtesy of R. Courtney and J. Lee.)

tion of an abrasion will enhance the effectiveness of treatment for the problem.

In the following sections of this chapter, a variety of corneal abrasions are defined and discussed. Where possible, the cause of the staining pattern and its management are also addressed.

HYPOXIA-INDUCED ABRASIONS ASSOCIATED WITH CONTACT LENSES

A number of abrasions occur as a result of corneal hypoxia under contact lenses (Table 7–2). Overwear abrasions (CCC) are caused by corneal hypoxia. The central corneal clouding[35] (Fig 7–5) and the edematous corneal formations (ECF)[29, 36] seen with polymethylmethacrylate (PMMA) contact lens wear are prototype examples of complications secondary to corneal edema.[58] Epithelial microcysts and vertical striae characterize hydrophilic contact lens overwear complications caused by inadequate corneal oxygenation.[65]

Polymethylmethacrylate Overwear Abrasion

Although a less frequently occurring problem since the widespread use of rigid gas-permeable (RGP) and hydrophilic soft lenses, a PMMA overwear incident is still a potential event.[26] After a day during which PMMA lenses are inadvertently worn for approximately 23 hours, a patient awakes with acute ocular pain after only a few hours of sleep. Additional symptoms may include extreme photophobia, excess tearing, hazy and reduced visual acuity, a significant foreign body sensation, and gross lens intolerance.

The probable course of events in this condition is as follows. The cornea has adapted to the reduced-oxygen environment under the PMMA lenses provided during the normal wearing period. Additional edema develops as the cornea is deprived of oxygen if lenses are worn for a longer period than is usual. The corneal nerves lose sensi-

TABLE 7–2.

Summary of Hypoxia-Induced Corneal Abrasions

Central corneal clouding
Edematous corneal formations
Polymethylmethacrylate overwear abrasion
Pseudodendrites
Corneal blotting
Microcysts
Microbubbles
Microdeposits

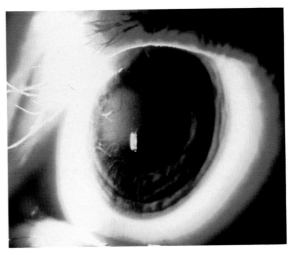

FIG 7–5.
Central corneal clouding associated with polymethylmethacrylate (PMMA) contact lens wear.

tivity[5] because of the prolonged hypoxic state during this longer wear period (see Chapter 5). Unaware of any problem on lens removal, the patient goes to sleep. As the corneal nerves regain sensitivity, the patient awakens to a sensation of acute ocular discomfort from an abrasion, as seen in Figure 7–6.

The treatment for overwear syndrome consists of discontinuing all contact lens wear during the wound healing process. Cold compresses and systemic analgesics are helpful to relieve symptoms. Optional pressure patching, prophylactic topical antibiotics, or bandage soft contact lenses are employed by some practitioners. Most abrasions

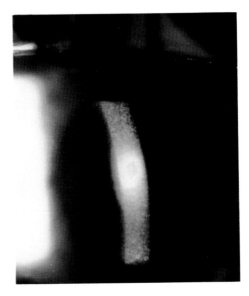

FIG 7–6.
Overwear abrasion associated with PMMA contact lens wear. (Courtesy of P. Blaze.)

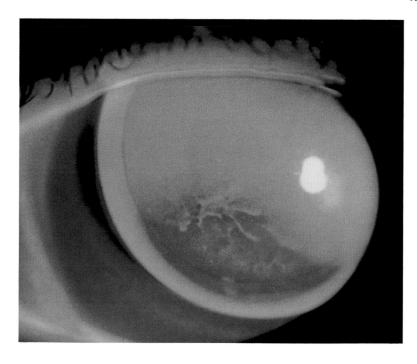

FIG 7–7.
Edematous corneal formation associated with long-term PMMA wear. (Courtesy of K. Lebow.)

of this origin heal uneventfully without complications, and some practitioners believe this occurs faster without patching. The pain usually resolves within 6 to 10 hours, but 3 to 7 days should be allowed for thorough corneal healing before resumption of contact lens wear. During the early stages of healing, the clinician may witness some negative staining in the areas of the abrasion. Refitting with a lens material transmitting more oxygen is the choice to prevent a recurrence of the condition. It is critical that the patient be reeducated on the importance of maintaining a sensible wearing schedule, thus avoiding further overwear incidents.

Edematous Corneal Formation and Epithelial Pseudodendrites

Differential diagnosis between a contact lens overwear problem, a contact lens chemical complication, or a viral ulcer may not be easy in certain cases. Dendritic formations of the cornea may be confusing to the clinician because of the diverse causes of these branching lesions.[42] Timely diagnosis and treatment may be paramount to the patient's future corneal health and visual status. The differential diagnosis between an ECF (Fig 7–7), a pseudodendrite (Fig 7–8), or a herpes simplex dendrite (Fig 7–9) will dictate the course of remedial action. Key diagnostic signs are the location of lesion and the staining effect of fluorescein or rose bengal.

An ECF is classically seen with long-term PMMA rigid contact lens wear.[13] This condition is associated with hypoxia and is seen as central corneal branching in the ep-

ithelium. This dendrite does not show true staining, instead fluorescein pools in an arborized pattern corresponding to branches of the lesion. This condition is resolved by refitting with an RGP material. Total resolution may be slow, and an occasional trace scar may be persistent for many months. In contrast, pseudodendrites may be associated with a herpes zoster[44] incident or more commonly as a complication of the use of soft contact lens care products containing thimerasol or chlorhexidine.[1, 42] These branch-

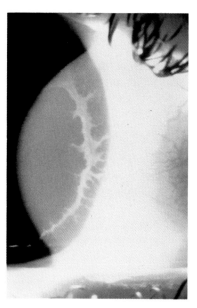

FIG 7–8.
Pseudodendrite formation related to thimerasol hypersensitivity. (Courtesy of P. Caroline.)

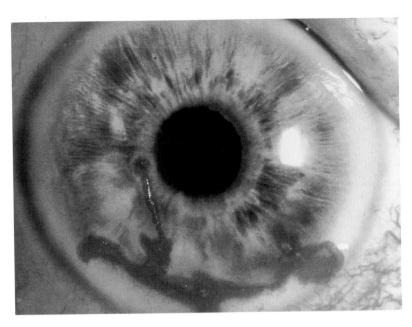

FIG 7–9.
Herpes simplex dendritic ulcer.

ing, serpentine lesions are plaquelike, usually more peripheral, bilateral, and stain faintly with fluorescein and rose bengal. Chemical hypersensitivity pseudodendrites require time to heal and future avoidance of thimerasol and chlorhexidine.[5] The true dendritic ulcer associated with herpes simplex is usually unilateral and stains deeply with fluorescein and rose bengal. It shows specific end bulbs with its branches. Decreased corneal sensitivity is a helpful symptom for the clinician's differential diagnosis. Medical treatment with newer antiviral agents is encouraging. Specific diagnosis and tentative treatment of a corneal dendrite may be difficult if multiple factors such as PMMA contact lenses, thimerasol products, and exposure to herpes simplex are presented. The clinician must assess corneal sensitivity, look for end bulbs, and concentrate on a very marked staining pattern to rule out the simplex ulcer before proceeding with any contact lens wear.[15] A differential diagnosis of ECF, pseudodendrite, and herpes simplex dendrite is given in Table 7–3.

Corneal Blotting

Corneal blotting has been observed with hydrogel contact lenses worn on an extended wear basis (Fig 7–10). Lin and Mandell[40] report blotting formations are best seen immediately after the eyes are opened following sleeping with lenses and suggest the condition usually disappears within 2 hours.

The blots are reportedly different from punctate staining; they are larger, more diffuse, and have a duller fluorescein appearance. The blot shapes are said to be round, with tails, crescents, or vertical or horizontal streaks attached. The condition is usually bilateral and should be differentiated from epithelial wrinkling or the corneal mosaic phenomenon. The proposed etiology suggests debris under the lens or tear chemistry as factors. Treatment consists of switching to daily wear soft lenses or RGP lenses for extended wear.

Hydrogel Microcystic Staining and Microdeposits (Microbubbles)

Observing a soft contact lens patient by slit-lamp biomicroscopy may reveal pits or depressions in the corneal epithelium (Fig 7–11). Positive and negative staining may be observed simultaneously in these areas. Bourassa and Benjamin[6] described this effect associated with nonmoving microdeposits embedded in the anterior corneal surface be-

TABLE 7–3.
Differential Diagnosis

	Lesion Location	Shape	Fluorescein Staining
Edematous corneal formations	Central cornea; unilateral	Branching twiglike	Negative pooling
Pseudodendrite	Peripheral cornea; bilateral	Plaquelike	Moderate
Herpes simplex	Unilateral	Classic branching with end bulbs	Deep stain

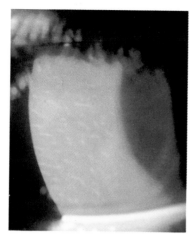

FIG 7–10.
Corneal blotting. (Courtesy of S. Lin and R. Mandell.)

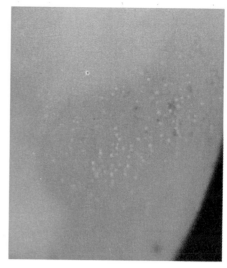

FIG 7–11.
Epithelial microcysts, positive and negative staining.

hind a soft contact lens. The fluorescein staining of these pits or microbubble depressions is similar to the larger bubble depressions seen commonly with rigid contact lenses but are much smaller than the dimple veil effect.

Microcysts as reported by Josephson[28] and Zantos[64] have similar appearance to microdeposits but differ in etiology. Bruce and Brennan[5] describe epithelial microcysts as translucent dots 15 to 50 μm in diameter. Microcysts occur as a result of hypoxia induced by contact lens wear and are found most commonly in extended wear (see Chapter 2). They may be resolved by refitting with a lens having greater oxygen transmissibility or reverting to a less demanding wearing modality.

from the use of devices or techniques of lens insertion and removal. These are summarized in Table 7–4.

Lens Removal Abrasion

Removing a contact lens from the eye can be a damaging experience. It is important that the wearer makes certain the lens is still on the corneal surface before attempting removal. Using a DMV or other suction removal device when the lens is absent can induce a serious abrasion as corneal tissue is removed instead of the lens (Fig 7–12).

MECHANICAL ABRASIONS

A multitude of contact lens–related abrasions occur as a result of damaged, defective, or poorly designed lenses, or

TABLE 7–4.
Summary of Mechanical Abrasions and Staining

Form	Lens Type
Lens removal	Rigid and soft
Poor edge design	Rigid
Accidental epithelial debridement	Soft
Lens cracks, chips, nicks, and tears	Rigid
Epithelial wrinkling	Rigid
Corneal wrinkling	Soft
Hydrogel "smile"	Soft
Superior arc	Rigid
Tinted soft lens impression ring	Soft
Furrow/limbal hypertrophy	Soft
Superior limbal epithelial seal off	Soft
Epithelial splitting	Soft
Dimple veil	Rigid

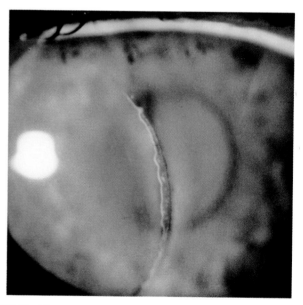

FIG 7–12.
Corneal abrasion caused by a DMV device pulling off epithelium rather than a contact lens. (Courtesy of K. Lebow.)

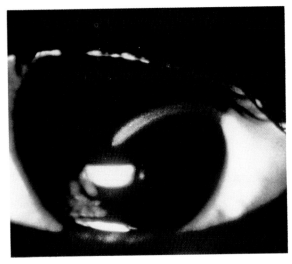

FIG 7–13.
Corneal laceration by a rigid contact lens turning on its edge during removal.

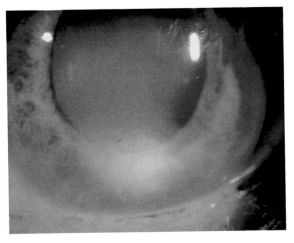

FIG 7–15.
Finger scrape corneal abrasion during soft contact lens removal.

A similar-appearing abrasion may occur when a rigid lens ejects only partially from the cornea. The resultant scraping or lacerating of the cornea occurs as the lens is pressed against the corneal surface (Fig 7–13).

In soft lens removal, the finger pinch abrasion or the finger scrape abrasion may occur as the wearer attempts to squeeze an absent lens between the thumb and index or middle finger. Occasionally a conjunctival abrasion or hemorrhage may occur from this procedure because of aggressive finger action (Fig 7–14). The scrape abrasion is typically seen on the inferior cornea and is the result of the wearer trying to wipe or slide the lens into the lower cul-de-sac when no lens is present on the cornea (Fig 7–15). More serious consequences can develop from the use of a fingernail to lift a lens off the cornea during routine lens removal (Fig 7–16,A). Although the fingernail abrasion or laceration may heal sufficiently to reduce pain and irritation, a recurrent corneal erosion may subsequently develop.[17] Fingernail abrasions can be very serious in aph-

akes, who because of poor vision may scrape large areas of the cornea, as shown in Figure 7–16,B.

In the absence of secondary infection, most other lens removal–related abrasions heal quickly without complications. Many authorities advise antibiotic prophylaxisis and pressure patching if the lesion is significant. Recurrent injuries of this nature can be avoided with patient re-education on removal techniques.

Abrasion Caused by Poor Lens Edge Design

The most common microabrasions related to edge design are those induced by rigid contact lenses. These abrasions are usually observed in the 3 and 9 o'clock areas of the cornea and conjunctiva and are one of the causes of peripheral corneal desiccation syndrome (Fig 7–17), which is covered in more detail in Chapter 9. Peripheral corneal desiccation or 3 and 9 o'clock staining is often the result of improper edge contour (Fig 7–18) or improper secondary curve selection or fabrication.[33]

Abrasion may occur as a result of the shearing action

FIG 7–14.
Conjunctival hemorrhage caused by finger squeeze soft contact lens removal technique. (Courtesy of M. Swearingen.)

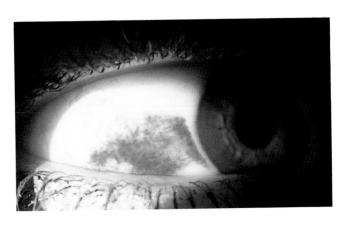

A

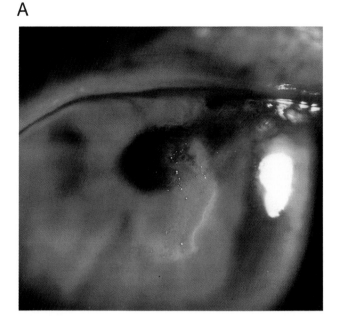

B

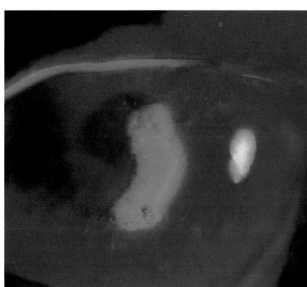

FIG 7–16.
A, large bandlike fingernail abrasion occurring during lens removal by an aphakic rigid gas-permeable (RGP) wearer. **B,** cobalt filter, fluorescein-stained corneal abrasion view of **A.** (Courtesy of R. Grohe.)

of the lens edge as it moves back and forth with changes in lateral gaze. It may also be caused by excessive lid gap with poor lens edge design or by inadequate lateral lens movement from limbus to limbus. Abrasions of this type may develop over a relatively short period of time and may be present as a chronic problem. The resolution of the problem may be achieved with modification or redesigning

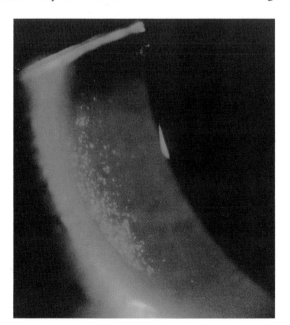

FIG 7–17.
Peripheral corneal desiccation (3 and 9 o'clock staining) seen with a hard contact lens.

of the lens periphery (see Chapter 9) or a change in the type of lens worn.

Accidental Epithelial Debridement

This traumatic condition is rare today with modern soft contact lens design. The typical scenario involved a tight-fitting, thick, low water content daily wear hydrogel lens left in the eye overnight. When this lens wearer awakens, attempts to forcefully pull the severely adhered lenses off the cornea would result in the accidental removal of large portions of the epithelium (Fig 7–19). This action would be accompanied by severe pain.[32, 47]

The problem of lens adherence or binding to the cornea is exacerbated by reduction in tear production during sleep and the consequent change in tear tonicity. The phenomenon was observed with certain specialty lenses, such as early silicone elastomer lenses, RGP and hydrogel lens combinations, and some early high water content extended wear hydrogel lenses.

Treatment requires (lengthy) lens discontinuance. When healing proceeds without complication, the patient may experience long-term apprehension regarding the resumption of contact lens wear.

Abrasion From Lens Cracks, Chips, Nicks, and Tears

Physical damage to a contact lens can produce a variety of abrasions. The appearance of the abrasion or stain will depend on the type of contact lens, the frequency and dura-

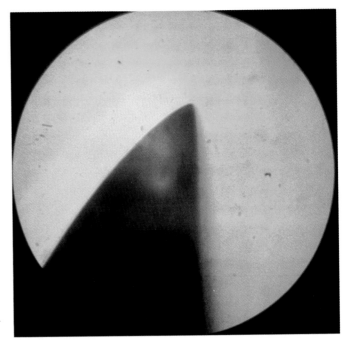

FIG 7–18.
Chisel-shaped rigid contact lens edge. (Courtesy of P. Caroline.)

tion of lens wear, and the location of the defect on or in the lens. A cracked or chipped rigid lens (Fig 7–20,A) may induce mild to severe abrasion or laceration of the corneal surface (Fig 7–20,B). Rigid lenses, which move considerably more than soft lenses in the eye regardless of the fit, may affect any portion of the cornea or conjunctiva (Fig 7–20,C–E). Abrasions caused by lens defects may appear as a diffuse pattern of tracking or linear scrapes or as varying degrees of lacerations or puncture wounds of the cornea (Fig 7–20,F).

The severity of the injury will dictate the specific mode of treatment. The cornea may quickly heal uneventfully after lens removal. Generally, defective lenses must be replaced, but occasionally a simple modification of the chipped edge of a hard lens will provide a temporary resolution of the problem after healing is confirmed. The more severe corneal damage will require therapeutic intervention with prophylactic antibiotics, a pressure patch, or both. Some situations might require the use of a bandage soft contact lens.

Abrasions seen with damaged soft contact lenses will not be as predictable. When a soft lens has a cut or tear in

FIG 7–19.
Accidental epithelial debridement induced by soft contact lens removal. (Courtesy of P. Caroline.)

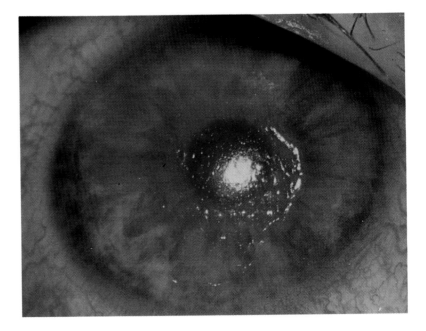

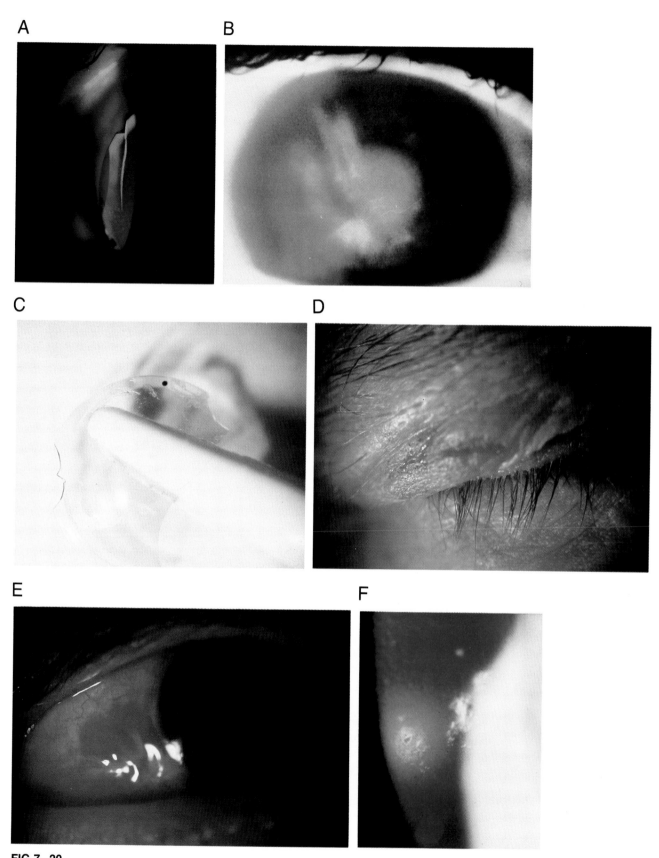

FIG 7–20.
Cracked-chipped rigid contact lens in situ **(A).** (Courtesy of M. Swearingen.) Diffuse corneal abrasion induced by the cracked lens **(B).** (Courtesy of M. Swearingen.) Fractured RGP lens retrieved from an aphakic patient **(C)** who was hit on the exterior lid by a tree branch **(D)** and subsequently experienced a corneal abrasion, lacerated conjunctiva, and subconjunctional hemorrhage **(E).** Puncture wound of cornea caused by damaged rigid lens **(F).** (Courtesy of A. Tomlinson.)

A

B

C

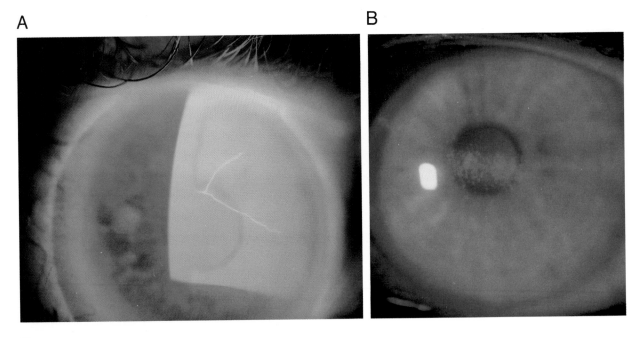

FIG 7–21.
A, torn soft contact lens in situ. **B,** diffuse scrape abrasion induced by torn soft contact lens. (Courtesy of A. Tomlinson.) **C,** vascularized infiltrative ulcer scar from an abrasion caused by continued wear of a torn soft contact lens. (Courtesy of M. Swearingen.)

the body of the lens (Fig 7–21,A), an appearance of a dull scrape stain pattern (Fig 7–21,B) may be seen. Symptoms may vary from a mild nonspecific ache to an obvious foreign body sensation that may continue after the lens is removed.

Lens tears or lens fractures may be very small and innocuous when observed in situ. However, the clinician must be diligent in finding these flaws because severe complications may develop (Fig 7–21,C). Most abrasions caused by soft lens defects are not severe and are remedied through immediate lens replacement without discontinuation of wear. However, the possibility of corneal damage

under a soft lens is another argument for all patients to have their corneas stained with fluorescein to confirm the amount and intensity of any abrasion present.

In contrast to RGP lenses, when a soft lens has a nick (Fig 7–22) or tear on the edge of the lens, it seldom causes corneal insult. Patients have been observed wearing nicked lenses for weeks or months without being aware that the lenses were damaged and needed replacement. No discontinuation of lens wear is required if the clinician observes no corneal staining from the nicked lens, but the damaged lens should be replaced.

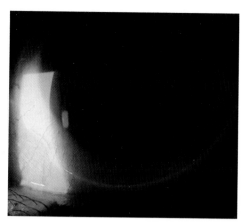

FIG 7–22.
Nicked soft contact lens.

Corneal Wrinkling or Anterior Corneal Mosaic

Anterior corneal mosaic as reported by Fischer in 1928 and by Schweitzer in 1967 may occur with normal or abnormal corneas, with and without contact lens wear.[4] The phenomenon of corneal wrinkles can be seen with both hydrogel and rigid contact lenses (Fig 7–23).[41]

Current opinion is that the condition is induced by mechanical forces imposed on the cornea by the weight of the lid and the contact lens. Bruce and Brennan[5] differentiate epithelial wrinkling associated with PMMA contact lens wear from corneal wrinkling related to hydrogel lens wear. Epithelial wrinkling is asymptomatic and recovers rapidly with lens removal. Epithelial wrinkling can also occur with thick RGP lenses. The corneal deformation is thought to be more serious, involves deeper corneal layers, and shows more pronounced folds. It can affect visual acuity and resolves much slower. With soft contact lenses, the resolution time may be correlated with the duration of lens

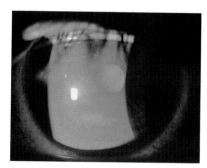

FIG 7–24.
Smile staining with soft contact lens wear.

wear. Switching from mid–water content, thin lenses to mobile nonhydroxyethylmethacrylate lenses has been reportedly effective.[49] Wrinkling seen with rigid lenses is probably caused by mechanical pressure inducing superficial corneal distortions and is found often in keratoconus. Clinicians must attempt to refit until the condition is resolved by having the patient use a different contact lens modality or discontinue lens wear if the wrinkles cause long-term corneal distortion or compromise.

Smile Stain Under Soft Contact Lens

The "smile" stain under the soft contact lens is observed as an inferior arc-shaped corneal abrasion, characteristically seen with specific types of hydrogel lenses (Fig 7–24). The lesion often may be vaguely seen biomicroscopically without fluorescein. Direct focal and retroillumination techniques while the patient is looking in an upward gaze allow better observation.

However, staining is very apparent when dye is instilled after lenses are removed.[54] The patient may be asymptomatic or may have mild complaints of dryness or irritation late in the day. Opinions on the etiology of this condition are discussed in detail in Chapter 9. Resolution is frequently achieved by changing the lens to a thicker, lower water content material.[45] No discontinuance of lens wear is necessary.

Superior Arc Stain

An arc pattern in which fluorescein is seen in the midperipheral region of the superior cornea is common with rigid lenses (Fig 7–25). Contributing factors in lens design are a base curve that is too steep, an optic zone too large, inadequate lens movement, or a poorly blended junction between the base and secondary curve. Some of these lens parameters can be modified to treat the condition, whereas base curve changes will require a new lens.[14]

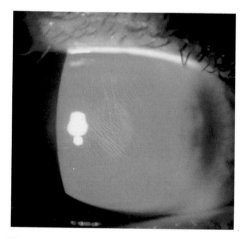

FIG 7–23.
Corneal wrinkling induced by mechanical factors of contact lens wear. (Courtesy of C. Abramson.)

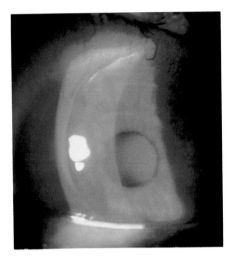

FIG 7–25.
Superior arcuate staining induced by a rigid contact lens.
(Courtesy of C. Abramson.)

Impression Ring Anomaly With Clear Pupil Tinted Soft Lenses

Although impression ring anomaly with clear pupil tinted soft lenses does not represent a true staining pattern on the cornea, it is mentioned in this chapter to provide information for differential diagnosis. The typical patient has very few symptoms other than a slight awareness of reduced quality of vision. The lens being worn is a specific brand of cosmetic color-enhancing, clear pupil, soft contact lens (Fig 7–26). Retinoscopy serves as the key diagnostic test for this condition. The clinician may observe a vague stationary ring or shadowlike reflex within the general region of the pupil that does not move with the blink. On removal of the lens the same shadowlike ring is observed. Keratometry may reveal some change in corneal curvature or minor distortion, depending on the area of depression. Some authors speculate that the back surface of the lens is

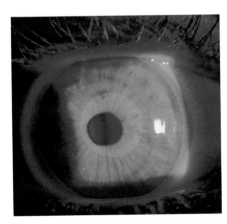

FIG 7–26.
Clear pupil, tinted (non–dot matrix) soft contact lens responsible for corneal impression.

altered in the area of the tint, causing an indentation at the junction with the clear pupil zone and that this is responsible for the corneal depression that occurs over time.

Specific treatment is indicated. Several days without lenses will allow the cornea to recover without any permanent indentation. In addition, the specific contact lens that induced the phenomenon should be replaced by an alternative design.

Furrow Staining and Limbal Hypertrophy

Furrow staining may be a variation of limbal epithelial hypertrophy in which the soft contact lens is thought to act as a tight bandage preventing normal sloughing of the epithelium (Fig 7–27,A). However, the furrow is more of a true stain effect because it remains after irrigation. Furrow staining is common in extended, hydrogel lens wear. Although the patient may be asymptomatic, groovelike furrows appear perpendicular to the limbus, as shown in Figure 7–27,B. Limbal hypertrophy, on the other hand, represents only a pooling of fluorescein in the heaped-up areas of the perilimbal cornea (Fig 7–28).[31]

No specific etiology has been substantiated, but a greater frequency of furrow staining has been observed with extended wear lenses that do not have optimum movement on blinking. Although more commonly seen inferiorly, superior limbal or circumlimbal occurrences can occur. Treatment by switching to a more free-moving lens design usually resolves the condition within 7 to 10 days. Ceasing extended wear by restricting the patient to only daily wear or refitting with RGP lenses may be necessary to prevent further complications. This condition again reemphasizes the value of staining an asymptomatic soft lens patient.

Superior Limbal Epithelial Staining

Superior limbal epithelial staining may be seen with a patient wearing high water content, extended wear soft contact lenses.[1, 47] The observation could occur during a routine follow-up examination, whereupon staining of the superior limbal cornea is evident (Fig 7–29). The eyes may appear quiet, with vision not affected and the patient asymptomatic. The condition is seen in the superior limbal region and is in the same area and has a similar appearance to epithelial splitting, but the lesion is less defined. This complication is considered to be caused by a sealing effect of the superior cornea by the contact lens and the upper lid.[52] It is seen more often with tight, high-riding lenses that show some degree of dehydration.

Treatment is provided by discontinuing lens wear until the lesion disappears. Many practitioners choose to refit with new lenses or a new design.

A B

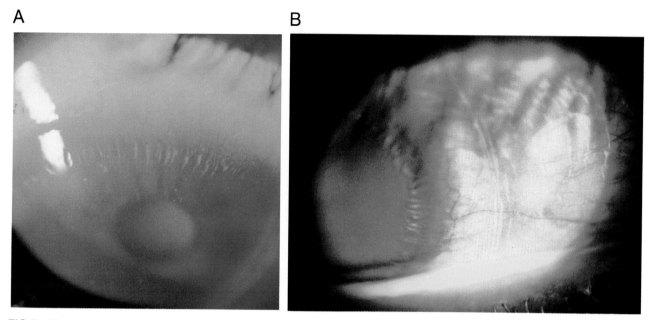

FIG 7–27.
A, furrow staining with soft extended wear contact lens. **B,** furrow staining and epithelial splitting secondary to an old hydrogel lens that was presumably dehydrated, resulting in base curve steepening. (Courtesy of R. Grohe.)

Epithelial Splitting

Epithelial splitting may be called superior epithelial arcuate lesion. It is a commonly missed defect in the superior limbal region of the cornea. It appears as a linear arc-shaped crack in the epithelium (Fig 7–30). Usually, the condition is not apparent until staining procedures are performed. Patients are usually asymptomatic and surprised when the anomaly is discovered. The borderline dry eye

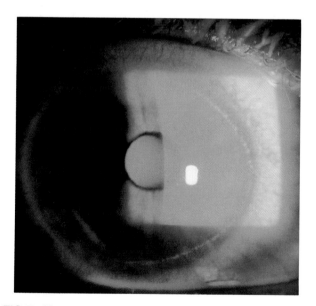

FIG 7–28.
Limbal hypertrophy observed with soft contact lens wear.

patient with this defect may experience occasional mild foreign body sensation after lens removal. Male presbyopes and wearers of high water contact lenses tend to be more likely to develop the condition.[20] Seldom observed clinically are signs of infection, hyperemia, or limbal infiltrates, but neovascularization may be an ultimate consequence if the condition does not resolve. The absence of rose bengal staining and bulbs on the ends of the splits help differentiate this condition from the dendrites in herpes simplex.[7, 16] Normal corneal sensitivity also exists. Opinions vary on the etiology of this condition and implicate hypoxia, edge design, giant papillary hypertrophy, superior limbic keratoconjunctivitis (SLK), foreign bodies, and toxic and infiltrative conjunctivitis.[12, 24]

Treatment usually consists of refitting with a different lens design or material, such as replacing lathe-cut soft lenses with molded or spin-cast design of different water content. Resolution often occurs within 1 week.

Dimple Veiling and Bubble Staining

Dimple veiling is found most often with rigid contact lenses but may be seen occasionally with soft contact lenses (Fig 7–31,A and B). The dimple veil is caused by bubbles depressing the cornea, giving it an appearance similar to a golf ball surface. These bubbles usually result from a poor-fitting relationship,[62] carbon dioxide accumulations under the lens, and inadequate lens movement (Fig 7–31,C). Both large and small bubbles have potential to cause dimple effects (Fig 7–31,D). The corneal dimples

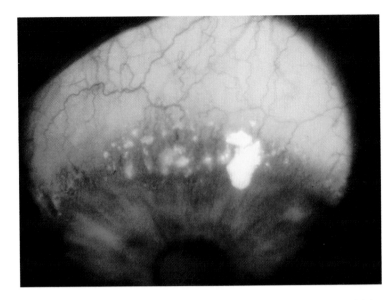

FIG 7-29.
Superior epithelial staining associated with soft lens wear. (Courtesy of Allergan Pharmaceuticals, Inc., Irvine, Calif.)

are usually well defined by fluorescein dye but do not absorb or represent true staining (Fig 7–31,E).

In that the dimples indicate a poor-fitting lens or inadequate metabolic function under the lens, redesigning the lens (by flattening curves or reducing diameter) or using different materials may provide a resolution. Several lens exchanges or skillful modifying of the existing lenses may be necessary and should proceed until no bubbles are observed. Proper follow-up is essential to confirm that the condition does not recur.

CHEMICAL ABRASIONS ASSOCIATED WITH CONTACT LENS WEAR

Abrasions of the ocular tissue from contact lens–related chemicals is common. The reason the condition occurs is

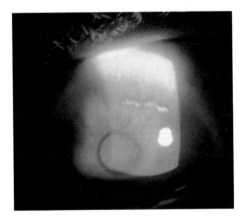

FIG 7-30.
Epithelial splitting associated with soft contact lens wear. (Courtesy of A. Epstein.)

related to the many contact lens care products available, the potential incompatibility of various products when used in conjunction, and the lack of patient understanding of proper sequence of use of products.[50] Other contributing factors include the inadvertent use of the wrong product, the accidental contamination of the lens surface by something transferred from the hands or fingers, or the use of outdated or contaminated care products. A summary of the factors related to chemically induced abrasions of the cornea is given in Table 7–5. Hypersensitivity to a specific agent or a toxic response can also be involved. Therefore, diagnosis of the exact cause is not always easy. Treatment may involve a trial and error approach.

Abrasion as a Result of Failure to Neutralize Hydrogen Peroxide Disinfection Solution

When a patient is switched from a one- to a two-step peroxide system using a neutralizing tablet, it is not always

TABLE 7-5.
Summary of Factors Related to Chemical Abrasion and Stains

1. Hydrogen peroxide
2. Surfactant cleaners
   a. Nonabrasive
   b. Abrasive
3. Enzyme cleaners
4. Preservatives
   a. Thimerosal
   b. Benzylkonium chloride
   c. Chlorhexidine
   d. Ethylenediamine tetraacetate
   e. Sorbic acid
   f. Polyaminopropyl biguanide
   g. Polyquaterium-1 (Polyquad)
   h. Ammonium chloride

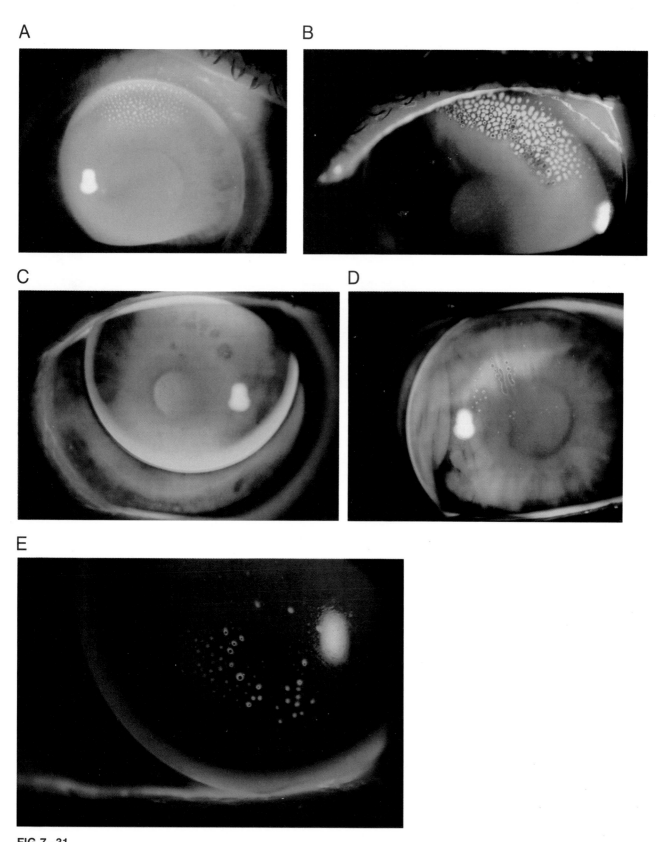

FIG 7–31.
A, dimple veil staining under rigid contact lens. (Courtesy of C. Abramson.) **B,** dimple veil staining under a soft contact lens. (Courtesy of K. Lebow.) **C,** nonwetting rigid contact lens. (Courtesy of P. Caroline.) **D,** large and small bubbles under rigid contact lens. (Courtesy of P. Caroline.) **E,** combined dimple veil and bubble staining under a daily wear RGP lens. (Courtesy of R. Grohe.)

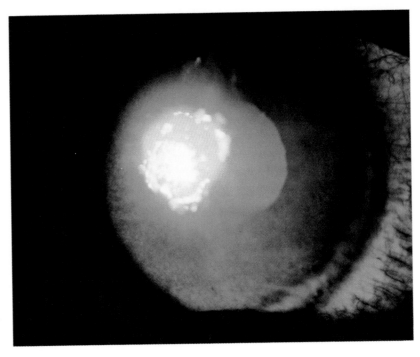

FIG 7–32.
Hydrogen peroxide abrasion of the cornea associated with improper neutralization. (Courtesy of P. Caroline.)

possible to achieve neutralization, especially among high water content (74%) lenses, by the time the lenses are placed on the eyes (Fig 7–32). A similiar problem may occur when hydrogen peroxide is incorrectly used to rinse lenses before insertion. Redness and irritation develop. This type of chemical abrasion requires several days of abstinence, frequent ocular lubricants, and cold compresses to resolve. After the cornea has cleared, resumption of contact lenses can proceed without event by replacing the

lenses and returning the patient to the previous hydrogen peroxide system.

Surfactant Cleaner Abrasion

Chemical staining (Fig 7–33,A), which could have been induced by an accidental exposure of the cornea to a surfactant cleaner applied to a rigid or soft contact lens, can be very severe and painful. The common scenario involves

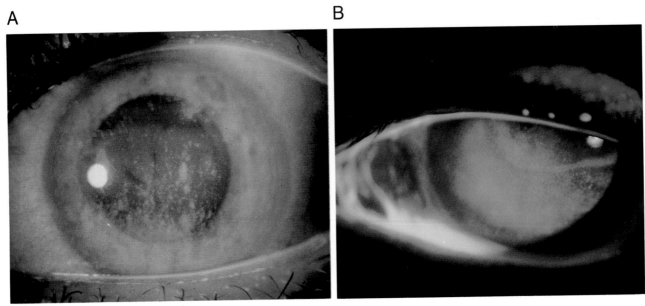

FIG 7–33.
A, surfactant cleaner abrasion. **B,** transcorneal keratitis staining secondary to inadvertent installation of an abrasive surfactant onto an aphakic eye. (Courtesy of R. Grohe.)

not rinsing a daily cleaner off a lens before insertion or mistakenly using a daily cleaner directly in the eyes (as a rewetting drop). A diffuse keratitis can develop where an RGP abrasive cleaner is inappropriately instilled into the eye, as shown in Figure 7–33,B. Treatment depends on the intensity of the wound. Most will heal within a few days and will be helped with lubricants, cold compresses, and lens discontinuance. The potential for secondary infection must be relayed to the patient, and antibiotic and anti-inflammatory medications should be considered.[6, 15] Prevention entails caution when contact lens care products are used. A common factor among surfactant-lubricating drop incidents is the tendency for patients to clean their lenses in the morning rather than at night after removal. Thorough verbal and written instructions to both new and experienced contact lens wearers are essential. Care product manufacturers should be encouraged to provide color-coded container caps to prevent such injuries by allowing easier identification of solutions.

Enzyme Exposure

Incomplete rinsing or incorrect neutralization of enzyme cleaners from lenses can result in residual enzyme causing painful corneal abrasions. This can occur when high water content soft lenses are left in the enzyme for an excessive period and placed in the eye without effective neutralization. In other cases, misdirected use of enzymes as surfactant cleaners or rinses before insertion have occurred.

A typical patient appears with moderate conjunctival infection and general symptoms of irritation and mild burning for several weeks, as shown in Figure 7–34. Treatment consists of lens removal and discontinuance of lenses. It is important to note that enzyme treatments, although traditionally used with soft lenses, are now gaining wider use with RGP lenses, so that these forms of abrasions may now be seen with such patients.

Staining Induced by Sensitivity to Preserved Solutions

Thimerosal has been indicted as the principal sensitizing preservative in many contact lens product hypersensitivity reactions,[5, 47] but sensitivity has also been attributed to other preservatives such as benzalkonium chloride (BAK), chlorhexidine gluconate, ethylenediamine tetraacetate (EDTA), sorbic acid, polyaminoprophyl biguanide (Dymed), polyquaterium-1 (Polyquad), and various ammonium chloride chemicals. Thimerosal hypersensitivity may show mild to severe conjunctivitis, superficial punctate keratopathy (SPK), bulbar and limbal follicles, subepithelial and stromal infiltrates, and neovascularization with continued exposure.[30, 33] The pseudodendrite formation discussed earlier is an example of another potential response to this chemical.

Reaction to BAK-preserved wetting and soaking solution can cause moderate, diffuse SPK staining as observed in the case of an RGP contact lens wearer (Fig 7–35). Symptoms may include reduced visual acuity, photophobia, discomfort, and reduced wearing time. In this case, treatment consisted of discontinuance of contact lens wear for 7 to 10 days. In some cases, simply changing to a non-BAK-preserved solution may suffice as treatment. Some studies indicate no uptake of BAK by RGP contact lens materials,[25] yet cases resolved by discontinuing BAK products are reported. Other studies evaluating BAK binding to RGP surfaces have been contradictory.[51, 61] If a patient is symptomatic, the best approach is to discontinue the use of any BAK-preserved solutions.

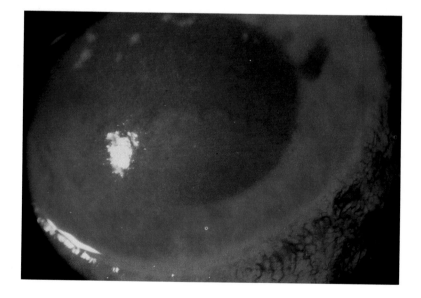

FIG 7–34.
Enzyme abrasion caused by incorrect product usage.

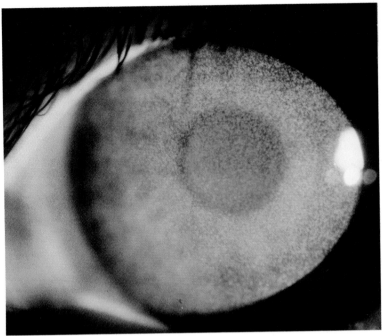

FIG 7–35.
Benzalkonium chloride preservative abrasion associated with RGP contact lens wear. (*Courtesy of K. Lebow.*)

Contact Lens Superior Limbic Keratoconjunctivitis

Superior limbic keratoconjunctivitis is often confused with giant papillary conjunctivitis, vernal limbitis, thimerasol hypersensitivity, and other types of conjunctivitis.[1] Although idiopathic SLK of Theodore has many similar signs and symptoms, the type induced by soft contact lens wear has no relationship to thyroid disease. However, thimerasol sensitivity may be a factor.[56] This complication of soft contact lens wear is limited to the superior cornea.[59] Symptoms of lens awareness, burning, itching, redness, photophobia, and intermittent mucous discharge are common.[47] Mild papillary hypertrophy, inflamed superior tarsal area, bulbar conjunctival staining, superior limbal hypertrophy, epithelial dulling, and punctate staining of the superior one third of the cornea are specific bilateral signs (Fig 7–36). As the condition becomes more severe, faint pannus, linear subepithelial opacities, more intense corneal staining, and reduced visual acuity may be observed.[5] The condition is not well understood and may become chronic for more than 1 year. Treatment dictates cessation of contact lenses, use of ocular lubricants, and possible use of topical corticosteroids. When the problem is resolved, resumption of contact lenses may be considered. The procedure of choice is to refit with RGP lenses and avoid preserved solutions where possible. The condition is discussed in more detail in Chapter 6.

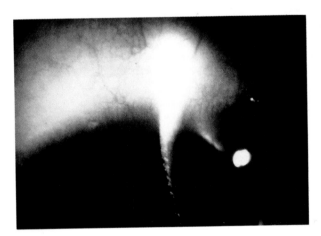

FIG 7–36.
Superior punctate keratitis associated with soft contact lens wear.

FOREIGN BODY ABRASIONS WITH CONTACT LENS WEAR

Corneal abrasions can be induced by foreign particles, tear film residues, or other substance on or under a contact lens. A list of the various causative factors is listed in Table 7–6. Treatment depends on the severity of the abrasion. It requires prompt lens removal, followed by irrigation of the foreign body, discontinuance of lens wear to allow for healing, and application of prophylactic or therapeutic topical medications. Pressure patching may need to be considered on an individual case basis.

TABLE 7-6.

Summary of Foreign Body Abrasions With Contact Lens Wear

Foreign body behind contact lens
Tear film residues or deposits
Dry streak staining
Lens calculi
Cosmetics

Foreign Body Under a Contact Lens

Foreign particles under soft and rigid contact lenses differ in their frequency, mode of entry, and form. A foreign body may occur under a rigid lens anytime after the lens is inserted during the period of wear. Tear pumping under the lens allows these particles to float freely under the lens, causing irritation, discomfort, lacrimation, and a track stain pattern (Fig 7-37). In more severe events, an actual laceration of the cornea may occur (Fig 7-38). In most cases, particles under hard lenses are quickly removed by the same mechanism that allows entry. However, particles under rigid lenses are much more irritating than particles under a soft lens.

Foreign bodies under soft lenses usually occur during insertion and less commonly during the wearing period. Although the snug hydrogel lens minimizes particles entering beneath the lens, a puncture or scraping abrasion may occur if a foreign body is present (Fig 7-39).

Abrasions From Tear Film Residues

Tear film deposits on contact lenses (Fig 7-40,A) may induce corneal staining (Fig 7-40,B). Debris in conjunction with dryness under the lens can cause scuff staining (Fig 7-40,C) with RGP lenses or a pitted stain with soft contact lenses (Fig 7-40,D). The diffuse type of corneal abrasion induced by deposits has a similar appearance with both rigid or soft lenses. Correction of the problem will require lenses to be rigorously cleaned (usually enzymatically) and occasionally rigid lenses polished and hydrogel lenses replaced. In most cases of deposit-induced abrasions, the severity does not require lenses to be discontinued for any significant period. However, patients should be reinstructed in the care of lenses. In chronic lens depositers, a switch to disposable daily wear soft lenses, the use of frequent lubrication with artificial tears, or the switch to a more deposit-resistant lens modality (Chapter 8) is advocated. Patients who wear RGP lenses should use an abrasive surfactant cleaner daily.

Dry Streak Staining

Dry streak staining is associated with rigid contact lenses and occurs as a radial pattern in the midsuperior corneal area beneath the lens (Fig 7-41). It is formed by mucoid debris that accumulates at the junction of the optic zone, producing tracks as the lens displaces downward during the blink. New lens lubricants, alternative surfactant cleaners, or changes in lens design may resolve the problem.

Abrasion From Lens Calculi

Specific to certain hydrogel contact lens materials, certain patients, and modes of wear, these lipid-protein-calcium deposits, often called jelly-bumps, or lens calculi, form on the anterior lens surface (Fig 7-42). Only as these deposits become widespread do patients express symptoms of reduced vision or lens awareness. However, an occasional abrasion is observed because of a puncturing through to the posterior surface or the inadvertent inverted insertion of the lens. Hansen[23] reports that the calculi may produce

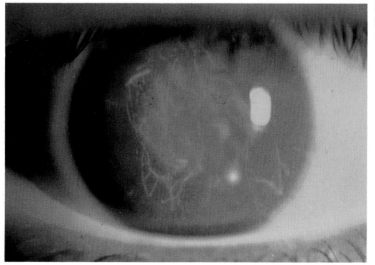

FIG 7-37.
Foreign body abrasion induced by brick dust under rigid contact lens. (Courtesy of A. Tomlinson.)

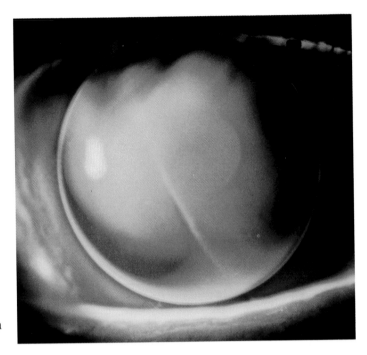

FIG 7–38.
Corneal laceration caused by broken glass under a rigid lens. (Courtesy of P. Caroline.)

corneal distortion, which is seen with retroillumination even if staining is not evident. Most common lens calculi occur with high water content soft lenses worn on an extended wear basis. Experience has shown that the same patients frequently form more calculi in one eye than the other. Improvements in lens care systems, lens designs, patient compliance, reduced extended wear use, daily wear disposables, and more frequent lens replacements have greatly reduced this problem.

FIG 7–39.
Diffuse foreign body abrasion under a soft contact lens.

ABRASIONS RELATED TO THE USE OF COSMETICS

The worlds of fashion and beauty create an interest in products that help people look their best. The use of cosmetics and the wearing of contact lenses fall into this category. Therefore, the clinician must expect various eye and facial cosmetics to be used by many contact lens wear-

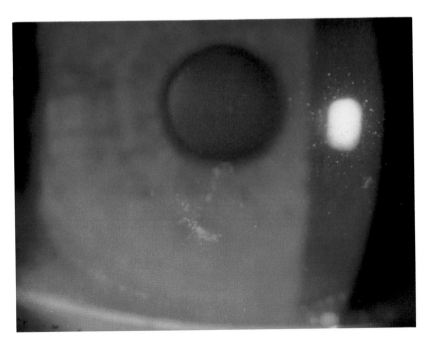

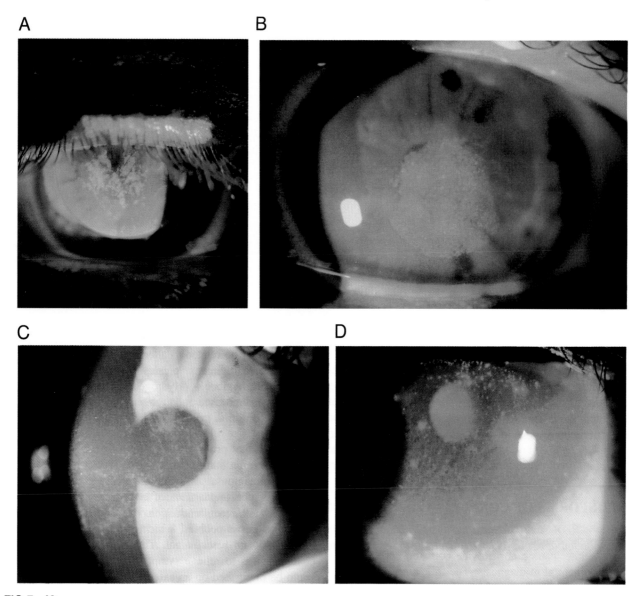

FIG 7–40.
A, lens film on both surfaces of a rigid contact lens. **B,** abrasion induced by lens film under a contact lens. (Courtesy of P. Blaze.) **C,** scuff staining under a rigid contact lens. (Courtesy of P. Caroline.) **D,** staining as a result of trapped debris under a soft contact lens.

ers. Unfortunately, the clinician must also expect to see complications of the two when they are used in combination. Mascara, eye shadow, eyeliner, facial powder, blusher, cleansing cream, moisturizer, highlighter, undereye cream, lip gloss, hair spray, cologne, nail polish, and various associated products are examples of cosmetics that may produce such complications.[34]

Mascara may induce the most common abrasions from cosmetics. Deposits or films on lenses, impregnated chemicals, and discoloration of lenses may occur with cosmetics (Fig 7–43,A). Symptoms of redness, itching, burning, dryness, blurred or transient vision, reduced lens toler-

ance, and foreign body sensation are common with patients using cosmetics. These problems and the need for frequent lens replacement because of the adverse effects of cosmetics can be minimized with some common sense and reasonable use of the products. Heavy eyeliner should not be applied close to the lid margin and tear prism junction. This will greatly reduce the amount of cosmetic residue in the tears. In addition, the sequence of cosmetic application may be modified to avoid ocular complications. The mascara brush injury shown in Figure 7–43,B would not have occurred if the patient's soft contact lens was in place at the time of mascara applications. The preferred daily se-

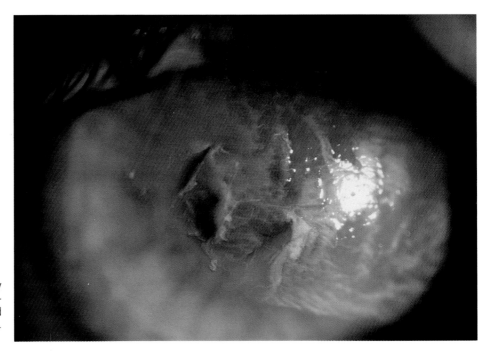

FIG 7–44.
Massive epithelial necrosis by cautery when a hair curling device was accidentally placed on the cornea. (Courtesy of R. Grohe.)

this phenomenon is common with daily wear. Seldom does the patient have any significant symptoms, but the appearance of this condition can be dramatic. The lens in situ may be fixed in place on the cornea and will not move even with a forced blink procedure. Retrolens debris that acts like a biological glue is often seen between the lens and corneal surface (Fig 7–48,A). When the lens is dislodged or removed from the eye, slit-lamp biomicroscopy will reveal an arc-shaped depression stain coincident with the position of the adhered lens edge (Fig 7–48,B). Man-

agement consists of discontinuing lens wear until the adhesion heals, with an initial goal of clearing any residual compression rings. Next, the lens should be modified to allow for greater edge clearance. If this does not eliminate the adhesion, refitting the patient with a slightly opposing fit (if originally fit steep, refit 0.50D flatter; or if originally fit flat, refit 0.25D steep) will usually reduce the problem. A final recourse may require refitting with a soft contact lens. The lens adhesion phenomenon is discussed further in Chapters 8 and 9.

FIG 7–45.
Filaments associated with soft contact lenses. (Courtesy of P. Caroline.)

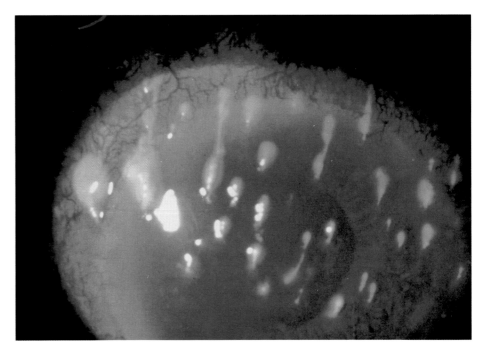

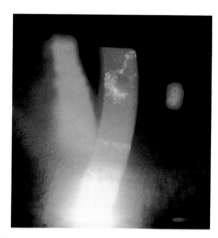

FIG 7–46.
Blotch stain associated with soft lens wear.

Postkeratoplasty Staining With Contact Lens Wear

Surgical grafting of tissue to resolve damaged, defective corneas or to correct highly ametropic conditions may require postsurgical contact lens therapy. The corneal surface beneath the contact lens may provide multiple staining formations. Commonly, a midperipheral circular stain coincident with the graft wound or scar is observable (Fig 7–49). Although this may not always represent true staining but merely fluorescein pooling, this area must be watched closely to avoid infection, ulceration, or other complications such as edema or neovascularization caused by mechanical or hypoxic effects of contact lens wear. The importance of staining as a diagnostic sign takes on greater significance because the graft zone frequently is devoid of any sensitivity until at least 3 years after surgery.[48] Large-diameter, RGP contact lenses should be the modality of

first choice with this type of patient.[10] Soft lenses in a piggyback combination with hard lenses or the RGP-center, soft-skirt combination lenses may also be useful.[9, 63]

Radial Keratotomy and Contact Lens Abrasion

Although radial keratotomy staining is not caused directly by contact lens wear, the use of contact lenses after the refractive procedure may exacerbate this associated complication.[2] Inclusion cysts may form along the incision line scars (Fig 7–50). These cysts could subject the eye to infectious ulceration, especially if the contact lens induces hypoxic or poor tear exchange. Large-diameter, RGP contact lens with optimum fitting to the peripheral cornea is the treatment of choice.[53]

Keratoconus Staining With Contact Lens Wear

The observation of staining in the keratoconic patient wearing contact lenses is usual with the use of rigid lenses. Abrasions of the cone are very common because of the physical alignment of the lens, the advancing status of the condition, deficiencies of tear lubrication, and the fragile nature of this area of the cornea. Swirl staining is typical of this condition (Fig 7–51). Occasional staining of the intermediate cornea may be induced because of poor fitting characteristics of the lens. Peripheral corneal desiccation is also common if limited lens movement is seen. Because of the chronic nature of keratoconus staining, it is important to routinely document its appearance with either a drawing or a photograph so that changes or progression of the condition can be easily assessed.[60] Treatment of these abrasions are important to prevent scarring. Use of soft hydro-

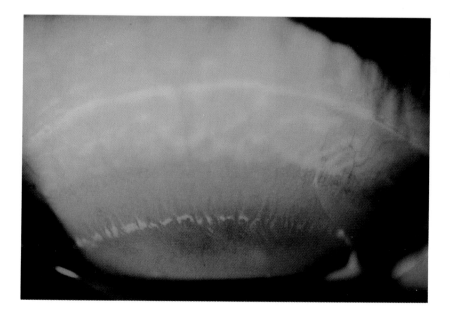

FIG 7–47.
Conjunctival compression stain observed in conjunction with peripheral limbal hypertrophy secondary to extended wear soft contact lenses.

A

B

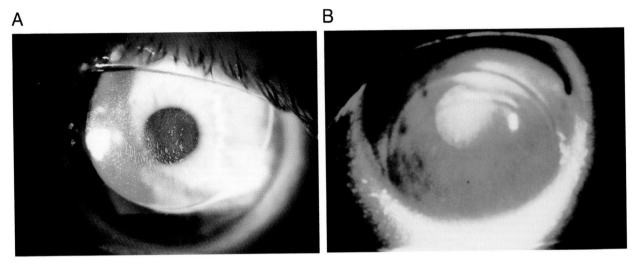

FIG 7–48.
A, adhesion substance under RGP contact lens. (Courtesy of M. Swearingen.) **B,** adhesion abrasion associated with RGP lens. (Courtesy of S. Zantos.)

philic contact lenses as a carrier in a piggyback system or as a temporary bandage can be effective. The hard-center, soft-skirt combination lens (Soft Perm, Sola Barnes Hind, San Diego, Calif.) is also a viable alternative in keratoconus.

Ultraviolet Abrasion With Contact Lens Wear

Overexposure to ultraviolet (UV) radiation is a common occurrence on the ski slopes and by the seaside or lakeside. The contact lens wearer who fails to provide ocular protection from the sun's rays may have photophobia, lacrimation, and difficulty opening the eyes late in the evening or may awaken in the middle of the night with a sore eye. This type of abrasion appears similar to staining seen with a chemical keratitis (Fig 7–52). Treatment entails discontinuance of contact lenses, cold compresses, and oral analgesics, as well as possibly topical prophylactic antibiotics and anti-inflammatories.[7, 15] Adequate healing may require 1 week before contact lens wear can resume. The frequency of this complication can be reduced with the use of newer contact lens materials with UV filters and consistent use of sunglasses.

WOUND HEALING

The abrasion has been detected. A tentative diagnosis and a pending course of action are determined. What takes

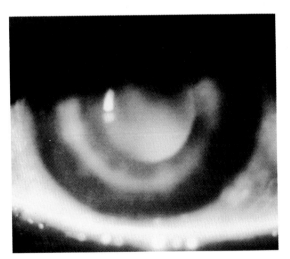

FIG 7–49.
Midperipheral corneal postkeratoplasty scar staining.

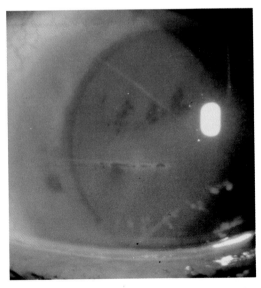

FIG 7–50.
Radial keratotomy scars depicting inclusion cyst formation. (Courtesy of P. Caroline.)

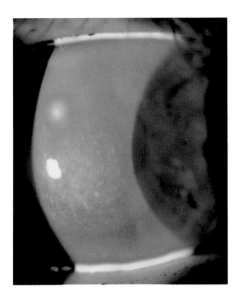

FIG 7–51.
Swirl staining of a keratoconic cornea associated with rigid contact lens wear. (Courtesy of P. Blaze.)

place at the site of damaged ocular tissue? A brief overview of wound healing is presented in this chapter to give a perspective of the healing process after a contact lens abrasion (Fig 7–53). Several factors affect the healing process of a corneal or conjunctival abrasion. The size, location, depth, and causitive agent of the tissue damage are relevant. Because of differences in metabolism, vascular proximity, and cell population, biochemical components at the trauma sight will dictate the specific healing response. Most central corneal abrasions of the epithelial tissue heal quickly if no complications develop.[55] This is particularly so when abrasions are confined to the epithelium and do not extend past Bowman's membrane and into the stroma (e.g., those of mechanical or hypoxic origin). However, deeper, traumatic, more extensive, or peripheral abrasions often require more time to resolve (e.g., following chemical injury). The healing process can be described as comprising three aspects: cell migration, cell division, and epithelial adherence (Fig 7–54). Reepithelialization of small wounds proceeds as the defect is covered by migration of adjacent epithelial cells. Then cell division takes place to thicken the cell layer. Larger wounds take longer to heal because of the need for more mitosis and cell development. The development of microvillae may be the key to cell adhesion to the underlying tissue (Fig 7–55)[8] and provides rapid wound healing. In recurrent corneal erosions,[17] the initial trauma apparently affects the microvillae. Laceration abrasions induce a complex process of healing involving an intricate biochemical and cellular response (Fig 7–56). A tissue plug develops in the wound, and healing proceeds in a timely manner if complications do not develop.

The process of wound healing of the cornea is a very complex, rapidly changing subject that requires the clinician to continually update and review current research.[32, 55] The present standard of care dictates precise judgment from practitioners as to the use of topical medication and pressure patching in the promotion of patient comfort, speed of healing, quality of healing, and prevention of secondary infection. Pharmacological treatment may consist of a short-acting cycloplegic and a topical antibiotic. The use of pressure patching is somewhat controversial. The goal of patching is to enhance comfort by minimizing upper lid movement, which may cause a scrapinglike action that could actually delay reepithelialization. Patching can also increase corneal temperature, thereby enhancing microbial growth. A balanced approach involves no patching for smaller abrasions but aggressive patching in cases of large abrasions or epithelial defects.[46] The use of a bandage effect contact lens is also a matter of judgment by the clinician.

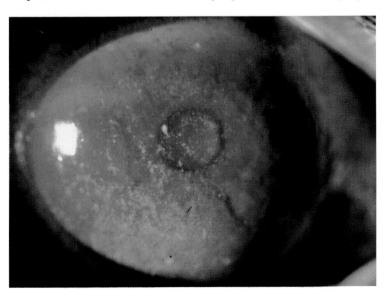

FIG 7–52.
Ultraviolet-induced corneal abrasion occurring in soft contact lens wearer after all-day exposure during snow skiing.

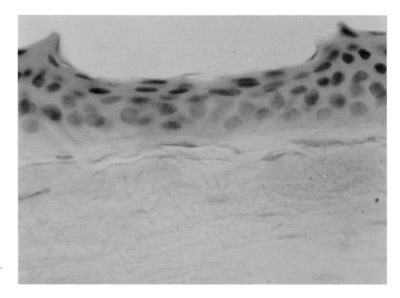

FIG 7–53.
Electron microscopic view of a corneal abrasion.
(Courtesy of P. Caroline.)

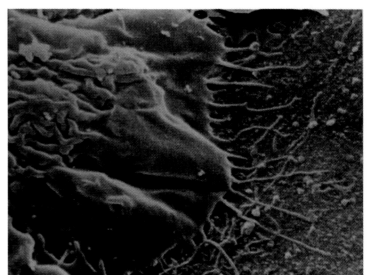

FIG 7–54.
Electron microscopic view of epithelial cell migration. (Courtesy of P. Caroline.)

FIG 7–55.
Electron microscopic view of epithelial microvillae. (Courtesy of P. Caroline.)

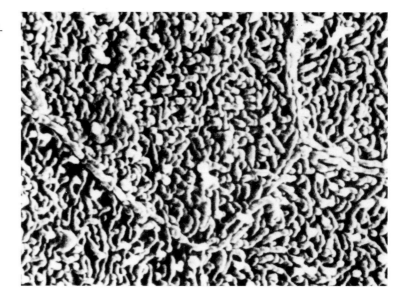

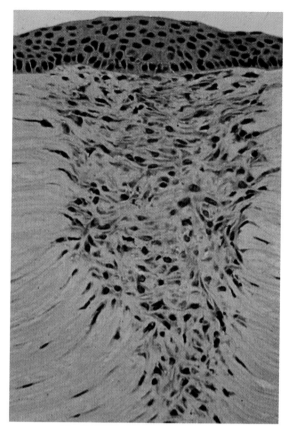

FIG 7–56.
Electron microscopic view of healed cornea laceration-abrasion. (Courtesy of P. Caroline.)

PERSPECTIVE

The detection of corneal or conjunctival abrasion by fluorescein is clinically invaluable. The use of various staining dyes and specific biomicroscopic procedures to visualize the traumatized ocular surface tissue expedites diagnosis and subsequent treatment. Taking the time to use these procedures is paramount to the well-being of the patient. The abrasion conditions depicted in this chapter should serve as a reference guide to the clinician. The greatest attention must be directed at the prevention of serious complications after corneal abrasion secondary to contact lens wear.

REFERENCES

1. Abel R, DePoalis M, Shovlin J: Superior limbic keratitis. *Int Contact Lens Clin* 1985; 12:572–585.
2. Anderson AE: A fundamental approach to post-RK contact lens fitting. *Contact Lens Forum* 1988; 13(12):46–48.
3. Andrasko G: Preliminary evaluation. *Contact Lens Spectrum* 1990; 5(9):40–42.
4. Bron A, Tripathi R: Anterior corneal mosaic. *Br J Physiol Opt* 1970; 25:8–13.
5. Bruce AS, Brennan NA: Corneal pathophysiology with contact lens wear. *Surv Ophthalmol* 1990; 35:25–60.
6. Bourassa S, Benjamin WJ: Microdeposits and associated epithelial surface pits with gel extended wear contact lenses. *Int Contact Lens Clin* 1980; 15:338–340.
7. Cantania LJ: *Primary Care of the Anterior Segment.* Norwalk, Conn, Appleton & Lange, 1988.
8. Caroline PJ: Micrographic study of wound healing. *Contact J Club* 1985.
9. Cohen EJ, Adams CP: Post-keratoplasty fitting for visual rehabilitation, in Dabezies OH (ed): *The CLAO Guide to Basic Science and Clinical Practice.* Orlando, Fla, Grune & Stratton, 1984, vol 2, pp 1–527.
10. Constad WH. Fitting post-op keratoplastic patients with RGP CLS. *Contact Lens Forum* 1988; 13(12):40–44.
11. Courtney RC, Lee JM: Predicting ocular intolerance by use of a filter system enhancing fluorescein staining. *Int Contact Lens Clin* 1982; 9:326–335.
12. Epstein AB: Epithelial splitting. *Contact Lens Forum* 1990; 15(10):66.
13. Epstein AB, Donnenfeld ED: Edematous corneal formations. *Contact Lens Forum* 1990; 15(8):32.
14. Fonn D, Gauthier C: Aftercare of RGP lens wearers. *Contact Lens Spectrum* 1990; 5(9):71–82.
15. Fraunfelder FT, Roy FH: *Current Ocular Therapy,* ed 3. New York, WB Saunders Co, 1990.
16. Forstot SL: Marginal corneal degenerations. *Int Ophthalmol Clin* 1984; 24:93–106.
17. Galbavy EJ, Mobilia EF, Kenyon KR: Recurrent corneal erosions. *Int Ophthalmol Clin* 1984; 24:107–131.
18. Goldberg JB: *Biomicroscopy for Contact Lens Practice,* ed 2. Chicago, Professional Press, 1984.
19. Goldberg JB: Dehydration of contact lenses. *Int Contact Lens Clin* 1990; 17:197–198.
20. Grant T, Terry R, Holden BA: Extended wear of hydrogel lenses, in Harris MG (ed): *Problems in Optometry: Contact Lenses and Ocular Disease.* Philadelphia, JB Lippincott, Co, 1990, vol 2, pp 599–622.
21. Grohe RM: RGP problem solving. *Contact Lens Spectrum* 1990; 5(9):82–83.
22. Guralnik DB: *Webster's New World Dictionary of American Language.* New York, Collins & World, 1978.
23. Hansen D: Corneal irregularities caused by patient non compliance. *Contact Lens Spectrum* 1990; 5(10):85–86.
24. Hine HA, Bach AT, Holden BA: An etiology of arcuate epithelial lesions incurred by hydrogels. *Trans Br Contact Lens Assoc* 1984; 4:48–50.
25. Hoffman WC: Ending the BAK-RGP controversy. *Int Contact Lens Clin* 1987; 14:31–35.
26. Holden B: Suffocating the cornea with PMMA. *Contact Lens Spectrum* 1989; 4(5):69–70.
27. Hum LG, Schwaderer KN: Filamentary keratitis associated with contact lens wear. *Int Contact Lens Clin* 1987; 14:117.
28. Josephson J: Microcysts. *Int Contact Lens Clin* 1979; 6:40.
29. Kame RT: Clinical management of edematous corneal formations. *Rev Opt* 1979; 116:49–71.

30. Kame RT: Adverse ocular response to soft lens solutions. *Contact Lens Forum* 1984; 9(1):97.

31. Kame RT: Limbal epithelial hypertrophy. *Int Contact Lens Clin* 1987; 14:453.

32. Kinosita S, Friend J, Thoft RA: Ocular surface epithelial regeneration and disease. *Int Ophthalmol Clin* 1984; 24:169–177.

33. Kline LN, DeLuca TF, Fishberg GM: Corneal staining. *J Am Optom Assoc* 1979; 50:353–357.

34. Koetting RA: Cosmetic complications of contact lens wear. *Int Ophthalmol Clin* 1981; 21:185–193.

35. Korb DR: Transparency with emphasis on the phenomenon of central circular clouding, in Haynes PR (ed): *Encyclopedia of Contact Lens Practice.* South Bend, Ind, Encyclopedia of Contact Lens Practice, 1962.

36. Korb DR: Edematous corneal formations. *J Am Optom Assoc* 1973; 44:246–253.

37. Korb DR, Herman JP: Corneal staining, subsequent to sequential fluorescein instillation. *J Am Optom Assoc* 1979; 50:361–367.

38. Laibson PR: Ocular adenoviral infection. *Int Ophthalmol Clin* 1984; 24:49–64.

39. Lasswell L: Slit lamp adaptation of Wratten filters. *Contact Lens Study Exchange,* August 1990, personal communication.

40. Lin ST, Mandell RB: Corneal blotting from extended wear. *Contact Lens Spectrum* 1991; 6(2):25–28.

41. Lowe R, Brennan NA. Corneal wrinkling caused by thin medium water content lens. *Int Contact Lens Clin* 1987; 14:403–406.

42. Mandel ER, Wagoner MD: *Atlas of Corneal Disease.* Philadelphia, WB Saunders Co, 1989.

43. Martonyi CL, Bahn CF, Meyer RF. *Clinical Slit Lamp Biomicroscopy,* ed 2. Mich, Time One Ink, 1985.

44. Olsen RJ: Herpes zoster. *Int Ophthalmol Clin* 1984; 24:39–48.

45. Osborn GN, Zantos SG: Corneal desiccation staining with thin high water content contact lenses. *CLAO J* 1988; 14:81–85.

46. Parrish CM, Chandler JW: Corneal trauma, in Kaufman HJ, Barron BA, McDonald MB, et al (eds): *The Cornea.* New York, Churchill Livingstone, pp 599–646. 1988,

47. Pettit TH, Meyer KT: Differential diagnosis of superficial punctate keratitis. *Int Ophthalmol Clin* 1984; 24:79–92.

48. Phillips AJ: Post-keratoplasty contact lens fitting, in Harris MG (ed.): *Problems in Optometry: Contact Lenses and Ocular Disease.* Philadelphia, JB Lippincott Co, 1990, pp 664–684.

49. Quinn TG: Epithelial folds. *Int Contact Lens Clin* 1982; 9:365.

50. Rodgin JI: *Pathology and Pharmacology of the Eye.* Chicago, Professional Press, 1983.

51. Rosenthal P, Chou MH, Salamone JC, et al: Quantitative analysis of chlorhexidine gluconate and benzalkonium chloride adsorption on silicone/acrylate polymers. *CLAO J* 1986; 12:43–50.

52. Schoessler JP: Superior epithelial abrasion with extended contact lens wear. *Int Contact Lens Clin* 1980; 7:46.

53. Shivitz IA: Fitting contact lenses after radial keratotomy. *Contact Lens Forum* 1988; 13(12):38–39.

54. Shulman PF: Clinical implications of arcuate staining with B&L Soflens. *Int Contact Lens Clin* 1977; 4:55.

55. Smolin G, Thoft RA: *The Cornea,* ed 2. Boston, Little, Brown & Co, 1987.

56. Stenson SM: Soft lens related SLK. *Contact Lens Forum* 1986; 11(12):22–24.

57. Stenson SM: Contact lenses a guide to selection, fitting, and management of complications. Norwalk, Conn, Appleton & Lange, 1987.

58. White PF, Miller D: Corneal edema. *Int Ophthalmol Clin* 1981; 21(2):3–12.

59. Wilson WM, Ostler HB: Superior limbic keratoconjunctivitis. *Int Ophthalmol Clin* 1986; 26:172–185.

60. Winegar W: A management overview of the keratoconus patient. *Contact Lens Forum* 1988; 13(12):28–34.

61. Wong MP, Dziabo AJ, Kiral RM: Adsorption of benzalkonium chloride by RGP lenses. *Contact Lens Forum* 1986; 11(5):25–32.

62. Zadnik K: A case of dimple veiling/staining. *Contact Lens Forum* 1988; 13(2):68–69.

63. Zadnik K: Post-surgical contact lens alternatives. *Int Contact Lens Clin* 1988; 15:211–220.

64. Zantos SG: Cystic formations in corneal epithelium during extended wear of contact lenses. *Int Contact Lens Clin* 1983; 10:114–117.

65. Zantos SG: Corneal infiltrates, debris and microcysts. *J Am Optom Assoc* 1984; 55:197.

66. Zantos SG, Zantos PO: Extended wear feasibility of gas permeable hard contact lenses for myopes. *Int Eye Care* 1985; 1:66–78.

67. Zuccaro VS: Rose bengal a vital stain. *Contact Lens Forum* 1981; 6(10):39.

PART III

Xerosis

Tear Film Changes With Contact Lens Wear

Alan Tomlinson, Ph.D., F.B.C.O.

The entire anterior ocular surface is covered by a tear film. This film has great versatility and is capable of adaptation to changes in its environment. However, these adaptations are not limitless, and in the presence of sufficient adversity, it displays a fragility that can lead to the eye being exposed to potential dangers and reductions in function.

A great deal of clinical observation and research has been directed toward determining the effect of contact lens wear on the corneal tissue (see Chapters 1–7). However, the most intimate contact (and possible effect) of the contact lens is on the preocular tear film. Although less attention has been directed in the past toward the effect of contact lens wear on the tear film, an emerging body of new information is being generated. An ideal contact lens would minimally disturb the normal, preocular tear film, but such a lens does not exist. Significant alterations do occur to the structure, composition, physiochemical properties, and dynamic behavior of the tear film as a result of contact lens wear. In this chapter the effects of contact lens wear on all these aspects of the tear film are discussed.

An intact tear film is essential for the health and correct visual function of the eye. The tear film has four principal functions.[138, 161] First, it provides a uniform optical surface for the cornea (the tear film filling in irregularities within the corneal tissue), and second, it flushes cellular debris and foreign matter from the cornea and the conjunctival sac. For the latter function, the tear film must provide lubrication for the anterior ocular surfaces. Third, the film provides the cornea with nutriment needed to carry out its normal metabolic activity, namely, dissolved oxygen from the atmosphere, which is the principal source of supply to the corneal epithelium and stroma (see Chapter 1). The final role of the tears is in a defense of the cornea, achieved primarily by the antibacterial activity of certain of its constituent proteins and enzymes.

STRUCTURE OF THE TEAR FILM

The tear film is classically described as a three-layer structure consisting of the anterior or superficial lipid layer, a central aqueous phase and the underlying mucus layer immediately adjacent to the corneal epithelium (Fig 8–1).[198] A more complete representation of the tear film, however, would require a six-layer model, as described by Tiffany,[178] which takes account of additional layers and interfaces (Fig 8–2). The average thickness of the tear film has been estimated as between 4 and 6 μm.[90, 131, 132] This film is thickest immediately after the blink and decreases during eye opening to a minimum of about 4 μm.[146] The tear film is thinnest over the ocular surface within the lid aperature. Along each lid margin the tears form a meniscus where the eyelid touches the globe, which extends along the entire upper and lower eyelids. Twenty-five percent of the exposed tear volume is contained in the tear meniscus.[91] Tears drain from the eye via the puncta, which dip into the lacrimal river formed along the tear meniscus. Reformation of the preocular tear film takes place with each blink as the compressed lipid layer

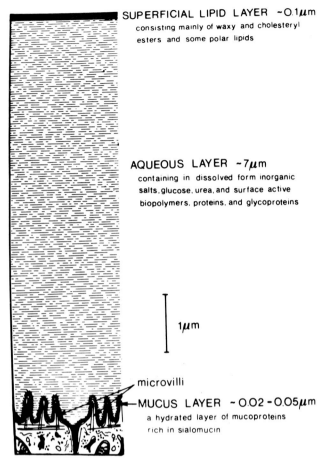

SUPERFICIAL LIPID LAYER ~0.1μm
consisting mainly of waxy and cholesteryl
esters and some polar lipids

AQUEOUS LAYER ~7μm
containing in dissolved form inorganic
salts, glucose, urea, and surface active
biopolymers, proteins, and glycoproteins

1μm

microvilli
MUCUS LAYER ~0.02-0.05μm
a hydrated layer of mucoproteins
rich in sialomucin

FIG 8–1.
The structure of the tear film drawn to scale. (From Holly FJ, Lemp MA: *Surv Ophthalmol* 1977; 22:69. Used by permission.)

SIX-LAYER TEAR FILM MODEL

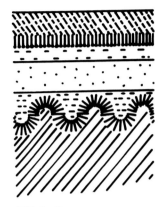

AIR

Oily layer
Polar lipid monolayer
Adsorbed mucoid

Aqueous layer

Mucoid layer
"Glycocalyx"
CORNEAL
EPITHELIUM

FIG 8–2.
A six-layer model of the tear film showing the additional layers and interfaces. (From Tiffany J: *J Br Contact Lens Assoc* 1988; 11:35. Used by permission.)

Zeiss.[138] A duplex structure has been ascribed to this film in which the outer layer consists of cholesterol esters and the inner layer a molecular film of phospholipids, fatty acids, and free cholesterol.[161] The functions of the lipid layer are to retard evaporation of the underlying aqueous layer[107, 141] and to form a barrier along the lid margins that retains the lid margin tear strip and prevents its overflow onto the skin.[138] This prevents surface contamination of the tear film with the highly polar lipids of the skin of the face; such contact would lead rapidly to breakup of the tear film.[90]

The most substantial component of the tear film is the middle aqueous phase, which comprises 98% of the total tear film thickness,[91] or 6 to 7 μm of its thickness.[138] This phase, secreted by the lacrimal gland and the accessory glands of Krause and Wolfing, contains many of the substances that provide the nutriments and defensive properties of the tears. It contains inorganic salts, glucose, and urea, as well as biopolymers, proteins, and glycoproteins.

The innermost layer of the tears immediately adjacent to the epithelial cells of the cornea is comprised of mucus (see Fig 8–1). This layer in its functional form comprises less than 0.5% of the total tear thickness, or less than 0.05 μm.[91] This layer of mucus glycoproteins is secreted by the more than 1.5 million Goblet cells of the conjunctiva and subsurface vesicles contained within this tissue.[161] The mucus layer serves several functions in the action of the tear film. The intimate relationship between the mucus layer and the microvillae and microplicae of the corneal epithelial cells helps to form the attachment of the tear layer to this underlying cellular structure.[138] It also provides a lubricant for lid action. Mucus threads within the tear film are the means of removal for entrapped debris,

between the two closed eyelids extends upward with the opening of the lid. This action drags the aqueous layer with it and effectively thickens the tear film. If blinking does not recur before the tear film thins as a result of evaporation, small black holes will be seen in the layer, which may lead to corneal or conjunctival drying. The rate at which this drying occurs is a measure of tear film stability.

STRUCTURE OF THE TEAR FILM IN CONTACT LENS WEAR

The tear film consists of distinct phases already described as three separate layers[198] or six if all the interposing interfaces are considered (see Figs 8–1 and 8–2).[178] The anterior or superficial phase, comprising about 1% of the total tear film thickness,[91] or 10 mμm,[161] is a layer of lipid derived principally from the tarsal (meibomian) glands of the lid margins and the accessory subaceous glands of the cells, and foreign bodies. Such intruders are entrapped within the mucus threads, which slowly migrate toward the edge of the lids and eventually to the caruncle before removal from the eye.[147] Little, if any, conjunctival mucus passes down the lacrimal drainage passages.[143] Holly and Lemp[95] have suggested that the epithelium of the cornea is hydrophobic and that covering by a surfactant such as mucus is necessary to render it wettable and to give a stable tear film. This assertion has been challenged by Cope et al.[32] who suggest that the structure of the cell membranes in conjunction with the presence of glycocalyx on the cell's surface makes the concept of cellular nonwettability unlikely (see Fig 8–2). Recent experiments on rabbit corneas[178] indicate that the corneal epithelium is highly wettable after the removal of mucus by acetylcysteine rinsing. However, mechanical wiping of the surface appears to be highly damaging and produces low wettability. This suggests that the lubrication function in which the mucus layer provides a buffer for lid movement over the anterior ocular surface may be its principal function. Alternative mechanisms for corneal epithelial wetting have been proposed. Dilley[36] has suggested that the glycocalyx of the corneal epithelium serves as an intermediary to the fixation of mucus to the epithelial surface. Liotet et al.[120] maintain that the surfacing agent for the corneal epithelium is the glycocalyx and not the mucus; therefore, the disappearance of goblet cells during dry eye syndromes is not the cause but the result of the dryness, epithelial cell integrity being an essential for the stability of the tear film.

The presence of a contact lens in the eye has dramatic effects on tear film structure. In recent years considerable interest has been focused on evaluating tear film structure in the presence of contact lenses using the technique of interference fringe patterns. This technique is often ascribed to a suggestion by McDonald,[134] although Koby[112] and Ehlers[41] had previously noticed diffuse patterns in tear film. McDonald[134] is credited with the suggestion that the principle of thin film phase shift to establish destructive interference patterns can be used to observe the thickness and nature of the tear film lipid layer.

Hamano,[72] Josephson,[103] Guillon,[68, 69] Forst,[48] and Doane[37] have used the noninvasive technique of interference fringe microscopy to qualitatively and quantatively assess the behavior and thickness of the lipid and aqueous phases of the tear film in normal and pathological ocular states and in the presence of contact lenses. The various applications of the technique have included high- and low-magnification camera systems,[68, 72] modified slit-lamp biomicroscopes,[48, 103] handheld instruments in association with slit lamps,[68, 69, 185] and high-speed video recording.[37]

Hamano[72] was the first to describe the typical surface patterns of tears using the interferometer technique. He described three categories of patterns as marmoreal, flow,

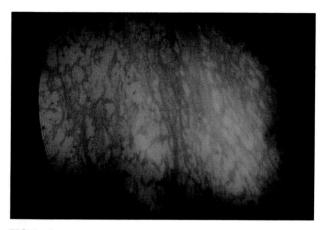

FIG 8–3.
Interference fringe pattern seen from the human tear film. This is the pattern described as marmoreal. (Courtesy of J. Josephson.)

and amorphous. These categories were extended to four by Guillon,[68] when he described a colored fringe pattern. In normal human eyes the marmoreal pattern occurs in the majority, 90% according to Hamano[72] and 60% according to Guillon.[68] This pattern appears as a marblelike structure seen with or without the presence of contamination (Figs 8–3 and 8–4). It appears gray and is said to be found in the presence of a lipid layer 13 to 70 nm thick. The amorphous pattern is the next most common, occurring in about 15% of patients, and indicates a thick, stable pattern. Its color is an even blue-gray and is indicative of a thick lipid layer 70 to 90 nm (Fig 8–5). The flow pattern[68] (Fig 8–6) has an incidence of approximately 10% and is easily recognizable by its wavy pattern, which is caused by the spreading of various lipids at different thicknesses across the surface. The lipid thickness is highly variable and in the range of 10 to 90 nm. The colored fringe pattern occurs in less than 5% of cases (Fig 8–7).[68] This pattern indicates higher lipid layer thicknesses ranging from 86 to 170 nm. Such patterns often show lipid films contaminated by mucus strands or lumps, which appear as dark spots in the film.

The type of pattern can indicate the suitability of the patient for contact lens wear. Patients with contaminated, marmoreal patterns often show excessive surface drying and deposit buildup when fitted with lenses, whereas patients with amorphous patterns show good tolerance for contact lens wear. Such patients, however, may show lipid deposition on soft lenses. Patients with flow patterns also show good tolerance to contact lens wear. Those with colored fringe patterns, which are indicative of excessive secretions by meibomian glands, may have chronic blepharitis and may be poor candidates for contact lens wear because of a predisposition to deposit formation.[68] Hamano[72] has observed that the pattern may change in the

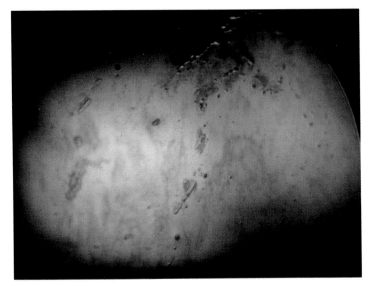

FIG 8–4.
A contaminated marmoreal interference fringe pattern. Contact lens patients with this type of pattern may show excessive surface drying and deposit formation. (Courtesy of J. Josephson.)

presence of contact lens wear. The most common pattern in the non–contact lens wearing eye, that of the marmoreal form, is less frequently seen, and the structureless amorphous pattern becomes dominant.[68] This pattern is seen to persist even after the removal of contact lenses, probably as a result of tear film instability induced by lens wear. Hamano[72] has observed that the interference fringe pattern is closely correlated with breakup time, the application of the contact lens changing the surface pattern of the tear film toward that of the amorphous type and shortening the tear breakup time. Because the interference fringe pattern may differ from the center to the periphery

of the cornea even in the normal non–wearing contact lens eye, Hamano[72] restricts his observations to the central portion of the cornea. It is perhaps significant that less stable patterns are seen at the corneal periphery, an area in which tear breakup is seen to occur first.

Observations made of the tear film, particularly the tear film over a contact lens, can be of interest because they give some indication of the presence of a lipid film and the thickness of the underlying aqueous layer. Where the lipid is broken, a wedge-shaped tear film will be produced and an interference fringe pattern observed. Fringes of equal thickness are equally spaced in straight lines par-

FIG 8–5.
Interference fringe pattern from the human tear film showing the amorphous pattern. Patients with this type of pattern show good tolerance for contact lenses. (Courtesy of Contact Lens Research Consultants, London.)

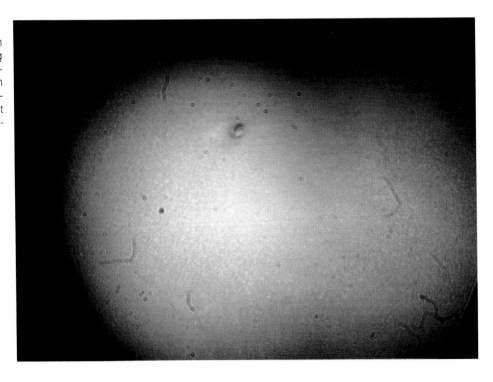

A

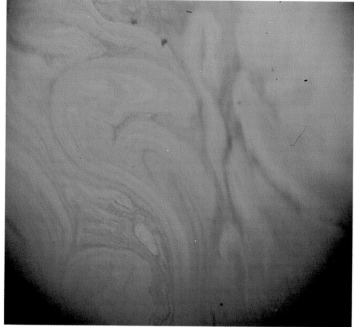

B

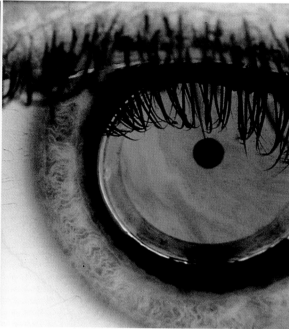

FIG 8–6.
Interference fringe pattern from the human tear film showing the flow pattern seen in high magnification in **A,** and in the low magnification view in **B** obtained with the handheld Tearscope (C-L-R-C). Patients with this pattern show good tolerance to contact lens wear. (Courtesy of Contact Lens Research Consultants, London.)

allel to the edge of the wedge and represent the increase in wedge thickness.[68] The color and separation of the fringes can be used as an indicator of the angle of the very thin wedge-shaped sheets that form in the tear film. When white light is used in the observation system, colored

fringes will be observed in the tear film. If the lipid layer is thinner than 86 nm, no interference colors will be present, but different lipid patterns in varying shades of gray will be distinguished. For greater lipid thicknesses, interference fringe patterns will be seen in the lipid layer

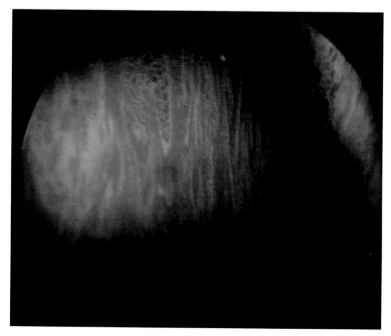

FIG 8–7.
Interference fringe pattern from the human tear film showing the color fringe pattern. These patterns are indicative of excessive secretion of the meibomian glands and are found in patients with chronic blepharitis and those who are poor candidates for contact lens wear. (Courtesy of J. Josephson.)

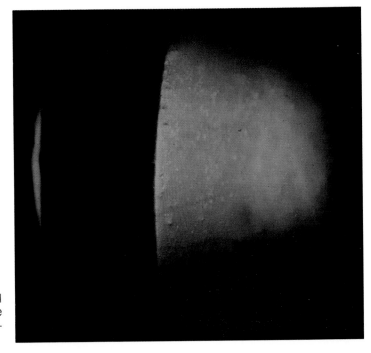

FIG 8–8.
The tear film on a hydrogel contact lens. A vertical line of colored interference fringes is seen near the anterior edge bevel of the lens. (Courtesy of J. Josephson.)

itself. In those situations where the lipid layer is broken or totally absent (i.e., contact lens wear), interference fringe patterns will be seen from the aqueous layer, which will allow an estimate of its thickness. Where the tear film thickness is greater, the interference fringe patterns will be seen to separate; where the tear film thickness is less, the fringes will be seen to come together and the color will be more intense.

Guillon[68] has described the appearance of the tear film in the presence of various types of contact lenses (Fig 8–8). On hydrogel lenses he has observed that a thin lipid layer is present most commonly in a marmoreal or flow pattern. The amorphous pattern is present in unfavorable cases of unstable prelens tear film. Of the different types of hydrogel lens materials, polyhydroxyethylmethacrylate (PHEMA) appears to have the most stable prelens tear film, whereas films on the front of higher water content polymers are thinner and less stable. Lens geometry is also thought to affect the prelens tear film on hydrogel lenses. Those of standard thickness and ultrathin lenses have thicker and more stable tear films than hyperthin lenses, where the lipid layer may not be visible. It has been noted that an increase in lens movement is highly disruptive to the prelens tear film observed by interference fringe techniques.

Guillon's[68] findings of a stable lipid layer on the anterior surface of hydrogel lenses is not confirmed by Young and Efron.[202] They report that the lipid layer was absent or very thin on hydrogel lens surfaces, with water content ranging from 36.5% to 85%. It was only in the higher water content lenses that lipid layers were seen at all. This is interpreted to be a benefit of the high water lens because the presence of the lipid layer would support a thicker aqueous layer on the anterior surface of such lenses.

On hard contact lenses, the prelens lipid layer is usually absent. The aqueous layer then seems to form a continuously thinning wedge that can be evaluated by the separation of fringes and their color to determine its actual thickness. It is probable that the edge of the hard contact lens acts as a barrier to the propogation of the superficial lipid layer over the surface of the thin unstable aqueous prelens tear film (Fig 8–9).[68] Guillon[68] has noted the presence of some superficial lipid layer on more wettable rigid gas-permeable (RGP) lens materials and on lenses of larger diameter. On such lenses the marmoreal appearance is more likely to be noted, indicating a relatively more stable tear film. The more stable tear film with larger-diameter RGP lenses is probably the result of lid coverage of part of the lens edge. This suppresses the breakup effect of the lens edge, creating a more normal tear meniscus and enhancing tear spreading on the anterior surface of the lens. This observation would argue for the fitting of RGP lens designs according to the Korb or superior positioning (lid attachment) fitting philosophy. The observations of Guillon[68] are somewhat at odds with those of Doane and Gleason,[38] who have observed, using video tear film interferometry, that the flow of the prelens tear film is usually toward the adjacent meniscus at the edge of the lid. This can occur even against gravity in the case of a lid attachment fit. They have noted that the most stable tear film occurs with interpalprebral fitting philosophies.

Bleshoy and Guillon[68] have modified the specular

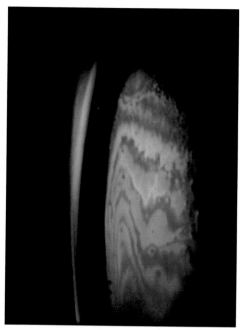

FIG 8–9.
The tear film over a rigid gas-permeable (RGP) lens. The tear film shows an incomplete lipid layer and colored fringe patterns from the aqueous phase of the tears. (Courtesy of Contact Lens Research Consultants, London.)

noncontact microscope to observe the mucus layer of the tear film in the presence of contact lenses. They note that on the corneal epithelial surface the absorption mechanism of the cells ensures a secure, but thin, mucus coverage that conforms to the underlying shape of the surface. On contact lenses, however, the mucus coverage was found to be thicker and more loosely attached in the case of hydrogel materials. On rigid corneal lenses, no mucus layer was visible, but during drying some remnants were seen as loose globules varying in size and attached to the surface. They concluded that contact lens materials are less easily wetted with tear film mucus and are more dependent on the spreading mechanism of lid action to maintain the presence of the film. Thus, any incongruities of lid to ocular and lens surfaces will lead to inadequate mucus spread and consequent tissue and surface drying.

Recent observations on high water content hydrogel lens materials by Guillon and Guillon[69] during extended wear cycles have noted significantly more stable and thicker tear films immediately on waking than during the open eye phase of extended wear. The presence of a more stable prelens (particularly lipid layer) tear film at waking might well account for the different rate of tear film evaporation noted at this time. Also, the greater thickness of mucus after overnight lens wear may well contribute to lens tightness and adhesion found in overnight wear of both hydrogel and RGP lens materials. This may be the

mechanism of adhesion instead of dehydration during overnight wear. Brennan et al.[11] have failed to demonstrate lens dehydration during sleep.

Forst[48] has described the color sequence observed during his microscopic observations of the structure of the tear film lipid layer. He has observed some lipid coverage of hydrogel and RGP lens materials. Further, Forst[48] has noted that the interference fringe patterns seen on contact lens patients are similar to those noted in heavy smokers; this may indicate a less stable tear film in such patients.

Other changes in the structure of the tear film as a result of contact lens wear has been studied by others.[201] Hayashi[79] has observed the mechanics of contact lens motion, and Conway and Richmond[28] have studied the pressures induced in the tear film between a hydrogel contact lens and the eye during the initial stages of blinking. It was found that the effects of soft lens deformation reduces the pressure on the tear film, especially when that tear film is thin. In a later study these same workers studied the motion of a contact lens toward the eye during the blinking process; the tear film thickness was increased, as was comfort to the patient with a decrease in the modulus of the lens material. Thus, lenses with a decreased modulus, for instance, a hydrogel lens, would give greater comfort and tear layer thickness than a hard contact lens with a higher modulus. Therefore, it is possible that hydrogel lenses maintain greater tear film thicknesses beneath them than do hard lenses during the blink.[29] Martin and Holden[127] confirmed that the force beneath the hydrogel lens was dependent on the elastic modulus of the material, as well as the thickness and bearing relationship of the lens. They found that the pressure beneath the contact lenses was negative with respect to the atmospheric pressure of the corneal apex and became less negative at the corneoscleral limbus.[127]

STABILITY OF THE TEAR FILM IN CONTACT LENS WEAR

For the tear film to provide the functions just described, it is important that it be stable and that the relative position of its various layers not be disturbed. The stability of the tear film may be disturbed in various pathological states[96, 130] or in the presence of contact lens wear.[91, 92, 172] Mechanisms by which the tear film is destabilized have been discussed by several workers, and it is important to review their various theories before a detailed discussion of the contact lens effects on tear film stability is supplied.

DISRUPTION OF THE NORMAL TEAR FILM

The disruption of tear film stability and the development of dry spots on the ocular surface were thought originally[140] to be caused by drying of small areas of the tear film because of discontinuity of the lipid layer.[140] This is unlikely, however, because dry spot formation by evaporation of the total thickness of the tear film would take more than 10 minutes.[91] This is considerably longer than the dry spot formation time in most humans, which is between 30 seconds and 1 minute. Holly[87] and Lemp et al.[116] advanced an alternative theory for the mechanism of tear film rupture based on the assumption that the lipids present at the tear-air interface migrate rather rapidly to the mucus-aqueous interface and eventually overwhelm the hydrophilic capacity of the mucus layer, thus creating localized areas of high hydophobicity on the corneal epithelium (Fig 8–10). These nonwettable areas increase until substantial tear film breakup takes place. These areas of nonwettability are not present in the normal eye, provided the blink mechanism is functioning. Because it usually takes 20 to 30 seconds to develop, the tear film is reestablished by the normal blink action of the lid passing across the anterior ocular surface and the maintenance of the normal relative positions of lipid and mucus layers. This reestablishment of the tear film layer, however, may not take place in the presence of abnormally unstable tear films, for instance, dry eye conditions, or in the presence of a contact lens (see later discussion).

The theories of Holly, although widely accepted, have been challenged recently by Sharma and Ruckenstein.[172] The dispute centers on the likelihood that a moderate increase in interfacial tension at a mucus-aqueous interface is sufficiently high to make the mucus layer nonwettable (especially because the tear-air interfacial tension is increased by the presence of lipids). In addition, they assert that the presence of lipids is not necessary for tear film rupture observed even in the event of complete obstruction of the meibomian gland openings.[96] Sharma and Ruckenstein[172] elaborate on a theory originally postulated by Lin and Brenner,[119] who ascribed the rupture of the entire tear film to van der Waals' dispersion forces acting on the aqueous tear film. Although these dispersion forces are unlikely to cause rupture of the entire tear film within the normally observed tear breakup time, Sharma and Rucken-

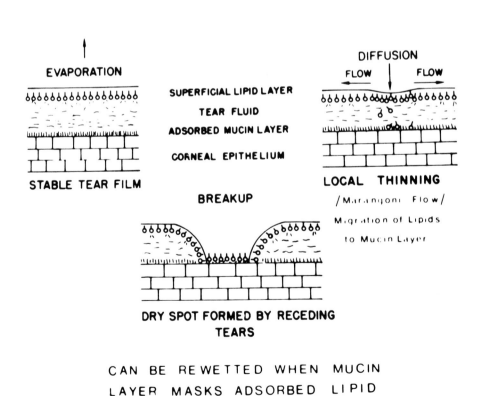

MECHANISM OF TEAR FILM RUPTURE

FIG 8–10.
The mechanism of dry spot formation. (From Holly FJ: *Am J Optom Physiol Opt* 1981; 58:324. Used by permission.)

stein[172] suggest an elaboration of the theory (Fig 8–11). This postulates a three-stage process of tear film breakup. The blink action exerts a sheer force across the thin tear film, which redistributes and smoothes the mucus layer on the corneal epithelium, masking any lipid contamination and the basic hydrophobic nature of the tissue. At this stage the overlying aqueous film is stable but is slowly thinning because of evaporation and drainage. After restoration the mucus layer begins to thin under the influence of the dispersion forces acting on it at several places where the film is initially somewhat thinner. If this process is not reversed by another blink, the growing interfacial perturbations cause mucus layer rupture within 15 to 50 seconds in a normal eye. The final stage of the process occurs when the aqueous film comes into contact with the exposed hydrophobic epithelium at various places where the mucus layer is ruptured. This, in turn, is responsible for the rapid, consequent rupture of the aqueous phase of the tears. This is described as a two-step, "double-film" mechanism of tear film rupture because it applies to breakup specifically at the mucus and aqueous phases of the tears.

Sharma and Ruckenstein's[172] postulate correlates the time of rupture to thickness of the mucus covering of the

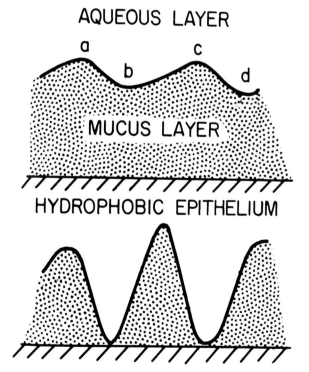

AQUEOUS LAYER
MUCUS LAYER
HYDROPHOBIC EPITHELIUM

FIG 8–11.
Mechanism of tear film rupture. The amplification of the interfacial nonhomogeneities takes place because of the dispersion forces. The mucus coating of the epithelium ruptures at points *b* and *d* where the film is locally initially thinned. (From Sharma A, Ruckenstein E: *Am J Optom Physiol Opt* 1985; 62:246. Used by permission.)

epithelium. After a blink is passed, a thin (0.02–0.04 mm) mucus layer is restored on the corneal epithelium. van del Waals' dispersion forces act on this mucus layer to destabilize it, resulting in its eventual rupture. This rupture exposes the underlying hydrophobic epithelium to the aqueous tear film. The aqueous phase of the tear film then breaks rapidly, resulting in lipid contamination of the cornea and the formation of increasingly large areas of nonwetting.

It is of interest in the light of this theory that recent work by Tiffany et al.[179] shows a negative correlation between the surface tension of the tears and a tear film breakup in normal and dry eyes. In such states, as well as in the presence of high surface tension, the tear film breaks up more rapidly. The surface tension was found to depend much more on the presence of soluble mucus in the tears than on the presence of tear proteins; when the mucus concentration was low, the surface tension was higher. Thus, in the presence of lower mucus concentrations, tear breakup times were reduced.

A new hypothesis on tear film stability is advocated by Liotet et al.,[120] who contend that the surfacting agent on the corneal epithelium is not mucus but the glyocalyx, the even spread of the tear film thus being the function of the cells of the corneal epithelium and not simply a result of mucus wetting of this tissue. Therefore, epithelial cell integrity is essential for the stability of the tear film, and the disappearance of goblet cells and the consequent disruption of the tear film during sicca syndromes are not a cause of dry eyes but a result of the dryness. According to the theory of tear film stability advocated by Liotet et al.,[120] the development of a dry spot on the cornea results from the interference with the corneal epithelial cells' capacity to synthesize glycocalyx and the consequent lack of specific sites of fixation for mucus proteins. Such an interference could occur from a physical trauma or nutritional deprivation resulting from contact lens wear.

An alternative hypothesis for the incompleteness or absence of mucus leading to dryness during contact lens wear has been offered by Versura et al.[193] These workers found a significant decrease in the mucus glycoconjugates in asymptomatic contact lens wearers, and they speculate that the contact lens could contribute to the failure of tear film stability by altering the production of mucus.

Also important in the stability of the tear film is the integrity of the lipid layer. The lipid is secreted by the meibomian glands at the lid margins. Alterations in the functions of these glands (meibomian gland dysfunction, or MGD), is associated with chronic blepharitis,[133] patient intolerance to contact lenses,[81] and hydrogel lens deposits.[81, 163] In those cases where gland production is reduced or alterations take place in lipid composition,[152] patients may complain of transient dry eye symptoms, lens intolerance unrelated to fit, and blurring of vision. First described by Henriques and Korb[81] in relation to contact lens wear, MGD may be effectively treated by prescribing lid scrubs and warm massages.[158] Effective treatment leads to increases in the tear film breakup time in contact lens patients, a testament to the improved tear film stability.[158]

It is clear from these discussions, as Fatt[46] has observed, that the physical properties promoting tear film formation and stability are not fully understood at this time. What has been observed clinically, however, is that the presence of the contact lens in the eye can severely disrupt tear film integrity and can lead to symptoms and signs of dry eye. As Holly[92] has pointed out, the contact lens can be considered an artificial device immersed in the bodily fluids (tear film) on the anterior surface of the eye. This device must be biocompatible with the fluids and the adjacent tissues to allow them to maintain the normal functions and avoid complications. The ideal contact lens would rest on a continuous aqueous tear film layer sandwiched between the lens and the epithelium and would be coated on its anterior surface with a continuous tear film complete with the superficial lipid layer. The stability and continuity of both the prelens and postlens tear films are important for contact lens wear without complications. For a lens surface to be thoroughly wettable with tear fluid, the water-material interfacial tension should be as low as possible and preferably near zero.[92] The more hydrophilic the surface of the contact lens, the more stable the prelens tear film. It is ironic, therefore, that even today's hydrogel lenses are not completely wettable,[92] and all hard lens materials are even less so. However, the presence of a mucus coat derived from the tear film on the anterior and posterior surface of a contact lens renders it considerably more wettable within a very short time after insertion into the eye.[9] It should be noted that water content of a hydrogel contact lens does not reflect its inherent ability to be wet by the tears, for example, frozen pure water has an interfacial tension that renders it less wettable with liquid water than many other substances. Hydrogel lenses depend as much on the polymer matrix as on the water content for their wettability, so high water content hydrogel lenses are not necessarily more wettable than low water content lenses.[89] Hard contact lenses have varying degrees of wettability, which have been measured by various authors.[168, 173] The three techniques employed by the contact lens industry for measuring the surface wettability of RGP contact lenses, namely, the Sessile drop test, the Captive Bubble test, and the Wilhelmy plate technique, have recently been criticized by Fatt,[46] who has developed a new method for measuring tear film spread and breakup on model eyes. The values claimed by all of these techniques of measurement of contact angle as a measure of lens wettability have lost much of their credibility by misuse in claiming greater biocompatibility for new contact lens materials. It is clear that a wide range of contact angles are acceptable for contact lens materials.[181]

In addition to the need for a certain basic surface hydrophilicity in a contact lens material, the stability of the tear film will also depend on other factors, including the edge design of hard contact lenses.[92] The edge design of the lens determines the shape and size and the degree of unsaturation in the tear meniscus around the lens and the drainage rate of the prelens tear film, a more rapid drainage rate leading to rapid prelens breakup.

When one contemplates the stability of the tear film around a contact lens, it is important to consider the different nature of the prelens and postlens films. The postlens tear film consists of aqueous tears that form a film between the corneal epithelium and the posterior surface of the lens. This fluid film possesses a positive pressure that tends to separate the two solid surfaces. This pressure is known as a *disjoining pressure*[34] and may be positive or negative, depending on the hydrophilicity of the two solid surfaces. If both surfaces are hydrophobic, the pressure is negative and the fluid film will be unstable and will rupture, allowing contact between the lens and the corneal epithelium.[88] However, if only one of the solids is hydrophilic, the disjoining pressure is positive.[92] Therefore, it is essential that either the corneal epithelial surface or the posterior surface of the contact lens should remain wetted by mucus to maintain a positive disjoining force between the surfaces and to avoid contact adhesion. A hard contact lens placed in the eye is susceptible to various hydrostatic forces in the tear film. On initial instillation, the lens traps tears to form a meniscus around the edge.[92] The negative pressure of the tear meniscus will eventually be counteracted by the positive disjoining pressure in the postlens tear film, but this pressure will tend to thin the tear film. For lenses fitted in contact with either lid, such as superior positioning lenses, the meniscus pressure around the lens edge will be equalized by tear flow toward the meniscus with lower pressure.

Any contact lens placed on the eye will almost immediately be covered by a mucus coat that improves wettability.[9, 92] Accumulation of protein deposits, however, particularly those denatured or heavily contaminated by lipids, will have a negative effect on tear film stability. The resulting decrease in tear film breakup time on the anterior surface of lenses produced by such accumulations will alternatively expose the lens to air aqueous solution during blinking. Holly[92] has commented that "no known solid surface can remain biocompatible when exposed to such rapidly changing, extreme surface chemical conditions." For the tear film to be constantly replaced by the blinking process, the lids must be in close apposition to the anterior ocular surface. This relationship is disrupted by the presence of a contact lens on the cornea. This loss of lid congruity can seriously affect the ability of the lid to renew the mucous layer during blinking.[118]

Sharma and Ruckenstein[172] suggest that premature rupture of the epithelial mucous layer during contact lens wear could result in the postlens film breakup for a non-wettable lens material and adhesion of the contact lens to the cornea. The excessive ocular discomfort and potential damage that can occur from stationary contact lenses on the eye, even those with the best oxygen transmission characteristics, were shown in the late 1970s with the silicone lens.[44] These problems led to the banning of this material for contact lens use in West Germany and Japan at that time.

MEASUREMENTS OF TEAR FILM STABILITY

The stability of the tear film has been measured clinically by assessing the time from the last blink to the breakup of the tear film. The breakup has been observed using different techniques. The earliest techniques used the instillation of fluorescein to enhance the ability to discriminate the break in the tear film layer (Fig 8–12). The average values obtained for breakup time in the fluorescein tear breakup test is 10 to 40 seconds for a normal group of subjects. Times less than 10 seconds are thought to be borderline, and those less than 5 seconds are clearly indicative of dry eye syndromes. Norn[146] observed that the breakup time

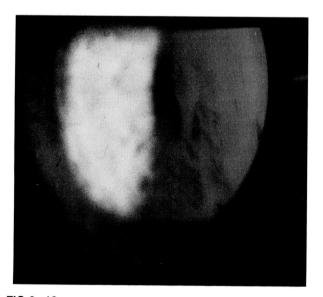

FIG 8–12.
Tear film breakup in a tear breakup time test carried out after fluorescein instillation.

averaged between 25 and 30 seconds in normal individuals but showed a wide fluctuation. He found the phenomenon not to be correlated with palprebral fissure width, intraocular pressure, or ambient humidity and temperature. Lemp et al.[116] found that the breakup time was very rapid (<10 seconds) in patients with dry eye syndrome. Lemp and Hamill[117] have later shown that the normal range of breakup times is dramatically affected by holding the lids apart and by instilling a local anesthetic. No relationship, however, was found between breakup time and age, sex, or corneal sensation. They found that the breakup time is reproducible in an individual eye.[117] Others,[191] however, have found the breakup time measured by this technique not to be a reproducible phenomenon, variations of 20 seconds or more being commonly found from one measurement to the next. An interesting variation is the low average tear breakup time found in the Indian population.[26] A mean value of less than 10 seconds has been reported in a "normal" population. This is explained by the low humidity, high temperature, and high incidence of trachoma in the patient population studied.

Mengher et al.[136] have found that the instillation of fluorescein in the conventional tear breakup tests reduces the precorneal tear film stability. This induced instability persisted for 10 to 20 minutes after the instillation. This led to the development of a noninvasive tear breakup test in which a grid pattern is projected onto the eye and the specular reflection observed with a biomicroscope.[137] Using this technique, Mengher et al.[137] measured the tear breakup time from the time of the last complete blink to the first observation of a disturbance in the clear reflex of the grid pattern on the cornea. This technique records longer values of breakup time, typically 40 to 150 seconds, with 80% to 85% of patients showing more than a 10-second breakup time. With this technique a noninvasive breakup time of less than 10 seconds is thought to be indicative of a dry eye state.

Hirji et al.[85] have described a similar adaptation to that of Mengher et al. for measuring noninvasively the "prerupture phase time"(Fig 8-13).

Other noninvasive tear breakup tests have also been developed. Patel et al.[156] used the keratometer mire image to observe breakup of the tear film. These workers recorded average values in the normal population of 18 seconds and found a reduction in their measurement (i.e., the tear thinning time [TTT]) of 3 seconds with the instillation of fluorescein. They also found diurnal variations in individuals[155] and reductions in stability with age.[157] Guillon[68] describes a technique using the handheld tear film interferometer to measure noninvasively the breakup time. Observations of the lipid film under the conditions of this test show breakup times in excess of 45 seconds in most normal patients. The technique can also be used to measure the ante-

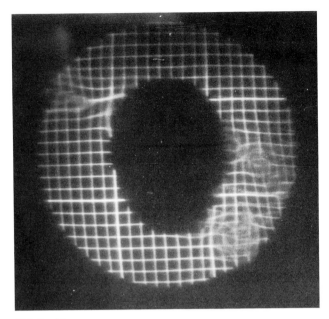

FIG 8–13.
The breakup of the tear film is seen as a distortion of a mire reflection in a noninvasive technique for measurement of tear film thinning time. Distortions of the mire image can be seen at the 10 and 4 o'clock positions in this illustration. (Courtesy of S. Patel.)

rior surface drying time on contact lenses. A method in which patients can observe their own precorneal tear film has been described by Yaeger and Gotz.[201] They adapted the technique originally described by Von Helmhotz in which the entoptic phenomenon of tear flow across the anterior surface of the corneal can be visualized.

EFFECT OF CONTACT LENS WEAR ON TEAR BREAKUP TIME

The wear of any type of contact lens reduces the time from the last complete blink to the first observation of tear breakup.[43] The first observations of the effect of hydrogel lens wear on tear breakup time were recorded by Klein and DeLuca,[111] who noted a large decrease in breakup time measurements with soft lens wear. They ascribed this to the interference with the mechanism by which mucin was spread over the cornea and by the contact lens disruption of the lipid layer, causing rapid increased evaporation. A similar effect was noted by Hamano,[72] who found a correlation between the reduced tear breakup time noted in contact lens wearers and the increased observation of the less stable amorphous patterns observed by biodifferential interference microscopy (Fig 8–14). Young and Efron[202]

noted low noninvasive tear breakup times with hydrogel contact lens wear. They found that the noninvasive tear breakup time was greater with higher water content lenses, though only significantly so in two pairs of lenses. This is mildly suggestive of greater tear film stability with the high water content hydrogel. Patel[154] has recorded short tear film thinning times with the wear of hydrogel lenses, averaging 6.1 seconds on the front of the lens (a reduction of almost two thirds in TTT). Barhgat[7] recorded a reduction of 58% in the mean breakup time immediately after the removal of hydrogel lenses. This reduction in tear breakup was still 42% after 6 hours following lens removal. This suggests very prolonged tear film instability induced by hydrogel lens wear. Short breakup time has been found to be associated with a predisposition to deposit formation.[121] Others,[26] however, found no correlation between contact lens wear and tear breakup time in an Indian population. But the average tear breakup time in the sample was less than 10 seconds. Therefore, more than three fourths of the samples studied in this population fell within the borderline dry eye category.

The problem of contact lens intolerance induced by relatively unstable tear films (low tear breakup times) was described by Andres et al.[5] These workers described categories of breakup times greater than 12 seconds as normal, 10 to 12 seconds as borderline, and less than 10 seconds as dry eye. They found that "a little" more than 2% of the normal patients developed contact lens intolerance, whereas more than 12% of the borderline patients had problems with contact lenses, and 86% of the dry eye patients, regardless of whether they wore a hard or soft lens, had problems. Their recommendation is that all patients with breakup times less than 10 seconds not wear contact lenses. Fanti and Holly[44] have pointed out, however, that consideration of the breakup time alone may not be reliable enough to use as a clinical predictor of contact lens intolerance in marginal dry eye states. They advocate also considering tear production, because a high tear production rate may offset the tendency for tear film instability. A short breakup or a low Schirmer test result by itself may not result in poor wearing performance, provided that the other factor, either tear production or tear film stability, is large enough to compensate for the deficiency. Fanti and Holly[44] propose the contact lens wetting value (W), defined as the sum of these two parameters where $W = F_1$ (breakup time) $+ F_2$ (Schirmer) and F_1 and F_2, are factors that are numerically equal to 1 with appropriate dimensions to render W dimensionless. They found that as long as the wetting value was more than 25 when breakup time was measured in seconds and Schirmer was measured in millimeters, the contact lens wearing performance was acceptable.

Comparison of percentages of BUT in central area
for experienced and inexperienced subjects.

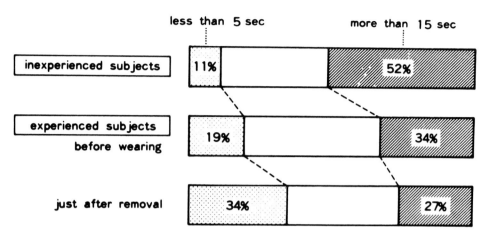

FIG 8–14.
The effect of contact lens wear on tear breakup time *(BUT)* can be seen by the increased number of short breakup times noted in experienced subjects compared with nonwearing (inexperienced) subjects. The effect of contact lens wear on rapid tear film breakup is seen to persist after lens removal. (From Hamano H: *Contact Intraocular Lens Med J* 1981; 7:205. Used by permission.)

EFFECT OF CONTACT LENS WEAR ON BLINKING

The maintenance of the corneal integrity is dependent in part on the proper reformation of the precorneal tear film by the blinking action of the eyelids. Improper blinking is known to cause changes in the structure and stability of the tear film.[2] The normal blink, in the absence of contact lens wear, averages about 12 blinks per minute,[17] shows marked variations between individuals, but remains relatively constant for the same individual. The average interblink time is 4.8 seconds, but all individuals show mixed interblink periods of longer and shorter duration. The type of blink is shown to vary between individuals, with about 80% showing complete blinks, 17% showing incomplete blinks, and 2.5% showing twitches.[17]

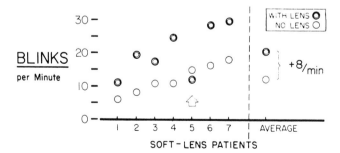

FIG 8–15.
The average blink rate and net change in patients before and after wearing soft contact lenses. On average, an increase of eight blinks per minute occurs as a result of the soft lens wear. (From Hill RM: *Int Contact Lens Clin* 1984; 11:366. Used by permission.)

It has been suggested that wearing a contact lens changes the blink in such a way that blinking is less frequent and more often only partial.[92] Systematic studies of blink in adapted hard and soft contact lens wearers, however, suggest that both groups show an increased number of complete normal blinks (from 12 to >20 blinks per minute) (Fig 8–15) with more regularity in the interblink period.[18] In a few cases, however, significantly poorer blinking is exhibited in the presence of contact lenses with greater incidence of incomplete blinks.[83, 84] It is perhaps the latter individuals who show the problems with contact lens wear that result from poor blinking (see Chapter 9), and it is these patients who need to carry out blinking exercises.[92]

TEAR PRODUCTION IN CONTACT LENS WEARERS

The physiological tear production rate is approximately 1 to 2 μL/min,[142, 160, 174, 200] with a turnover rate of about 16% of the total volume per minute. Tear flow has been found to decrease with age[35] but is not affected by the sex of the individual.[80] In the absence of reflex tearing, there appears to be no diurnal variation in tear production rate.[80] Jordan and Baum[102] have shown tear production to be significantly decreased in the presence of topical anaesthesia. Mishima[140] has suggested that tear tonicity may have a role in the regulation of tear flow such that increased tonicity leads to increased flow to protect the cornea from the harmful effects of the changes in osmolarity. Tear secretion has been found to be reduced in cases of obstructed tear passages.[145] In such a situation it might be expected that there would be increased tear production in the presence of increased tear evaporation, but this does not appear to be the case.[189]

Tear production has been most frequently measured by the use of the Schirmer tear test,[70] but this is notoriously unreliable and poorly reproducible.[199] Holly et al.[94] have modified the test to improve its reliability. Hamano et al.[73] described a variant on the conventional technique in which phenol-impregnated cotton thread is substituted for the filter paper strip of the Schirmer test. Flow rates have also been measured using tear-absorbing substances.[144, 204] Recently fluorophotometric techniques have measured the rate of decay of fluorescein instilled into the precorneal tear film (Fig 8–16).[142, 149, 160] Some of these tests have been used to measure the rate of tear production in contact wearers. Hard contact lenses produce an initial rise in reflex tearing in unadapted patients, but this rapidly decreases with adaptation to lens wear. In spite of the anticipation that in those situations contact lenses would reduce tear production as a result of decreased corneal sensitivity (secondary to anoxia), there have been no clear findings of abnormal tear production rates in contact lens wearers. The general finding with soft contact lenses is a normal tear production rate.[73, 149, 160, 175] Similar findings have been recorded for RGP and polymethylmethacrylate (PMMA) lens wearers.[73] It appears, therefore, that the osmolarity changes in the tear film recorded during contact lens wear[63] are more likely to be caused by increased tear evaporation with contact lenses[186] than by changes in tear production during wear.

TEAR FILM COMPOSITION CHANGE WITH CONTACT LENS WEAR

The changes in the composition of the tear film as a result of contact lens wear are confused and contradictory. The effects on the tear film function and the health of the eye have not been fully described. However, it is known that alterations in tear composition are influenced by lens wear by the way in which the lens affects the production and elimination of tears from the eye and by the changes induced in the metabolic and barrier functions of the corneal epithelium. The changes depend on the stage of contact lens wear. Most of the changes that have been observed take place during the "adaptation" to contact lens wear.

The initial wear of a contact lens changes the rate of reflex tear production because of stimulation of the anterior ocular surface and lids. The increased volume changes the concentration of various elements of the tear film. This effect is most striking with the adaptation to hard contact lenses and to a lesser degree with soft lens wear. The adaptational changes usually include an initial decrease in concentration of certain components, which is followed by an eventual restoration to baseline levels or even slight elevations at the end of the period. Such changes have been reported for tear chloride,[170] tear sodium,[123] tear potassium,[139] cholesterol,[203] and total tear protein.[8, 13] Callender and Morrison[13] report the decrease in tear protein concentration during the initial stages of contact lens wear (Fig 8–17). This effect is transient and related to the initial increase in reflex tearing at this stage. An interesting

FIG 8–16.
This fluorophotometric technique (Fluorotron) measures tear production by observing the rate of decay of fluorescein instilled into the precorneal tear film. More rapid tear production results in rapid decay of fluorescence from the tear film.

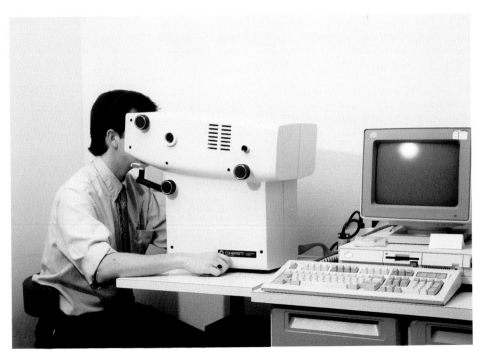

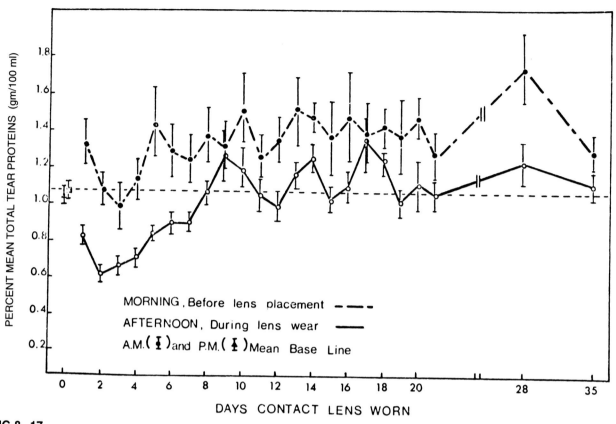

FIG 8–17.

A graphical representation of the mean tear protein concentrations for eight subjects measured during the first 35 days of contact lens wear. A decrease in tear protein concentration is seen, which is transient in nature and related to the initial increase in reflex tearing at this stage. (From Callender M, Morrison PE: *Am J Optom Physiol Opt* 1974; 51:939. Used by permission.)

observation of this study is that they found an elevated prelens application protein tear level throughout the study (even after adaptation to lenses had occurred). This phenomenon may be accounted for by the increased morning desquamation of epithelial cells and the presence of inflammatory cells in the normal sleep situation,[86] which add protein to the tear film. Alternatively, it may simply represent an altered blood-tear barrier function as described by Lundh et al.[124]

When tear protein levels in contact lens wearers are considered, particularly during the adapation to lens wear, it is important to make a distinction between the proteins derived from the lacrimal gland and those derived from serum. Lacrimal gland proteins (tear-specific prealbumin, lysozyme, and lactoferrin) tend to maintain the same level of concentration during reflex tearing. The serum-derived proteins, on the other hand, albumin, IgG, and transferrin, are reduced in concentration when reflex tearing is produced by initial contact lens wear. Other short-term compositional changes that result from lens wear include an increase in the glucose levels of the tear film during the initial stages of soft lens wear.[108] This difference is thought to be the result of the mechanical irritation causing

an increase in lacrimal gland flow, which, in turn, produces increased washout of glucose from the epithelial cells of the cornea because of the lowering of the normally very high diffusion resistance of these cells. A similar process probably accounts for increased tear lactate dehydrogenase (LDH) levels after hypoxia in humans.[58] Zschausch et al.[205] reported changes in glucose pyruvate and lactate concentrations in the tear film of contact lens wearers similar to the concentrations in those patients who experience mechanical injury. Therefore, the metabolite concentration in the tear film may be a measure of the mechanical effect of contact lenses.[205]

The longer-term compositional tear changes taking place during contact lens wear are incompletely described in the literature. Farris[45] found no differences in long-term wearers of both hard and soft lenses for tear lactoferrin, lysozyme, and albumin. Similar absence of change in lysozyme concentrations are confirmed by others.[97, 194] Tear calcium levels in established contact lens wearers appear to be slightly elevated[99] but not significantly so compared with controls. Vinding et al.[194] disclosed a significant decrease in secretory IgA levels in soft lens daily and extended wearers, a finding that may partly explain the greater exposure to infectious corneal and conjunctival complications experienced by these patients. Tear levels of serum albumin and serum IgG appear to increase in contact lens wearers,[124] which may indicate an altered blood-tear barrier function in these patients. Jones and Sack[101] measured the IgG/IgA ratio in the tear films of contact lens patients. Because this ratio increases dramatically during inflammation, the finding that a consistent (although not statistically significant) increase in IgG/IgA ratio in patients showing heavy deposits on soft contact lenses may be reflective of an immune specific lens response or the enhanced titer of tear IgG resulting from an inflammatory process. The finding of a significant increase in the ratio in high water content, extended soft contact lens wearers may indicate that these patients are experiencing a greater degree of inflammatory or immune stress. Temel et al.[177] report an increase in tear IgA levels in hard contact lens patients compared with controls but no significant increase in tear IgA levels of soft lens wearers. They believe that the continuous mechanical stimulation of conjunctiva alters the level of tear immunoglobulins in hard lens wear.

Changes have also been noted in mucous production in contact lens wearers. Greiner et al.[65] have described a change in the conjunctival mucous system in which an increase in the number of non–goblet epithelial cells with mucous secretory vesicles (the so-called second mucous system) have been observed in contact lens wearers. They found that the number of goblet cells remains unchanged but they produce different amounts of glycosidic residues, which may be a response to contact lens wear. It is possible, therefore, that the contact lenses contribute to the failure of tear film stability by altering the production of mucus. The increased production of mucus in contact lens–wearing patients may result in increased lens deposits, which, in turn, perpetuates a vicious circle in which further insult to the conjunctival surface results in another increase in mucus production. Allansmith[3] described this as "a spiral of increasing problems in the contact lens wearer."

Several workers have used techniques of tear film compositional analysis as noninvasive techniques from monitoring corneal epithelial metabolic state in contact lens wearers. Masters[128] describes a novel optical method based on the intrinsic fluorescence of cellular-reduced pyridine nucleotides to determine the partial pressure of oxygen dissolved in the aqueous tear layer of the precorneal tear film. This technique, known as *corneal redox fluorometry,* has the potential for providing important information about the normal corneal physiology and biochemistry during contact lens wear. Wilson et al.[197] uses the light scattering properties of the superficial cells of the corneal epithelium to indicate changes in corneal transpar-

ency. An increase in light scatter from this "anterior bright band" can be used to indicate deficiencies in epithelial bathing medium, because only healthy corneal epithelial cells supplied with an adequate precorneal film can maintain their transparency.

Fullard and Carney[55] have developed a technique in which the enzymes or carbohydrate metabolism, LDH, and malate dehydrogenase (MDH), has been measured. The primary source of these enzymes in the tear film is believed to be the corneal epithelial cells, the conjunctival cells making only a small contribution. The LDH/MDH ratio has been chosen as an index of change in epithelial cell activity as a result of hypoxia induced by eyelid closure and contact lens wear. These circumstances, called *anaerobic isoenzyme patterns,* result in increased LDH activity in the tissue.[58, 64, 98] The tear LDH/MDH ratio was chosen because it proved to be a more reliable parameter than individual activity of either enzyme; the absolute levels of tear LDH or MDH activity were found to be strongly dependent on tear flow rate.[54] The tear LDH/MDH ratio as a function of time of day is dependent on a smooth diurnal curve, in which the ratio is elevated after overnight eyelid closure and drops to a stable minimum 3 hours after waking.[55] Fullard and Carney[57] have suggested the use of the noninvasive tear enzyme activity test to measure the biochemical changes occurring within the corneal epithelium as a result of the relative hypoxia experienced during contact lens wear. The possible causes of the elevation of the tear LDH/MDH ratio under anaerobic conditions have been suggested as unbinding of intracellular M-type LDH within epithelial cells and increased cell membrane permeability, both processes occurring in response to reduced cellular energy under the more hypoxic conditions found in lid closure or contact lens wear.[55]

To investigate the effects of oxygen deprivation on tear enzyme activity, Fullard and Carney[56] placed subjects in gas goggles into which humidified gas mixtures were passed for up to 2 hours. These conditions provided the eye with levels of hypoxia up to 5% by volume of oxygen. Oxygen deprivation was found to cause an increase in the tear LDH/MDH ratio, which occurred several hours after the onset of hypoxia (Fig 8–18). This experiment established that the critical level of between 1% and 2% was necessary for a significant increase in the tear LDH/MDH ratio and that corneal hypoxia was responsible for the increased level of LDH, causing a rise in the LDH/MDH ratio. Therefore, the relative hypoxia on eyelid closure found during sleep results in an increased LDH/MDH ratio in part because of the reduction in oxygen supply to the corneal epithelium. However, the authors[56] note two important differences between their gas goggle experiment and the effect of overnight lid closure. First, the changes

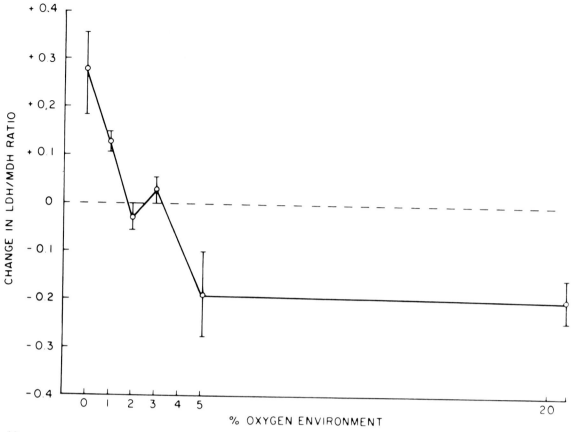

FIG 8–18.
Change in the lactate dehydrogenase/malate dehydrogenase (LDH/MDH) ratio in response to corneal exposure to reduced oxygen tension. This change is determined from the LDH/MDH ratio (for all subjects) found immediately before and after the test period and over the 4.5 to 7.5 hours after cessation of the test. (From Fullard RJ, Carney LG: *Acta Ophthalmol* 1985; 63:678. Used by permission.)

in total tear protein with oxygen deprivation were insignificant and showed no correlation with tear enzyme changes. Second, the tear enzyme ratio changes even with 2 hours of total anoxia, were not as great as those occurring after overnight closure. Other closed lid environmental factors may be important in determining the effect of lid closure on epithelial function. Thus, the prediction of extended wear lens performance in terms of oxygen availability may be of limited value because this parameter accounts for only part of the total stress on the corneal epithelium.[58]

A later study using tear enzyme activity to assess the corneal response to contact lens wear learned that after short-term wear of contact lenses, the tear LDH/MDH ratio was elevated.[57] The magnitude and time course of this elevation was influenced by the type of contact lens worn, its fit, and the duration of wear (see Fig 8–19). The effect of contact lens wear, the resulting relative hypoxia, did not occur for several hours after the commencement of contact lens wear, typically in the afternoon hours. As seen in Figure 8–19, the greatest change in the LDH/MDH ratio was

produced by steep fitting PMMA lenses worn for the longest period of time (5 hours). Alignment fitting and flat fitting PMMA lenses with greater tear pump facility produced less change in the ratio. The nonpumping, but more transmissible, soft lens materials produced even less change than flat fitting PMMA lens.

Physicochemical Properties of the Tears in Contact Lens Wear

The physical properties of the tears in contact lens wear that have received the most attention are osmolarity and pH.

The normal human tear pH has been shown to fluctuate diurnally, being lowest (most acidic) immediately on waking in the morning, with a slight but definite alkaline shift as the day progresses.[14] The value for normal tear pH has been measured variously from 6.93 to 7.83,[6, 14, 25, 27, 47, 148] the position of measurement and technique accounting for this range. The effect of contact

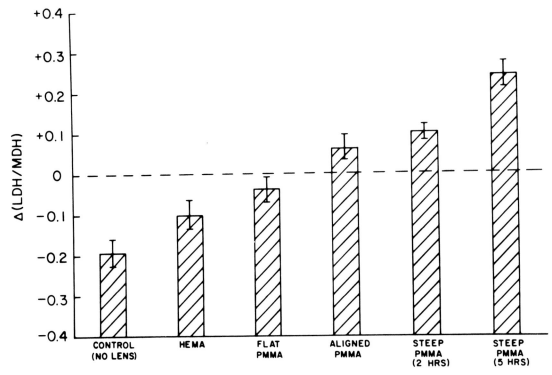

FIG 8–19.
The change in LDH/MDH ratio in response to the wearing of contact lenses. This change is determined from the mean LDH/MDH ratio (for all subjects) found between 8:00 A.M. and 10:00 A.M. and that over 6.5 to 9.5 hours after commencement of contact lens wear. Control data (no lens wear) over the same time period are also shown. Steep-fitting polymethylmethacrylate *(PMMA)* lenses are seen to produce a greater change in the ratio than flatter fitting PMMA or hydroxyethylmethacrylate *(HEMA)* contact lenses. (From Fullard RJ, Carney LG: *Acta Ophthalmol* 1986; 64:216. Used by permission.)

lens wear has been measured by a group of investigators with inconsistent results. Carney and Hill[16] found no difference between the tear pH of patients wearing PMMA lenses and their nonwearing baseline value. This is a little surprising because the impermeable lenses might have been expected to exert an effect on pH as a result of alterations in corneal metabolism. The same workers[15] found a decrease in pH with closed eye, hydrophilic lens wear; however, values were within the range reported for non–lens wearing eyes in the closed eye state.[14] No consistent trend in tear pH with lens wear was found by Browning and Foulks.[12] However, in a comparison of aphakic and fellow phakic eyes, a higher value was found in the aphakic eye.

Other groups of workers do report decreases in the pH of the tears in contact lens wearers. Hamano[71] found a reduction in pH and a consequent shift toward more acidic tear film in both hard and flexible lens wearers after 1 hour. Similar findings have been reported by Andres[6] and by Chen and Maurice[25] (Fig 8–20). It has been suggested that the change is caused by the relative hypoxia[6] or the trapped CO_2 in the post–lens tear film.[25] Chen and Maurice[25] point out, however, that because the value of pH

normally recorded in this postlens tear film is within the physiological range of values (7.3), any disturbance of the epithelial or endothelial cells of the cornea under contact lenses found in long term (extended wearers) cannot be ascribed to the acid environment of the tear film at the tissue surface.

Lattimore[114] has measured the pH of the anterior surface of hydrogel lenses at various stages in their wear. The pH of the lens, surface was found to increase from 6.99 with a new lens, to 7.43 after wear of lenses of up to 7 days. This suggests that the pH decrease and CO_2 trapping or buildup under soft lenses may lead to a pH gradient existing within the matrix of the hydrogel lens. This pH gradient would then create layers of varying water content and refractive index within the structure of the lens. This may account for some of the changes in visual function experienced by patients wearing hydrogel contact lenses.[114] The general finding that the pH of the tears is altered in a relatively minor way by contact lens wear is probably a testament to the buffering ability of the tear film.

Tear osmolarity is a critical factor in contact lens wear because it affects both corneal hydration and the fluid dynamics of hydrophilic contact lenses. Tear osmotic

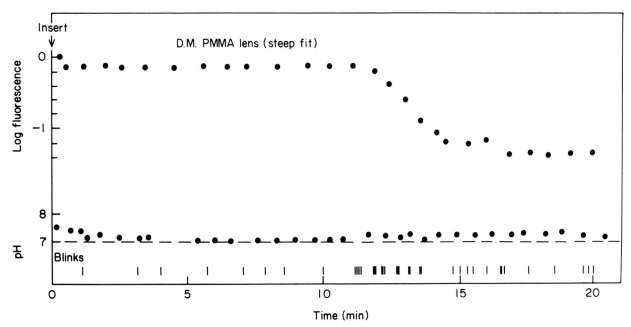

FIG 8-20.
The pH in the precorneal tear film is measured under a contact lens by a fluorescent probe. The change in total fluorescence and pH under a PMMA contact lens in one subject is shown. Note the falling concentration of pyranine on rapid blinking but no change in pH. The general finding that pH of tears is altered in a relatively minor way by contact lens wear is probably a testament to the buffering ability of the tear film. (From Chen FS, Maurice DM: *Exp Eye Res* 1990; 50:251. Used by permission.)

pressure has been found to increase with contact lens wear.[45, 63, 71, 126] An increase in tear osmolarity is reported in daily hard lens wear and for soft lens extended wear but not for daily soft lens wear.[45] This may signify a relation between corneal sensation and tear osmolarity. Gilbard et al.[63] suggested a mechanism for increased tear film osmolarity in contact lens wearers that proposes that decreased corneal sensitivity leads to a reduction in tear production. This reduced tear production rate in contact lens patients combined with the increased evaporation rate observed in all contact lens wearers[186] would lead to a lower volume of tear fluid in the eye and a consequent increase in tear osmolarity. Previously Jordan and Baum[102] had demonstrated that topical anaesthesia decreases tear secretion rates in humans by up to 75%. Similar results are reported by Gilbard and Dartt.[62] Values of the tear osmolarity in nonwearers and daily soft lens wearers have been recorded at 308 mOsm/L, whereas it is increased to approximately 317 mOsm/L in daily wear hard lens patients and extended wearers of soft lenses.[45] Additional evidence for Gilbard's theory is found in a study of aphakic contact lens wearers.[45] Farris[45] found in these patients that the osmolarity averaged 321 vs. 307 for phakic patients of the same age (Fig 8–21). This suggests a relationship between corneal sensation, which is reduced as a result of the cataract surgery, and osmotic pressure in these patients.

Tear Evaporation During Contact Lens Wear

The majority of the tears are eliminated from the eye by drainage through the puncta into the nasolacrimal duct and sac. This mechanism is not affected by contact lens wear. However, lenses produced significant effects on the evaporation mechanism of tear elimination. Tear evaporation from rabbit and human eyes has been measured by a variety of techniques.[74, 165, 186, 195] A wide range of values from 4 to 41×10^{-7} g/cm^2/sec have been recorded in normal eyes, with variation in measurement the result of individual variations in tear evaporation rate and differences in technique. Tear evaporation accounts for between 10% and 40% of the total elimination of tears from the eye under nonreflex conditions.[82, 138] It is not related to the rate of tear production measured by Schirmer test results[24] or by scanning fluorophotometry[189] and does not appear to be affected by sex or the age of the individual.[61, 165]

The lipid layer on the anterior surface of the tear film is necessary to inhibit the loss of tears from the eye by evaporation.[100, 141] In the absence of the protective lipid layer, the rate of evaporation is increased between 10 and 20 times.[141] Contact lenses have been found to increase the rate of tear film evaporation,[24, 186] probably as a result of mechanical disruption of the lipid layer of the tears (Fig 8–22). Tomlinson and Cedarstaff[186] reported an increase

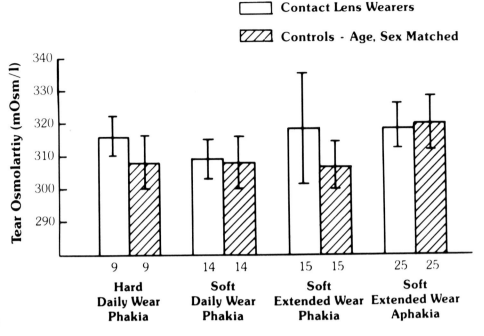

Contact Lens Wearers

Controls - Age, Sex Matched

Contact Lens Wearers and Age/Sex Matched Controls

FIG 8–21.
Tear osmolarity in contact lens wearers and age-sex matched controls without contact lens wear. (From Farris RL: *CLAO J* 1986; 12:106. Used by permission.)

in evaporation with all types of contact lenses measured. These included 38% and 70% hydrogels, silicone elastomer, PMMA, and modified PMMA hard lenses. Hamano et al.[74] found an increase in tear evaporation by their measurement technique only in soft lens wearers. Some of their wearers showed an initial increase in tear evaporation that returned to normal sometime later; a higher increase was noted in higher water content soft lens wear. They found no significant increase in PMMA or silicone lens wear. However, their technique was highly invasive, requiring a probe to be placed on the anterior ocular surface to encircle the cornea. This disruption of the integrity of the tear film probably accounted for their results. Only in soft lens wearers did additional tear film evaporation apparently occur as a result of an additional contribution from water loss from the lens substance. When comparisons of evaporation in soft lens wearers are made by a less invasive technique of measurement,[23] no significant difference in the tear evaporation rate increase (compared to the naked eye) is found, with water contents from 38% to 70% (Fig 8–22). In fact, the water content of the soft lens is thought to contribute little to the total water loss from the anterior ocular surface in these circumstances.

In situations where the lipid film of the tears has been found to be thicker and more stable,[69] as in the morning on eye opening after sleep, the tear evaporation rate is significantly reduced (Fig 8–23).[185] This initial decrease in tear evaporation is sustained for only a short period before the level returns to its normal (higher) value for the rest of the day. The morning low in tear evaporation rate indi-

cates a significant change in tear film chemistry at this time. The thicker lipid and mucus components of the tears found after the closed eye period of sleep may well affect the initial open eye situation in extended contact lens wear and be responsible for lens adhesion (see Chapter 9).

Rolando and Refojo[164] found a higher tear evaporation rate in keratoconjunctivitis sicca, a finding contested by Hamano et al.[74] However, Rolando and Refojo[164] maintain that increased evaporation may be a factor in pathological dry eye and suggest a syndrome of increased tear evaporation that can produce a paradoxical "wet, dry eye." A similar situation can occur in patients wearing contact lenses. The contact lens acts as a provocation and turns the marginal into a fully manifest dry eye, in fact, producing a contact lens syndrome of increased tear evaporation.

The method by which dryness during contact lens wear is most frequently combated is by the use of artificial tear supplements instilled into the eye. It is perhaps paradoxical, therefore, that an increase in tear evaporation rate has been measured after the instillation of eye drops.[165, 190] Both artificial tear and saline solutions produce this increase. It appears that a disruptive effect on the lipid layer occurs as a result of instillation. An increase in tear evaporation occurs initially after the instillation of the drop and persists for a period of time before returning to the normal level. If this persistence continues for too long, the beneficial effects of the extra fluid volume in the eye may be offset by continued loss of fluid by evaporation after all the excess fluid has been drained or evaporated off the eye. In such a situation there may be a "rebound dry eye effect" that could

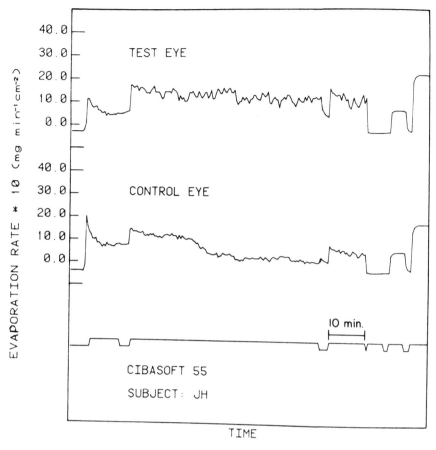

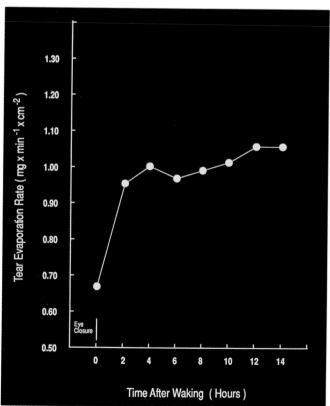

FIG 8–22.
The tear evaporation rate measured before, during, and after the wear of a hydrogel (38% water content) contact lens on the test eye. Elevations of tear evaporation rate are seen on insertion of the contact lens, an elevation continued after the removal of the lens. Throughout these measurements, the control eye wore no contact lens. The upper trace shows readings at three stages: during the initial baseline readings, during the wear of the contact lens, and after lens removal. These correspond to the first three deflections on the lower trace. (From Tomlinson A, Cedarstaff TH: *J Br Contact Lens Assoc* 1982; 5:141. Used by permission.)

FIG 8–23.
The average evaporation rate for a group of subjects measured at 2-hour intervals for 14 hours during the waking phase of the diurnal cycle. An initial low tear film evaporation rate is seen on waking (at zero time). This rapidly rises to a level within 2 hours, which is maintained for the remainder of the waking day. (From Tomlinson A, Cedarstaff TH: *J Br Contact Lens Assoc* 1992 (in press). Used by permission.)

lead, ultimately, to the patient experiencing more symptoms than occurred before drop instillation. Some concern has been expressed about the use of certain preservatives (particularly benzalkonium chloride) to preserve artificial tear solutions because it may cause disruption of the lipid layer. It appears that in the concentrations used in commercially available artificial tear supplements, this is not a significant concern.[188]

TEAR FILM DEPOSITS ON CONTACT LENSES

A wide variety of complex surface deposits have been observed on contact lenses. The components of these deposits are derived primarily from the tear film. The effect of these deposits is to disrupt tear film,[115] cause corneal staining, decrease lens comfort, increase wearer dissatisfaction[166] and frequency of lens replacement,[76] and lead to discontinuation of lens wear. Tear film deposition may be responsible also for minor ocular complications such as hyperemia, allergic or giant papillary conjunctivitis,[4] and severe complications, including microbial keratitis.[52, 159, 180, 196] Most of the attention of clinicians and researchers has been directed toward a study of tear film deposits on hydrogel contact lens materials.

Tear Film Deposits on Hydrogel Contact Lenses

The nature of deposits on hydrogel contact lens surfaces reveals the source of most of the material to be the components of the tear film: primarily lipids and proteins.[76, 106, 109, 110, 115] Kleist[109, 110] first described the basic lens deposits and classified them as organic and inorganic by visual appearance under microscopy. In samples of lenses examined and classified in the laboratories of Allergan Pharmaceuticals, Inc. worldwide, the relative incidence of the different types of deposit have been described.[109, 110, 192]

Protein Films

Protein films (Fig 8–24) are seen as thin semiopaque, white superficial layers covering all or parts of the lens surface.[30, 109] Occasionally they appear as clear and transparent layers or as colored film. They consist of mucus proteins, albumen, globulins, glycoproteins, mucin, and lysozyme.[78, 106] Sack et al.[167] described the nature of the in situ lens–bound protein layer as primarily denatured lysozyme. In addition to the predominant lysozyme contaminant found on daily and extended wear hydrogel lenses, Sack et al.[167] also reported the presence of lactoferrin, immunoglobulins, albumin, and glycoproteins. All of these tear constituents are found more commonly on ionic than nonionic hydrogel lens polymers. In most cases higher concentrations are found in extended wear materials. Leahy et al.[115] isolated, using gel electrophoresis, a large number of proteins on lens deposits that begin accumulating within 1 minute after lens application and increase progressively during wear. These proteins included lysozyme, albumin, lactoferrin, IgE, and IgA. The amount of lysozyme found on the lens surface is affected by the disinfection systems involving heat,[109] the lens surface drying during the interblink period, a low blink rate, a low tear

FIG 8–24.
A protein film on a hydrogel contact lens is seen as a thin, semiopaque, white superficial film covering all parts of the lens surface. This consists of mucus proteins, albumen, globulins, glycoproteins, mucin, and lysozyme. (Courtesy of Allergan Pharmaceuticals, Inc., Irvine, Calif.)

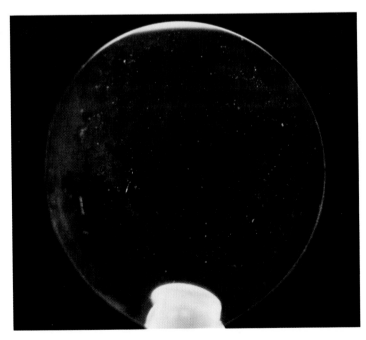

volume, and rapid tear breakup time.[113] Hosaka et al.[97] observed that most of the deposits occurring on hydrogel lens surfaces are found on the anterior rather than the posterior surface; in fact, only minimal quantities of deposit are found on the latter. This reinforces the importance of tear film discontinuity and the alternate drying and wetting of the anterior lens surface as a factor in deposition formation.

Kleist[109] first reported protein films to have an incidence of about 20% in hydrogel lens wearers in the United States, but later studies[192] placed the incidence at 33%, with variations as high as 40% in Europe. This form of deposit can lead to diminished visual acuity and comfort and staining of the cornea. Allansmith et al.[4] suggested that the presence of protein films on hydrogel lenses can be a factor in the mechanical and autoimmunological causes of giant papillary conjunctivitis secondary to contact lens wear (see Chapter 11).

Protein films on hydrogel lenses can be prevented by the scrupulous use of a surfactant cleaner immediately on removal of the lens from the eye. However, the more extreme forms require the use of strong oxidizing agents, which may also cause damage to the contact lens polymer.[42] A safer and more effective method of prevention and removal is the use of the enzyme papain.[122]

Lipids

Lipid deposits are frequently seen on hydrogel lenses[109] as a clear or slightly milky white film and are probably derived from the meibomian gland secretions, which provide the most anterior layer of the tear film (Fig 8–25). These lipids are easily removed from the lens by use of surfactant cleaners.

Lens Calculi

Kleist[110] also described the presence of inorganic films on hydrogel lenses. These films are potentially more damaging to the surface because heavy inorganic films may penetrate the lens matrix. These films appear in several forms, the most dramatic of which is lens calculi, which have alternatively been described as "jelly bumps," "mulberry-like growths," "barnacles," or calcium deposits. These deposits form on the anterior surface of the lens and contain calcium phosphate as a compact insoluble crystalline growth that can penetrate the lens surface (Fig 8–26). This form of deposit is frequently associated with protein and lipid films on the same surface. Hart et al.[76] reported that "jelly bump deposits" are composed primarily of lipids and are found mainly on high water content, extended wear hydrogel lenses. Clinical observations have indicated that several factors may predispose patients to lipid deposition in the formation of the lens calculi described by Hart et al.[76] These include dry eye syndromes,[40] incorrect blinking,[75] lipid-rich tear films,[77, 104] the use of diuretics[167] and oral contraceptives,[33] and MGD.[75] Kleist[110] reports lens calculi occur in about 13% of all lenses, ranging from 10% to 19% in various countries.[192] It occurs on those lenses that are chemically or thermally disinfected. This type of deposit appears to be specific to patients with a particular tear chemistry.[39, 60] The presence of lens calculi requires the lens to be replaced.

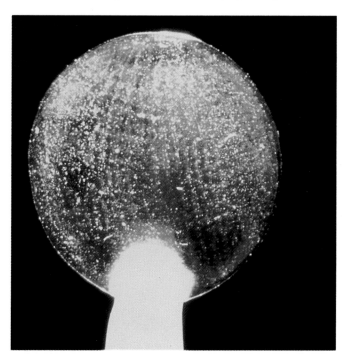

FIG 8–25.
Lipid deposits are frequently seen on hydrogel lenses as a clear or slightly milky white film and are probably derived from the meibomian gland secretions. (Courtesy of Allergan Pharmaceuticals, Inc., Irvine, Calif.)

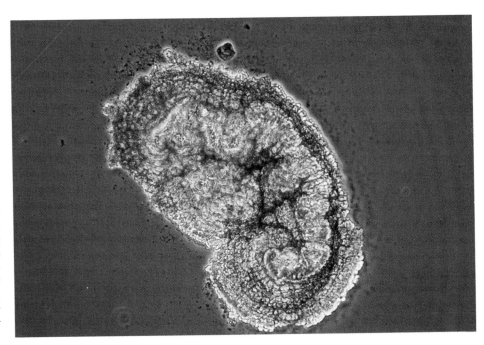

FIG 8–26.
A lens calculi is seen in phase contrast microscopy (magnification ×100). These deposits form on the anterior surface of hydrogel lenses and appear as compact, insoluble crystalline growths that can penetrate the lens substance. They are alternatively described as jelly bumps, mulberry-like growths, barnacles, or calcium deposits. (Courtesy of Allergan Pharmaceuticals Inc., Irvine, Calif.)

Calcium

Calcium carbonate deposits may also be seen in some hydrogel lenses[1] as crystalline growths with a definite needle-like form.[110] These crystals consist largely of calcium carbonate, which enters the surface of the lens, causing permanent damage to the structure (Fig 8–27). This form of deposit occurred in just less than 4% of the lenses analyzed by Kleist[110]; variations ranged from 3.5% to 8%.[192]

Calcium phosphate may also appear as a milky white deposit on hydrogel lens surfaces. Such deposits are seen in about 9% of cases (Fig 8–28)[110] with variations from 5% to 25%,[192] the higher incidence being related to the use of phosphate-buffered lens solutions.

One of the concerns of allowing deposits to accumulate on the surface of any contact lens is that it provides a possible site for attachment of bacteria and other microorganisms.[4, 52, 129, 180] Fowler et al.[52] suggest that the lens coating permits bacteria to accumulate and attach in the same way that it does to other mucus-covered nondesquamating surfaces. The proliferation of bacteria attached to the coating on hydrogel lens surfaces (Fig 8–29) may be a risk factor in extended wear contact lenses in which the in-

FIG 8–27.
Calcium carbonate deposits may be seen on some hydrogel lenses as crystalline growths. These crystals consist largely of calcium carbonate, which enters the surface of the lens, causing permanent damage to the structure. These deposits are seen here in phase contrast microscopy (magnification ×100). (Courtesy of Allergan Pharmaceuticals Inc., Irvine, Calif.)

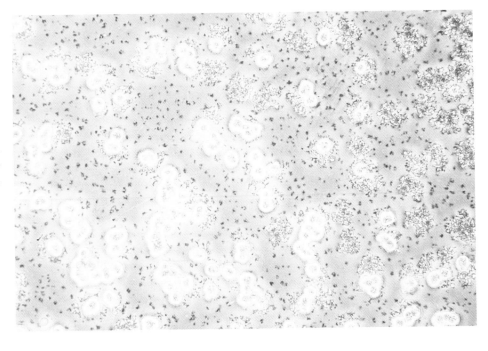

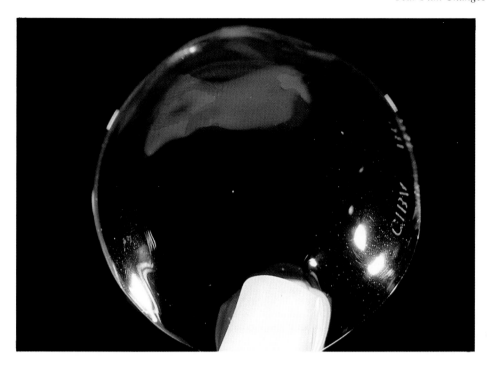

FIG 8–28.
Calcium phosphate appears as a milky white deposit on hydrogel lens surfaces, seen here in macroview. (Courtesy of Allergan Pharmaceuticals, Inc., Irvine, Calif.)

cidence of ulcers have been found to be significantly higher than that of daily wear (see Chapter 12).[160, 169]

Similar attachment of bacteria to RGP lens surfaces in which the integrity of the surface has been disrupted because of cracking and crazing of worn lenses has been reported by Grohe et al.[67] The accumulation of bacteria in the surface crevices of such lenses may pose a risk for infection.

The method of formation of deposits on hydrogel lens surfaces has been studied in vitro using artificial tears or standardized protein solutions.[20–22, 78] The differences in the composition of the solutions used in these experiments

compared with tear solutions and the differences in the environment in which the lens is placed during these in vitro experiments make extrapolation of the data to the in vivo situation difficult. In addition, in the eye a contact lens is exposed to constant drying and wetting and shear forces as a result of lid action during the blink process. All of these factors make the results on deposit formations in vitro of limited interest to the contact lens practitioner. Two studies have looked at in vivo processes of lens deposit on hydrogel surfaces. Fowler and Allansmith[49] observed that deposits formed on hydrogel lens surfaces in 30 minutes to 8 hours. They report coverings of up to 50% of the anterior

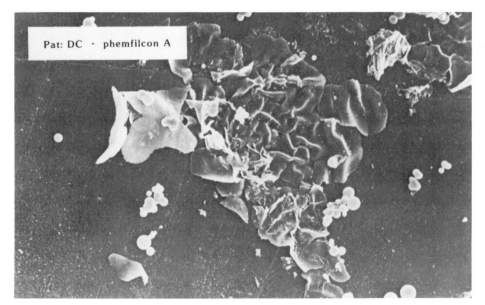

Pat: DC · phemfilcon A

FIG 8–29.
Staphylococcus epidermidis bacteria (round objects) are seen attached to exfoliated epithelial cells and deposits on the anterior surface of a 55% water content hydrogel lens.

lens surface with scattered cell membrane–like and mucuslike materials, with mucuslike materials on top of cells in places within 30 minutes of wear. Eight hours after onset of wear, 90% of the lens was covered with complex coatings. They observed that routinely worn lenses exhibited up to 90% of surface coverage. These deposits were found to remain even after professional cleaning of the lens. Fowler and Allansmith[49] did not identify the composition of the lens deposit. A later study by Leahy et al.[115] examined the deposits on new lenses worn from 1 minute to 8 hours. The morphology and composition of the deposits were analyzed by histological staining, light microscopy, scanning electronmicroscopy (SEM), sodium dodecyl sulfate, polyacrylamide gel electrophoresis with silvernitrate staining, and immunofluorescence microscopy. Specific proteins were found on individual lenses after as little as 1 minute of wear; increasing amounts of protein deposits were found as the wearing time increased. The rates and amount of deposition were found to be dependent on lens water content and the ionic characteristics of the material; less dependence was found on the individual patient's tear chemistry.

Factors Affecting Amount of Lens Deposition

In an attempt to control the amount of lens deposits occurring on hydrogel lens surfaces, practitioners need to be aware of the factors that influence the amount of deposit on lenses. This knowledge will allow them to choose the appropriate lens material for individual patients to avoid excessive accumulation. A number of studies have attempted to identify factors that influence the amount of deposits, these are: (1) lens water content, (2) lens surface chemistry, (3) patient's tear chemistry, and (4) lens surface integrity.

Lens Water Content
Fowler et al.[53] confirmed the widely held impression that the water content of hydrogel lenses significantly affected the amount of deposits. Examination of lenses by SEM showed that the higher water content lenses had more deposits on the surface than those with lower water content. Deposits on high water content lenses were found to be multilayered, covering the entire surface, and had a convoluted complex morphology reminiscent of the deposits seen on extended wear lenses. Tomlinson and Caroline[183] confirmed these findings in a study of various water content hydrogel materials (Fig 8–30). However, they pointed out the influence of tear chemistry in certain individuals able to wear high water content lenses and not show excess of deposits. It was suggested, however, that for patients categorized as "heavy depositers," lenses of only medium or low water content materials should be prescribed. The difficulty in the clinical situation is defining, before fitting, the patient with the propensity for heavy deposit accumulations. Leahy et al.[115] confirmed the tendency for the rate of deposit accumulation on hydrogel lenses to be affected by water content of the lens but disagreed that it is radically affected by individual patient tear chemistry.

Lens Surface Chemistry
Sack et al.[167] highlight the issue of whether it is the water content of the hydrogel lens, the surface chemistry (ionic nature) of the lens material, or both that actually determine the amount of deposit bound to the lens surface. Several contradictory theories have been advanced on this issue.[59, 93, 125, 162, 176] When this mechanism is evaluated, it is important to appreciate the interrelationship that exists between hydrogel water content and the ionic binding capacity of the material. Parker[153] and Stone et al.[176] suggested that hydrogels can be classified into three groups based on the water content and matrix chemistry of the polymers. These groupings are low water content nonionic hydrogels (e.g., polymacon, and crofilcon), high water content nonionic hydrogels (e.g., lidofilcon), and high water content anionic hydrogels (e.g., PHEMA copolymers). Sack et al.[167] suggest that the relationship of polymer

FIG 8–30.
The deposits seen on three different water content HEMA lenses worn by the same patient. A relatively clean 38% water content lens *(left)*, a slightly more heavily contaminated 55% HEMA lens *(center)*, and a heavily contaminated 70% HEMA material with multilayered deposits *(right)*. The figure illustrates the effect of water content on the tendency for tear film deposits to accumulate on hydrogel lenses.

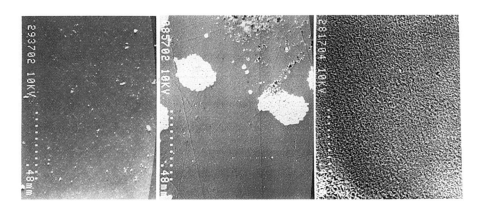

structure to biofilm formation is determined principally by the ionic binding capacity rather than the water content of the material. Their results agree with those of Stone et al.[176] on anionic PHEMA copolymer lenses; they found the lens-bound protein layer to be thick and consisting of loosely bound lysozyme, whereas on the nonionic hydrogels, the surface is much thinner and consists of a mixture of denatured tear proteins. Tomlinson and Caroline[176] offer support for the importance of surface chemistry in findings that a mid–water content (55% Elite Hydrowave, San Diego, Calf.) ionic hydrogel lens polymer could be as free of deposits as a low water content nonionic material when the mid–water content lens is chemically treated to change its surface chemistry (Fig 8–31).

The results of Sack et al.[167] suggest that the presence of methacrylic acid anions within the PHEMA copolymer allows this group of hydrogels to function in the same way as a cation exchange, absorbing more of the basic tear constituents. Therefore, acidic matrix lenses would be particularly prone to cationic species–reduced spoilage. These conclusions would lead to the recommendation that in patients with a propensity to lens deposition that materials of low water content nonionic nature would be preferred. A lens of this type, the crofilcon A material (CSI), is frequently thought to be the "cleanest" lens available. This lens does compare well with mid–water content hydrogel lenses in comparative analyses of surface deposition.[53, 105, 182, 183] However, as may be anticipated from a

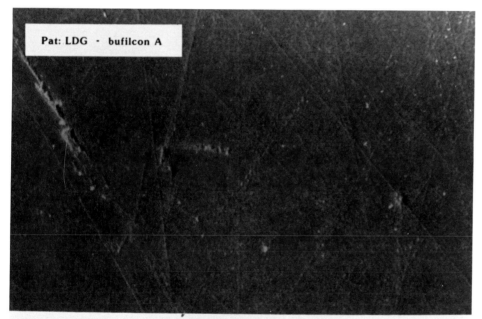

Pat: LDG · bufilcon A

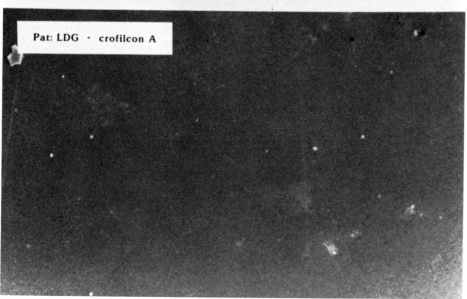

Pat: LDG · crofilcon A

FIG 8–31.
The effect of surface chemistry of hydrogel contact lenses on deposit formation illustrating that a mid–water content lens *(top)* can be as free of deposits as a low water content nonionic material *(bottom)* when the midwater content lens is chemically treated to change its surface chemistry. (From Tomlinson A, Caroline PJ: *J Br Contact Lens Assoc* 1989; 12:9. Used by permission.)

consideration of the surface chemistry of the lens materials, direct comparisons of crofilcon with other low water content nonionic lens materials[115, 187] find similar amounts of deposits on all of the lenses studied.

The results of Leahy et al.[115] showing large differences in deposition on mid–water content disposable lenses, Acuvue (Johnson & Johnson, Jacksonville, Fla.) and crofilcon A (CSI), support the conclusions of Sack et al.[167] that protein deposition is dependent on the ionic capacity of the lens material. Therefore, although a disposable lens provides the advantage of convenience, in view of the relatively greater amounts of protein found on such lenses after only a relatively short time of wear, it cannot be assumed that there is less potential for immunological response to the disposable lens than is the case with conventional lens types.

Patient's Tear Chemistry

Contact lens practitioners are well aware of the propensity for certain patients to build up heavy deposits on hydrogel lenses, whereas others wearing the same lens type may be almost free of deposits and their complications. This would suggest the strong influence of the individual patient's tear chemistry on lens deposition (Fig 8–32). Tomlinson and Caroline[183] have shown widely variable amounts of deposit on the same high water content nonionic material worn by a group of patients (surface coverage varied from 2% to 100% of the lens area). The

FIG 8–32.
The effect of individual patients' tear chemistry on deposit formation on hydrogel lenses. Three different patients wore the same mid–water content HEMA lens. Light, medium, and heavy deposits are seen from scanning electron microscopy photographs obtained from patients *DH, PV,* and *AT.* The surface appearance of an unworn mid–water content lens is also shown *(control).* (From Tomlinson A, Caroline PJ: *J Br Contact Lens Assoc* 1989; 12:9. Used by permission.)

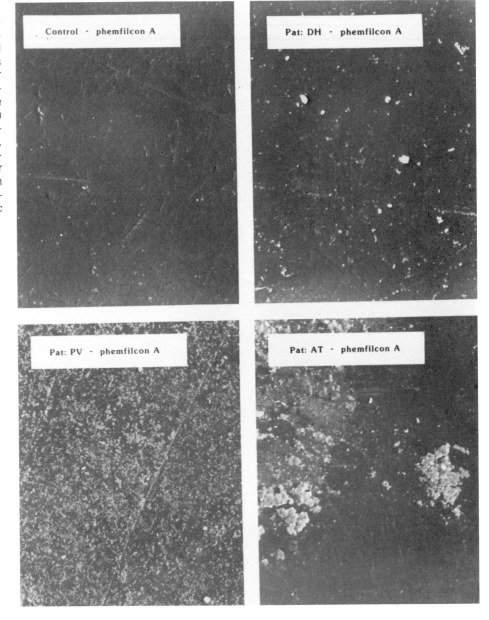

high or low amount of deposits seen on the high water content material is reflected on other lenses worn by the same individuals such that a heavy depositor on the high water content lens shows similar high deposits on low water content nonionic (highly resistant) lenses. This led the authors to recommend as an important patient selection criterion for high water content hydrogel lens wear a knowledge of the patient's tear chemistry (i.e., patients with low deposits being suitable for the high water content materials). The view of the importance of tear chemistry on the choice of the suitable lens materials for a patient is supported by Doughman et al.,[40] who found three times the incidence of heavy deposition in patients with dry eyes and Sack et al.[167] and Boonstra et al.[10] Leahy et al.[115] oppose its importance by contending that the water content and ionic character of the material are of more influence than the relative protein concentrations of the baseline tear film into which lenses are placed.

Lens Surface Integrity

The smoothness of the surface of hydrogel lenses appears to affect their propensity for lens deposits (Fig 8–33). Matas et al.[129] were the first to observe that scratches on the surface of hydrogel lenses appear to collect deposits. This was confirmed by later studies[19, 51]; Fowler and Gaertner[51] found that lathe or polishing marks on the lens surface provided a site for lens deposition, and the potential for binding of bacterial microorganisms to the surface led to the recommendation that lenses without polishing marks (molded lenses) should be considered in the fitting of patients with heavy depositing characteristics.

Deposits on Other Contact Lens Materials

Relatively few studies have considered the types of deposits occurring on contact lens materials other than hydrogels, but the lens analysis study carried out by Allergan Pharmaceuticals, Inc.[151] describes deposits found on other forms of lenses.

Polymethylmethacrylate

Examination of PMMA lens surfaces indicate the most common deposit is lipid. Some films, however, often contain proteins from the tears.[151] These surfaces are cleaned relatively easily with surfactant and enzymatic cleaning systems. Of all the hard contact lens materials, PMMA is the least susceptible to deposition from the tear film.[50]

Cellulose Acetate Butyrate

Lipid is the only deposit found on cellulose acetate butyrate (CAB) gas-permeable contact lens material.[151] They are easily removed with surfactant cleaners, but where they are a recurrent problem in specific patients, they may

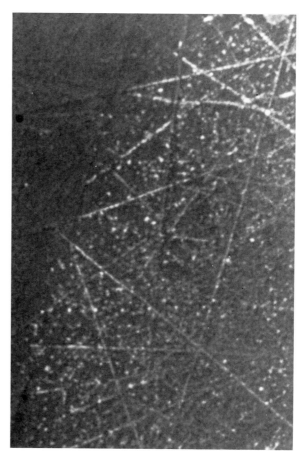

FIG 8–33.
The propensity for deposits to form in surface irregularities of hydrogel lenses. In the area of lens deposition, the pattern of surface scratches on the lens is defined by deposit formation.

indicate MGD. In some cases the lipid deposition on CAB materials is a more significant problem than occurs with silicone-acrylates (Fig 8–34).[171]

Silicone-Acrylates

Protein films are the main deposits found on silicone-acrylate (PMMA-Siloxane) copolymer RGP contact lenses (Fig 8–35).[50, 151, 171] These may be found in association with lipid. Surfactant cleaning may remove the latter, but protein films usually require the frequent use of enzymatic cleaners. Fowler et al.[50] noted that these RGP lens materials are considerably more susceptible to deposits than PMMA, often becoming coated with multilayer deposits within a couple of months of wear despite routine cleaning with surfactants. The problem of protein deposits on silicone-acrylate materials increases with the silicone content of the material. Protein deposits are a particular problem in the higher Dk materials and are a limiting factor in the design of these copolymers for extended wear. In some cases of higher Dk silicone-acrylate materials, cracking and

A   B

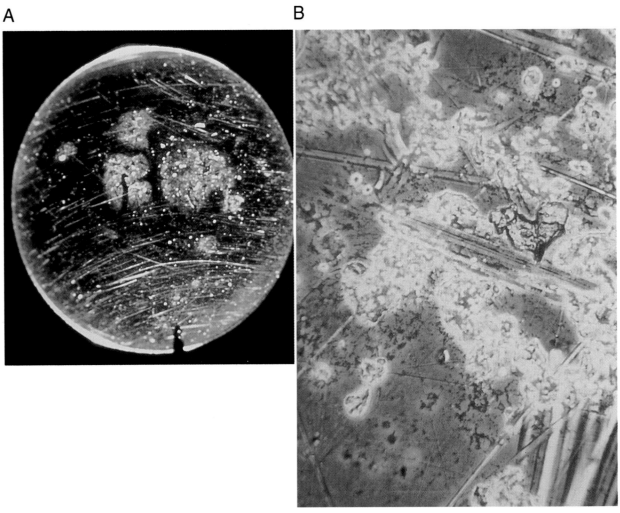

FIG 8–34.
Lipid deposits on cellulose acetate butyrate RGP lenses in macroview **(A)** and by phase contrast microscopy **(B).** (Courtesy of Allergan Pharmaceuticals, Inc., Irvine, Calif.)

A   B

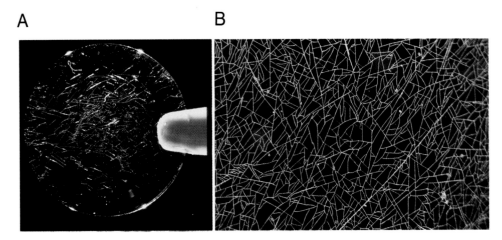

FIG 8–35.
Protein deposition on a silicone-acrylate RGP lens in macroview **(A)** and phase contrast microscopy **(B).** The cracking and crazing phenomenon associated with these lenses after extensive deposition and long-term wear is illustrated in **B.** (Courtesy of Allergan Pharmaceuticals, Inc., Irvine, Calif.)

A
B

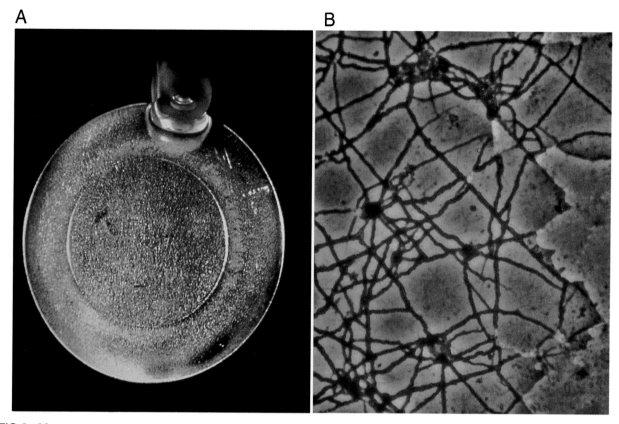

FIG 8–36.
Heavy protein and lipid deposits on silicone lenses **(A).** Accumulation of the protein film eventually leads to cracking and breakup of the surface treatment necessary to make these lenses hydrophilic **(B).** (Courtesy of Allergan Pharmaceuticals, Inc., Irvine, Calif.)

crazing of lenses have been linked to deposition (Fig 8–35). Inorganic materials such as calcium and magnesium salts have also been found on silicone-acrylate lenses.[171]

Fluoro–Silicone Acrylates

This form of RGP contact lens material is the most wettable and resistant to tear film deposition.[135] These lenses may attract protein and lipid film deposits, but they provide the better alternative than silicone-acrylate. Interestingly, the deposit resistance of different fluoro–silicone acrylate materials in which the fluorine content was varied was not found to be concentration dependent for fluorine levels greater than 20%.[184]

Silicone

Silicone failed as a generally fitted contact lens material in part because of its consummate ability to develop heavy protein and lipid deposits (Fig 8–36).[151] The protein film accumulated and eventually cracked in a crazed pattern that led to the development of rough surfaces and a breakup of the surface treatment necessary to make these lenses hydrophilic.

SUMMARY

The relation of a contact lens to the tear film is an extremely intimate one and one in which the lens affects the tear film and the tear film the lens. This chapter has attempted to cover this complex interaction and to detail the compromises on tear film integrity and complications of contact lens wear that can result.

REFERENCES

1. Abbott JM, et al: Studies in the ocular compatibility of hydrogels: IV. Observations on the role of calcium in deposit formation. *J Br Contact Lens Assoc* 1991; 14:21–28.
2. Abelson MB, Holly FJ: A tentative mechanism for inferior punctate keratopathy. *Am J Ophthalmol* 1977; 83:866–869.
3. Allansmith MR: Immunologic effects of extended-wear contact lenses. *Ann Ophthalmol* 1989; 21:465–467.
4. Allansmith MR, et al: Giant papillary conjunctivitis in contact lens wearers. *Am J Ophthalmol* 1977; 83:697–708.

5. Andres S, et al: Factors of the precorneal tear film break up time (BUT) and tolerance of contact lenses. *Int Contact Lens Clin* 1987; 14:103–107.

6. Andres S, et al: Tear pH, air pollution, and contact lenses. *Am J Optom Physiol Opt* 1988; 65:627–631.

7. Bahgat MM: Precorneal tear film changes due to soft contact lens wear. *Indian J Ophthalmol* 1985; 33:177–179.

8. Balik J, Kubat Z: Changes in tear proteins concentration in patients wearing gel contact lenses. *Optician* 1968; 155:205–207.

9. Benjamin WJ, Piccolo MG, Toubiana HA: Wettability: A blink by blink account. *Int Contact Lens Clin* 1984; 11:492–498.

10. Boonstra A, Van Haeringen N, Kijlstra A: Human tears inhibit the coating of proteins to solid phase surfaces. *Curr Eye Res* 1985; 4:1137–1145.

11. Brennan NA, et al: Dehydration of hydrogel lenses during overnight wear. *Am J Optom Physiol Opt* 1987; 64:534–539.

12. Browning DJ, Foulks GN: Tear pH in health, disease, and contact lens wear, in Holly FJ (ed): *The Preocular Tear Film in Health, Disease, and Contact Lens Wear.* Lubbock, Tex, Dry Eye Institute, 1986, p 954.

13. Callender M, Morrison PE: A quantitative study of human tear proteins before and after adaption to non-flexible contact lenses. *Am J Optom Physiol Opt* 1974; 51:939–945.

14. Carney LJ, Hill RM: Human tear pH diurnal variations. *Arch Ophthalmol* 1976; 94:821–824.

15. Carney LG, Hill RM: Tear pH: Hydrophilic lenses and the closed eye. *Int Contact Lens Clin* 1976; 3:30–31.

16. Carney LG, Hill RM: Tear pH and the hard (PMMA) contact lens patient. *Int Contact Lens Clin* 1976; 3:27–30.

17. Carney LG, Hill RM: The nature of normal blinking patterns. *Acta Ophthalmol* 1982; 60:427–433.

18. Carney LG, Hill RM: Variation in blinking behavior during soft lens wear. *Int Contact Lens Clin* 1984; 11:250–253.

19. Castillo EJ, et al: Characterization of protein adsorption on soft contact lenses: I. Conformational changes of adsorbed serum albumin. *Biomaterials* 1984; 5:319–325.

20. Castillo EJ, et al: Protein adsorption on hydrogels: II. Reversible and irreversible interactions between lysozyme and contact lens surfaces. *Biomaterials* 1985; 6:338–345.

21. Castillo EJ, Koenig JL, Anderson JM: Characterization of protein adsorption on soft contact lenses: IV. Comparison of in vivo spoilage with the in vitro adsorption of tear proteins. *Biomaterials* 1986; 7:89–96.

22. Castillo EJ, Koenig JL, Anderson JM: Protein adsorption on soft contact lenses: III. Mucin. *Biomaterials* 1986; 7:9–15.

23. Cedarstaff TH, Tomlinson A: A comparative study of tear evaporation rates and water content of soft contact lenses. *Am J Optom Physiol Opt* 1983; 60:167–174.

24. Cedarstaff TH, Tomlinson A: Human tear volume, quality and evaporation: A comparison of Schirmer, tear breakup time and resistance hygrometry techniques. *Ophthalmic Physiol Opt* 1983; 3:239–245.

25. Chen FS, Maurice DM: The pH in the precorneal tear film and under a contact lens measured with a fluorescent probe. *Exp Eye Res* 1990; 50:251–259.

26. Chopra SK, George S, Daniel R: Tear film break up time (B.U.T.) in non-contact lens wearers and contact lens wearers in normal Indian population. *Indian J Ophthalmol* 1985; 33:213–216.

27. Coles WH, Jaros PA: Dynamics of ocular surface pH. *Br J Ophthalmol* 1984; 68:549–552.

28. Conway HD, Richman M: Effects of contact lens deformation on tear film pressures induced during blinking. *Am J Optom Physiol Opt* 1982; 59:13–20.

29. Conway HD, Richman M: The effects of contact lens deformation on tear film pressure and thickness during motion of the lens towards the eye. *J Biomech Eng* 1983; 105:47–50.

30. Cook J, et al: Determination of proteins associated with hydrophilic contact lenses over three months of wear. *Optom Vis Sci* 1989; 66:88.

31. Cook J, et al: Investigation of mucin deposition on hydrophilic contact lenses. *Optom Vis Sci* 1989; 66:88.

32. Cope C, et al: Wettability of the corneal epithelium: A reappraisal. *Curr Eye Res* 1986; 5:777–785.

33. De Vries KA: Contact lenses and "the pill." *Contact Lens Forum* 1985; 10(11):21–23.

34. Derjaguin BV: Propulsive forces between charged colloid particles and the theory of slow coagulation and stability of lyophobe solutions. *Trans Farad Soc* 1940; 36:203–215.

35. DeRoetth A Sr: Lacrimation in normal eyes. *AMA Arch Ophthalmol* 1953; 49:185–189.

36. Dilly PN: Contribution of the epithelium to the stability of the tear film. *Trans Ophthalmol Soc UK* 1985; 104:381–389.

37. Doane MG: An instrument for in vivo tear film interferometry. *Optom Vis Sci* 1989; 66:383–388.

38. Doane MG, Gleason W: Further investigation of factors affecting contact lens wetting [abstract]. *Invest Ophthalmol Vis Sci* 1988; 29(ARVO suppl):279.

39. Dohlman CH, Boruchoff A, Mobilia EF: Complications in use of soft contact lenses in corneal disease. *Arch Ophthalmol* 1973; 90:367–371.

40. Doughman DJ, et al: The nature of "spots" on soft lenses. *Ann Ophthalmol* 1975; 7:345–348, 351–353.

41. Ehlers N: The precorneal film: Biomicroscopical, histological and chemical investigations. *Acta Ophthalmol* 1965; 81(suppl):21–34.

42. Eriksen S: Cleaning hydrophilic contact lenses: An overview. *Ann Ophthalmol* 1975; 7:1223–1226, 1229–1232.

43. Faber G, et al: Effect of hydrogel lens wear on tear film stability. *Optom Vis* 1991; 68:380–384.

44. Fanti T, Holly FJ: Silicone in contact lens wear: III. Physiology of poor tolerance. *Contact Intraocular Lens Med J* 1980; 6:111–119.

45. Farris RL: Tear analysis in contact lens wearers. *CLAO J* 1986; 12:106–111.

46. Fatt I: Observations of film breaking on model eyes. *J Br Contact Lens Assoc* 1990; 13:20–32.

47. Fischer FH, Wiederholt M: Human precorneal tear film pH measured by microelectrodes. *Graefes Arch Ophthalmol Clin Exp* 1982; 218:168–170.

48. Forst G: Observation of two structures of the tear film lipid layer. *Ophthalmic Physiol Opt* 1988; 8:190–192.

49. Fowler SA, Allansmith MR: Evolution of soft contact lens coatings. *Arch Ophthalmol* 1980; 98:95–99.

50. Fowler SA, et al: The surface of worn siloxane-PMMA gas permeable lenses: A scanning electron microscopy study. *CLAO J* 1987; 13:259–263.

51. Fowler SA, Gaertner KL: Scanning electron microscopy of deposits remaining in soft contact lens polishing marks after cleaning. *CLAO J* 1990; 16:214–218.

52. Fowler SA, Greiner JV, Allansmith MR: Attachment of bacteria to soft contact lenses. *Arch Ophthalmol* 1979; 97:659–660.

53. Fowler SA, Korb DR, Allansmith MR: Deposits on soft contact lenses of various water contents. *CLAO J* 1985; 11:124–127.

54. Fullard RJ: Tear enzymes as biochemical indicators of corneal dysfunction. Doctoral thesis, Melbourne, University of Melbourne, 1982.

55. Fullard RJ, Carney LG: Diurnal variation in human tear enzymes. *Exp Eye Res* 1984; 38:15–26.

56. Fullard RJ, Carney LG: Human tear enzyme changes as indicators of the corneal response to anterior hypoxia. *Acta Ophthalmol* 1985; 63:678–683.

57. Fullard RJ, Carney LG: Use of tear enzyme activities to assess the corneal response to contact lens wear. *Acta Ophthalmol* 1986; 64:216–220.

58. Fullard RJ, Carney LG, Hum T: Enzymes of carbohydrate metabolism in human tear fluid, in Holly FJ (ed): *The Preocular Tear Film in Health, Disease, and Contact Lens Wear*. Lubbock, Tex, Dry Eye Institute, 1986, p 529.

59. Gachon AM, Bilbaut T, Dastugue B: Adsorption of tear proteins on soft contact lenses. *Exp Eye Res* 1985; 40:105–116.

60. Gasset AR, Lobo L, Houde W: Spot formation and other abnormalities in hydrogel contact lenses. *Int Contact Lens Clin* 1975; 2(2):64–68.

61. Giesbrecht K, Tomlinson A: The aging tear film evaporation. *J Br Contact Lens Assoc* (in press).

62. Gilbard JP, Dartt DA: Changes in rabbit lacrimal gland fluid osmolarity with flow rate. *Invest Ophthalmol Sci* 1982; 23:804–806.

63. Gilbard JP, Gray KL, Rossi SR: A proposed mechanism for increased tear-film osmolarity in contact lens wearers. *Am J Ophthalmol* 1986; 102:505–507.

64. Goodfriend TL, Sokol DM, Kaplan NO: Control of synthesis of lactic acid dehydrogenases. *J Molec Biol* 1966; 15:18–31.

65. Greiner JV, Allansmith MR: Effect of contact lens wear on the conjunctival mucous system. *Ophthalmology* 1981; 88:821–832.

66. Greiner JV, et al: "Second" mucus secretory system of the human conjunctiva [abstract]. *Invest Ophthalmol* 1979; 8(suppl):123A.

67. Grohe RM, et al: RGP surface cracking: part II. Microbial concerns. *Contact Lens Spectrum* 1987; 2(9):40–46.

68. Guillon JP: Tear film structure in contact lenses, in Holly FJ (ed): *The Preocular Tear Film in Health, Disease, and Contact Lens Wear*. Lubbock, Tex, Dry Eye Institute, 1986, p 914.

69. Guillon M, Guillon JP: Hydrogel lens wettability during overnight wear. *Ophthalmic Physiol Opt* 1989; 9:355–359.

70. Halberg GP, Berens C: Standardized Schirmer tear test kit. *Am J Ophthalmol* 1961; 51:840–842.

71. Hamano H: Fundamental researches on the effects of contact lenses on the eye, in Rubin M (ed): *Soft Contact Lens Clinical and Applied Technology*. New York, John Wiley & Sons, 1978, p 135.

72. Hamano H: The change of precorneal tear film by the application of contact lenses. *Contact Intraocular Lens Med J* 1981; 7:205–209.

73. Hamano H, et al: A new method for measuring tears. *CLAO J* 1983; 9:281–289.

74. Hamano H, Hori M, Mitsunaga S: Measurement of evaporation rate of water from the precorneal tear film and contact lenses. *Contacto* 1981; 25(2):7–14.

75. Hart DE: Lipid deposits which form on extended wear contact lenses. *Int Contact Lens Clin* 1984; 11:348–362.

76. Hart DE, et al: Spoilage of hydrogel contact lenses by lipid deposits. Tear-film potassium depression, fat, protein, and alcohol consumption. *Ophthalmology* 1987; 94:1315–1321.

77. Hart DE, Tidsale RR, Sack RA: Origin and composition of lipid deposits on soft contact lenses. *Ophthalmology* 1986; 93:495–503.

78. Hathaway R, Lowther GE: Appearance of hydrophilic lens deposits as related to chemical etiology. *Int Contact Lens Clin* 1976; 3:27–35.

79. Hayashi TT: Mechanics of contact lens motion. Doctoral thesis, Berkeley, University of California, 1977.

80. Henderson JW, Prough WA: Influence of age and sex on flow of tears. *Arch Ophthalmol* 1950; 43:224–231.

81. Henriques AS, Korb DR: Meibomian glands and contact lens wear. *Br J Ophthalmol* 1981; 65:108–111.

82. Herold W: Die verdunstungsrate der Tranenflussigkeit beim Menschen verglichen mit einem physiokalischen Nmmodell. *Klin Monatsbl Augenheilkd* 1987; 190:176–179.

83. Hill RM: The quantitative blink. *Int Contact Lens Clin* 1984; 11:366–368.

84. Hill RM: Contact lens perspective. New York, Professional Press/Fairchild, 1988, p 55.

85. Hirji N, Patel S, Callander M: Human tear film prerupture phase time (TP-RPT)—a non-invasive technique for evaluating the pre-corneal tear using a novel keratometer mire. *Ophthalmic Physiol Opt* 1989; 9:139–142.

86. Holden BA, et al: The closed eye "cesspool" [abstract]. *Am J Optom Physiol Opt* 1987; 64(suppl):49P.

87. Holly FJ: Formation and rupture of the tear film. *Exp Eye Res* 1973; 15:515–525.

88. Holly FJ: Biophysical aspects of epithelial adhesion to stroma. *Invest Ophthalmol Vis Sci* 1978; 17:552–557.

TABLE 9–1.

Types and Causes of Dry Eye*

Aqueous deficiency	
Keratoconjunctivitis sicca	Infections, e.g., trachoma, mumps
Sjögren's syndrome	Trauma, e.g., irradiation, chemical
Congenital alacrima	burns
Riley-Day syndrome	Drugs, e.g., antihistamines,
Sarcoidosis	anticholinergics, β-adrenergic
Leukemia, lymphoma	blockers
Amyloidosis	Inflammation of lacrimal gland
Hemochromatosis	ducts by any other source

Mucin deficiency	
Vitamin A deficiency	Chronic conjunctivitis, e.g.,
Ocular pemphigoid	trachoma
Stevens-Johnson syndrome	Chemical burns

Lipid deficiency	
Congenital disorders	Meibomian keratoconjunctivitis

Lid resurfacing problems	
Eyelid abnormalities	Bell's palsy
Conjunctival abnormalities	Contact lens wear
Nocturnal lagophthalmos	

*From Lowther G, Malinosky V: *Dry Eye: A Clinical Overview.* Alcon Laboratories, 1988. Used by permission.

TABLE 9–2.

Systemic Medications Associated With Dry Eye and Ocular Surface Disease*

Antihistamines
  Hay fever medications
  Sleep medications
Antihypertensives
  β-Blockers
  Diuretics
  Methyldopa
Antiparkinsonian agents
Antiperspirants
Antitussives
Belladonna alkaloids
Chemotherapeutic agents
Opiates
Psychotropics
  Benzodiazepines
  MAO inhibitors†
  Phenothiazines
  Tricyclic antidepressants
Salicylates

*From Polak BCP: *Doc Ophthalmol* 1987; 67:115. Used by permission.
†MAO = monoamine oxidase.

wear rigid gas-permeable (RGP) wearers[98] and at 83% of extended wear RGP patients.[33]

WHY DO CONTACT LENSES INDUCE DRY EYE?

It is appropriate at this time to review the material discussed in Chapter 8 to determine the aspects of the interaction of contact lenses with the tear film that lead to the problem of dry eye: (1) thinning of the tear film, (2) loss of lid conformity, (3) lipid layer rupture, (4) corneal drying as a result of soft lens dehydration, and (5) change in the blink.

In addition to these more obvious causes of dry eye in contact lens wear are all of the subtle effects of lens wear on tear film described in the preceding chapter. Any of these singularly or in combination may exacerbate an already difficult situation in which marginal tear chemistry is trying to cope with the presence of contact lens on the anterior ocular surface.

Thinning of the Tear Film

The meniscus formed at the edge of hard contact lens draws fluid from its surroundings, producing a "black line," which is seen around the lens and indicates local thinning of the tear film.[37] This can result in 3 and 9 o'clock staining in the presence of a hard lens and reduced

tear breakup time in the presence of both hard and soft contact lenses.[45, 81] This is a problem particularly where tear breakup time is already reduced; such patients are categorized as having marginal dry eye (Fig 9–1).[2]

Loss of Lid Conformity

The physical presence of the lens can displace the lid away from the globe. This results in poor mucus spreading across the globe and areas of drying on the anterior ocular surface.

Lipid Layer Rupture

The presence of a contact lens on the eye, regardless of type, reduces the integrity of the lipid on the prelens tear film.[29, 31] Increased tear evaporation rate has been found with all types of contact lens.[103]

Corneal Drying due to Soft Lens Dehydration

Hydrogel lenses that show high evaporation from the anterior surface (e.g., thin or high water content) will draw fluid from the corneal substance, resulting in characteristic inferior, superior, or central punctate staining.[35]

Change in the Blink

Patients may change the nature of their blinks during contact lens wear,[37] leading to a greater incidence of incom-

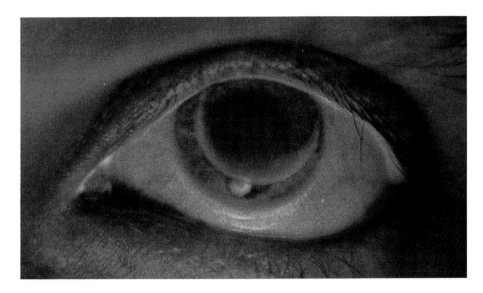

FIG 9–1.
Thinning of the tear film (stained with fluorescein) around the edge of a rigid gas-permeable (RGP) contact lens occurs as a result of the meniscus formed at the edge of the lens drawing fluid from this area. Darker areas at the edge of the lens indicate local thinning of the tear film.

plete blinks, which exacerbates the problems of resurfacing and tear film reestablishment.

CORNEAL COMPLICATIONS

The most common corneal complications of contact lens–induced dry eye are the phenomena of 3 and 9 o'clock staining with hard contact lenses and corneal desiccation in hydrogel contact lens wear.

3 and 9 O'clock Staining

Description

Staining of the cornea in regions immediately adjacent to the limbus is a common finding in hard contact lens wearers. This phenomenon has been variously described as juxtaposition staining,[5] persistent nasal and temporal stippling,[27] peripheral corneal desiccation,[43, 98] 4 and 8 o'clock staining,[3] or (most frequently) 3 and 9 o'clock staining.[3, 5, 11, 14, 27, 33, 36, 43, 51, 91, 93] This phenomenon is manifest as various densities of staining in the nasal and temporal regions of the cornea. This staining varies from a diffuse light staining with no coalescence,[93] through marked coalescence with deep penetration into the epithelial tissue, to significant loss of epithelial tissue. Extreme cases of chronic staining that have persisted for considerable amounts of time can lead to vascularized limbal keratitis (VLK), which includes corneal vascularization, scarring, and hyperplasia.[28]

Various grading systems have been used to describe the severity of 3 and 9 o'clock staining. Both Schnider[93] and Henry et al.[33] use five-point scales to describe the con-

dition. Schnider's system is illustrated in Figure 9–2. Henry's system[33] describes the phenomenon simply in terms of its appearance where 0 = not present, 1 = diffuse punctate staining, 2 = mild density, 3 = moderate density, and 4 = opacification or neovascularization. Such systems are useful for clinicians in grading the appearance in-office.

The phenomenon described by Grohe and Lebow[28] as vascularized limbal keratitis (VLK) represents an extreme form of the process graded by these systems. It is a complication of extended and, only occasionally, of daily RGP contact lens wear involving the cornea, limbus, and conjunctiva. Because of the inflammatory nature of the phenomenon, it is named VLK.[28] The four stages of this condition progress from a point where the systems of Schnider[93] and Henry et al.[33] leave off. Stage 1 VLK exhibits epithelial chafing with varying degrees of microsuperficial punctate keratitis (SPK) and heaping of hyperplastic corneal or limbal epithelium (or both). Stage 2 is characterized by the occurrence of the inflammatory response. During this hyperemic phase there is increased lens awareness and the eye is red. At stage 3, there is moderate conjunctival hyperemia because of the greater infiltrative reaction and expansion of the overlying corneal staining. A vascular leash emanating from the conjunctiva and across the edematous limbus leads to the raised epithelial mass (Fig 9–3). In stage 4, symptoms increase dramatically with photophobia and significant discomfort, including pain whenever the lens edge comes into contact with the elevated peripheral corneal mass. Significant conjunctival hyperemia and staining is often associated with an erosion of the elevated hyperplastic epithelium. In the most severe cases of 3 and 9 o'clock staining, the peripheral stroma begins to thin and a dellen is formed (Fig 9–4).[63]

A

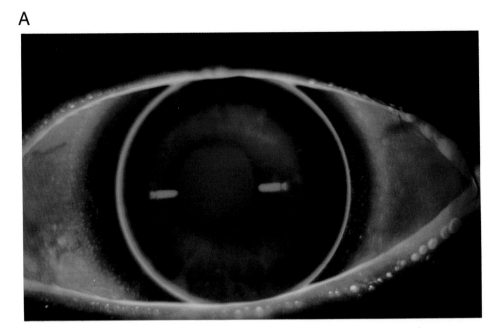

B

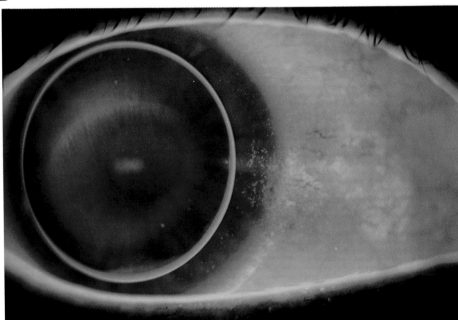

FIG 9–2.
Three and 9 o'clock staining is shown graded according to the system of Schnider.[93] Grade 0 is the absence of staining and is the situation in which the cornea wets well. **A,** grade 1 staining shows diffuse light staining with no coalescence; this requires no intervention. **B,** grade 2 staining shows light coalescence but the absence of fluorescein penetration into the deeper layers of the epithelium. Patients with this condition should be observed at follow-up visits.

Incidence

Three and 9 o'clock corneal staining is the most common complication of hard lens wear.[33, 93] Henry et al.[33] described the condition in 53% of patients fitted with extended wear RGP lenses. Solomon[98] reported the phenomenon occurring with both PMMA and RGP lenses worn for daily wear. It is more pronounced with prolonged lens wear but has been noted within the first month of wear by some observers.[59] Schnider et al.[93] found that patients with extended wear RGP lenses are more likely to experience the phenomenon than those in daily wear (Fig 9–5).

Causes

Lens Edge Abrasion or Chafing.—It has been suggested that excessive friction of the lens edge against limbal area can cause this phenomenon,[14, 27] making it more common in active eye turners and patients with corneal toricity. An

C

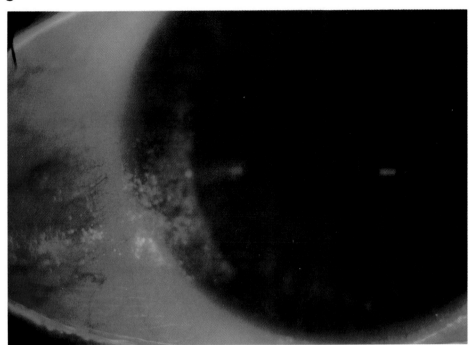

D

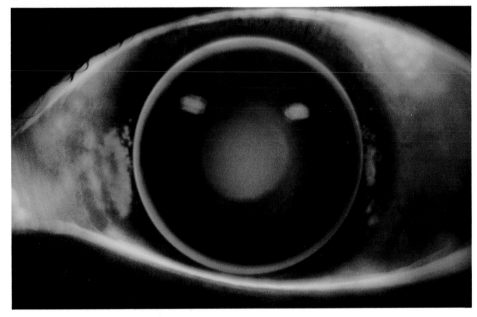

FIG 9–2 (cont'd.).
C, grade 3 staining shows marked coalescence with some deep penetration of fluorescein into the deeper epithelial layers. Such an appearance may lead to modification of the fit, design, or wearing schedule. **D,** grade 4 staining shows complete coalescence and extensive loss of epithelial cells. In such instances, lenses should be removed and epithelial regeneration should take place before refitting the patient. (Courtesy of C. Schnider.)

excessively loose lens might also be a cause of this problem.

Enlarged Lid Gap.—The enlarged lid gap caused by the presence of the contact lens is also thought by many to be a physical cause of 3 and 9 o'clock staining.[5, 11, 27, 47, 98] The loss of conformity of the lid to the anterior ocular surface may cause poor lubrication of the surface because of insufficient mucus spreading,[93] as well as other phenomena associated with tear film breakup (see Chapter 8). Many of the strategies of treating the condition aim at reducing the separation of the lid and eye by changes in the peripheral edge design of the contact lens.

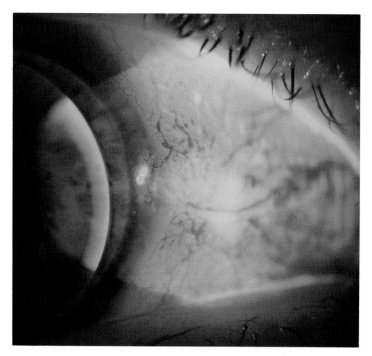

FIG 9–3.
An extreme form of peripheral corneal desiccation occurs in the condition of vascularized limbal keratitis described by Grohe and Lebow.[28] This inflammatory condition shows moderate conjunctival hyperemia and a vascular leash emanating from the conjunctiva and crossing the edematous limbus. (From Grohe RM, Lebow KA: *Int Contact Lens Clinic* 1989; 16:197. Used by permission.)

Tear Film Breakup With Contact Lens Wear.—The breakup of tear film caused by meniscus forces around the edge of the lens[37] may be responsible for the cornea being exposed in this area. This effect, combined with the general loss of tear film integrity during contact lens wear (see Chapter 8), makes the cornea much more vulnerable to drying. The consensus of opinion on the cause of the 3 and 9 o'clock staining favors corneal desiccation as the major cause of the loss of epithelial tissue.[11, 28, 33, 43, 47, 51, 95, 98]

Marginal Dry Eyes.—The phenomenon of 3 and 9 o'clock staining appears to occur more frequently in patients who have marginally dry eyes because of either insufficiency of lacrimation or poor quality of tears, leading to instability and rapid tear film breakup.[5] It has been shown that the phenomenon is more pronounced in patients taking medications that precipitate dry eyes, such as antihistamines, diuretics, and oral contraceptives.[27, 98]

Poor Blinking.—Infrequent or incomplete blinks have been suggested by several authors as the cause of 3 and 9 o'clock staining.[5, 14, 27, 51, 91] Whether poor blinking is the actual cause or just a factor that exacerbates a marginally dry eye or is a problem of a poorly designed lens is open to question. Korb and Korb[51] demonstrated the importance of blinking by showing that discontinuing wear of lenses in unilateral wearers caused significant improvement in 3 and 9 o'clock staining in both eyes. It was suggested that the presence of the contact lens in one eye provoked poor blinking that resulted in corneal drying of both

corneas. Sarver and Nelson[91] found that patients with the poorest blink habits were the ones showing the greatest 3 and 9 o'clock staining. Many clinicians suggest performing regular blink exercises to help reduce the problem of 3 and 9 o'clock staining.[14] Although alleviating the problem temporarily, unfortunately, good blinking habits are rarely relearned in the presence of a contact lens. Other strategies that avoid the problem are often more effective.

Lens Binding.—Lens binding, or adherence, to the cornea after overnight wear of RGP lenses can exacerbate 3 and 9 o'clock staining because of disruption of the tear layer where the lens indents the cornea (Fig 9–6).[100] Cases of peripheral ulceration in severe 3 and 9 o'clock staining secondary to RGP lens adhesion have been reported.[92]

Management

Effective management of 3 and 9 o'clock staining can be achieved by a number of strategies. A comprehensive review of these can be seen in Figure 9–7. Most of the lens-related strategies address the design of the edge of the hard contact lens in an attempt to reduce the gap between the lid and the cornea to maintain the integrity of the tear film in this region. The consensus of opinion favors a decrease in edge lift.[3, 11, 36, 95, 98] Holden et al.[36] demonstrated that edge lifts of 0.08 mm produce significantly reduced amounts of corneal desiccation (6%) compared with those found with 0.1-mm (43%) and 0.12-mm (100%) edge lifts. The lower edge lift design reduces the peripheral tear volume, decreases the gap in the periphery between the lid

A

B

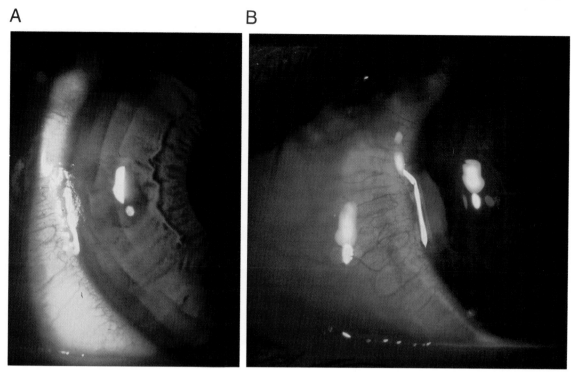

FIG 9–4.
In the most severe cases of 3 and 9 o'clock staining, the peripheral corneal stroma becomes thinned and a dellen is formed. This appears as a white opacification of the peripheral cornea **(A),** which shows extensive staining with fluorescein **(B).** (Courtesy of K. Lebow.)

FIG 9–5.
The phenomenon of 3 and 9 o'clock staining is found to occur more frequently in patients wearing extended wear RGP lenses than those in daily wear. (Courtesy of C.M. Schnider.)

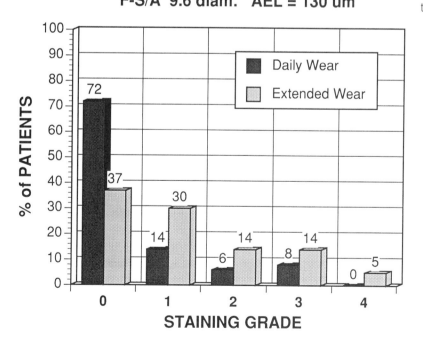

3 & 9 O'CLOCK STAINING
EXTENDED vs. DAILY WEAR
F-S/A 9.6 diam.   AEL = 130 um

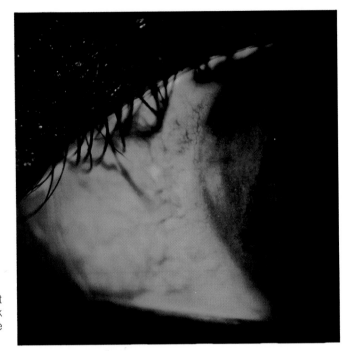

FIG 9–6.
Lens binding, or adherence, to the cornea after overnight wear of an RGP lens can exacerbate 3 and 9 o'clock staining because of disruption of the tear film where the lens indents the cornea. (Courtesy of K. Lebow.)

and the cornea, and minimizes the irritative interaction between the lid and the lens, thus avoiding poor blinking habits.[43] To achieve a low edge lift, a tricurve or tetracurve design with a steeper and narrower peripheral curve, such as a 11.5-mm radius and less than a 0.2-mm width, is desirable.[10] An aspheric design RGP lens offers the advantage of providing this type of edge lift.[10] The thinning of the anterior lens surface at the edge by the incorporation of a spherical CN bevel on the peripheral portion of lens will also help to reduce the lid gap even further.[5, 7, 43] Thicknesses of 0.1 to 0.12 mm are recommended.[11]

Others[93] have suggested that lower edge lifts will not solve the problem of 3 and 9 o'clock staining, particularly in extended wear RGP fitting, and advocate lenses with wide and relatively flat edge curve designs. However, their

studies do not cover the lower edge lift designs (around 0.10 mm) recommended earlier.

The base curve of the contact lens has also been suggested as a parameter that can be modified to reduce 3 and 9 o'clock staining. Steeper or aspheric designs are thought preferable to minimize tear breakup and avoid lid incongruities.[3, 43]

The diameter of the lens has also received attention. Some practitioners suggest an increase,[11, 93, 98] others a decrease, in lens diameter to avoid 3 and 9 o'clock staining.[3] However, larger-diameter RGP lenses combined with low edge lift designs and, in some cases, a "steeper than K" fitting relationship have been found to be common factors in the VLK that can occur secondary to peripheral corneal dessication.[28] It appears that when such lenses are

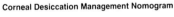

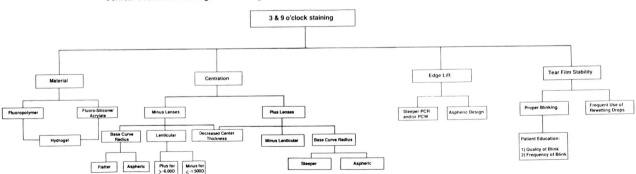

FIG 9–7.
Nomogram outlining the management of corneal desiccation. The changes in contact lens materials, design, and enhancement of tear film stability are listed. (From Jones DH, Bennett ES, Davis LJ: *Contact Lens Spectrum* 1989; 4(5):63. Used by permission.)

worn for extended wear, they alter the tear meniscus and create a desiccation and mechanical traumatic effect at the limbus that causes chafing of the epithelium and sets into motion a process of, as yet, undefined vasogenic response. For these reasons, large-diameter, low edge lift designs should be used with caution in extended wear RGP lens fittings.

The effect of many of the parameter changes just described is to alter the lens centration and change the fitting philosophy adopted in cases of 3 and 9 o'clock staining. Henry et al.[33] have shown a relationship between the frequency of the condition and lens position. They found that a superior- to central-fitting lens tucked under the upper lid resulted in considerably less corneal desiccation (38%) than interpalpebral fits (57%). Inferior decentering or low-riding lenses result in the greatest amount of staining (73%). For this reason, the avoidance of low-riding lenses is encouraged.[33, 94, 95, 98] Indeed, it has been shown that a low-riding lens is a factor in adhesion found in extended wear RGP lens fits. To avoid a low-riding lens and to give the desired superior positioning fit, one should use, for minus-powered contact lenses, a slightly flatter than K base curve radius selection.[43] This flat fit allows greater control of the lens position by the upper lid.[50] The problem of good lens centration with plus lenses is more difficult because of the greater lens mass. As a result, a smaller-diameter lens[6] that is lenticulated and made from a lower specific gravity material such as silicone-acrylate or *t*-butyl styrene may be preferred.[102]

The choice of lens material may also help to offset the problem of 3 and 9 o'clock staining in other ways. Materials that maintain more stable tear film on the front surface of the lens reduce the problem.[43] Rigid gas-permeable lens materials containing fluoro-silicone-acrylate may provide better tear film integrity and better wetting properties than those lenses containing silicone-acrylate alone.[34]

Persistent corneal desiccation caused by the 3 and 9 o'clock staining phenomenon presents a significant hazard to the health of the cornea by opening the way for corneal infection. Frequent monitoring of patients who wear RGP contact lenses is necessary to prevent the sequelae associated with the condition. The frequent absence of symptoms can result in significant corneal compromise before the patient is aware of any problem. Practitioners are advised to avoid or alleviate the problem as early as possible during the care of the patient.

Corneal Desiccation With Hydrogel Contact Lenses

Disturbances of the corneal epithelium secondary to hydrogel contact lens wear are well documented in the literature. Multiple causes of these patterns of staining are discussed in Chapter 7. A form of localized corneal desic-

cation with hydrogel lenses is described by several authors.[17, 35, 46, 47, 79, 108, 109] Various names have been given to the phenomenon, including pitting stain,[46] inferior arcuate staining,[108] epithelial fractures,[17] epithelial erosions,[35] and corneal desiccation staining.[79, 109]

Description

The drying staining generally occurs in the central,[17, 35, 79] superior midperipheral,[35, 46] or the inferior, midperipheral region of the cornea.[35, 47, 108] It is said to be more likely to occur in the inferior portion of the cornea because that is the area of the lens most frequently exposed because of lid position.[108] Others disagree, maintaining that staining is more commonly found in the central corneal epithelium,[35] because this part of the cornea is more exposed and contains more fragile epithelium than the periphery.[70] The staining can vary in degree from light, punctate staining through progressive confluent patches of epithelial cell loss, to erosions that include the full thickness of epithelium (Fig 9–8).[35] Patients with this problem are often asymptomatic until the level of epithelial loss increases, at which stage, pain and burning sensations may be reported, with an increase in limbal redness.[35] The incidence of the problem has been reported to be about one third of patients wearing hydrogel lenses.[46] This is consistent with practi-

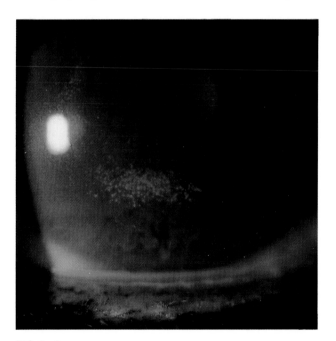

FIG 9–8.
Corneal desiccation with hydrogel contact lens wear is seen as punctate or confluent patches of epithelial cell loss usually in the midperipheral region of the cornea. It is thought to be caused by lens dehydration as a result of evaporation of the anterior lens tear film. This, in turn, causes fluid to be drawn from the corneal structure and loss of epithelial cells. (Courtesy of J. Dougal.)

tioner surveys, which determine the level of dry eye symptoms among soft contact lens patients to be between 20% and 30%.[80]

Causes

Earlier reports of the phenomenon[46, 47] describe the mechanical action of the midperipheral regions of the contact lens as being the cause of the staining. In addition, lens thickness, exposure of the lower half of eye as a result of lid position, and stagnation of tears beneath the lens were also thought to be implicated.[47] Definitive work by Holden et al.[35] and Osborn and Zantos[78, 80] clearly indicate the phenomenon to be related to lens thickness and water content. Most observers have noted the phenomenon as occurring in thin hydrogel contact lenses.[17, 35, 46, 47, 80, 108] Significantly, it has been found to occur particularly in thin, high water content lenses.[35, 79, 80] Holden et al.[35] suggest an etiology for the condition that links lens dehydration and thinning or loss of the postlens tear film with resulting mechanical damage or desiccation of the underlying epithelium. They postulate that evaporation of the anterior lens tear film draws water from the back of the lens to the front and ultimately fluid from within the corneal structure.

The erosion seen on the cornea coincides with both the thinnest portion of the contact lens and the area where the tear film is probably thinnest or least stable.[35] Andrasko[1] has shown that thin lenses dehydrate more than thicker lenses. As a result, decreasing the thickness of high water content hydrogel lenses to obtain optimum levels of oxygenation for the cornea during extended wear is not possible because of the corneal desiccation that would result. Therefore, the corneal desiccation phenomenon represents a limiting factor on the design of high water content lenses for extended wear.[79] Holden et al.[35] and Zantos et al.[109] have noted that the phenomenon is more likely to occur in low humidity environments than those in which humidity is high. This observation supports the corneal desiccation theory advanced by Holden et al.[35] In addition, Holden et al.[35] observed that in high-humidity environments, levels of lipid buildup on the front surface of hydrogel lenses are greater so that the tear film is more consistent and stable. This would act as an inhibitor to evaporative drying of the cornea. The importance of lens mobility on corneal staining under hydrogel lenses has also been considered by Holden et al.[35] and Zantos et al.[109] Holden et al.[35] found the phenomenon to be linked to lens immobility but thought that this was not a principal factor in its etiology. Zantos et al.[109] found no relationship to lens movement.

Zadnick and Mutti[108] suggest that the corneal desiccation with hydrogels is caused by a combination of metabolic and desiccation mechanisms. The area of the cornea involved, midway between the center and limbal region, is the area where the tear film is least actively exchanged with routine blinking. The tear film over the staining can therefore become filled with debris, become stagnant, and contain material toxic to the corneal epithelium.

Management

Fortunately, corneal drying with hydrogels is easily reversible. The disappearance of even confluent staining can occur within 2 hours of lens removal.[109] Management of the condition usually involves the use of thicker, lower water content hydrogel lenses for daily wearers. Patients who use extended wear who wish to continue with the modality should be refitted with mid–water content, thicker hydrogel lenses in preference to extended wear with thin, low water content lenses or even high water content lenses.[109] Increasing the lubrication in the eye or cleaning the lens more adequately may alleviate the problem by increasing the exchange of fresh tears, decreasing the amount of debris collecting under the lens, and replenishing the tear film.[108] Because deposit problems may occur with lens drying, disposable daily or extended wear contact lenses offer the advantage of reduced exposure to heavily contaminated lens surfaces.

PREDICTION TESTS FOR DRY EYE

Correct patient selection is an important technique in preventing contact lens–induced dry eye. It has been suggested that the dry eye is the most important cause of patient dissatisfaction and unproductive chair time in the practice of contact lenses, especially when it is not diagnosed and explained to the patient.[12] If it is possible to detect a marginal or borderline dry eye patient before contact lens fitting, many of the complications discussed earlier may be avoided.

Dry eye patients often have a clinical history in which lengthy fitting and different solutions have been tried by a number of practitioners. Such situations indicate a likely diagnosis of dry eye, which may be confirmed by the correct prediction test. A number of tests have been employed in an attempt to define, on the basis of inadequate tear physiology, the patient with "dry eye contraindications" to contact lens wear.

Tear Production Tests

Schirmer Test

Originally introduced by Schirmer in 1903, this relatively simple in-office procedure has been widely used to measure tear production rates. A standardized Schirmer tear test kit was introduced by Halberg and Berens[30] in 1961. This kit uses a strip of filter paper 5 by 30 mm bent 5 mm from the end and placed under the lower lid in a slightly temporal position.

In the Schirmer I test, the patient looks up and blinks normally for 5 minutes before the strip is removed and the wetted portion (beginning at the fold) is measured. An average (normal) Schirmer response is more than 22 mm of wetting; dry eye patients show averages of 7.6 mm of wetting during the 5 minutes. To avoid the irritation experienced during this test affecting the results, some practitioners prefer to use a 1-minute period for measurement.[74] The results obtained with this technique are multiplied by 3. An alternative form of the Schirmer I test is carried out using a local anesthetic (proparacaine). This *basal secretion test* is meant to record the amount of tear production in the absence of reflex tearing. Interpretation is similar to that with the unanesthesized Schirmer test described earlier.

In the Schirmer II test, a deliberate attempt is made to instigate reflex tear secretion. An anesthetic is applied to the eye, and the amount of wetting of the Schirmer strip is recorded after the deliberate irritation of the nasal mucosa in this eye. A reduced reflex lacrimal secretion is indicated if the wetted portion of the strip is less than 15 mm.[62] Dry eye patients in Schirmer tests are normally considered to be the patients with less than 5 mm of wetting in the 5-minute test. Holly[38] in his survey of 300 eye care professionals found the Schirmer test to be applied in a little more than one half of all cases of suspected dry eye, with most practitioners using the Schirmer II test.

Phenol Red, Cotton Thread Test

In this test devised by Hamano et al.,[32] a 70-mm thread impregnated with phenol red is inserted over the lower lid in a similar way to the Schirmer test strip. The testing time is only 15 seconds and is carried out with the eyes closed. Absorption of tears by the thread is measured by the amount of thread that is turned from red to yellow because of the pH of the tears. This test, which is less irritating than the Schirmer, produces much more reliable results.[4] The disadvantages of this procedure are that the thread has a relatively low absorption capacity, and in some cases it is possible for individuals to secrete tears at a higher rate than can be absorbed by the thread.[62] The test is designed to measure the residual volume of tears in the cul-de-sac and not the actual tear volume of the eye.[32] With this test the average wet length for normal patients is 16.7 mm, with a range from 3 to 48 mm. Values of less than 9 mm of wet thread are said to be diagnostic of dry eye.

Fluorophotometry

The most accurate method of measuring tear volume and tear turnover is fluorophotometry (see Fig 8–16).[71] In this technique a small quantity of sodium fluorescein is applied to the inferior conjunctiva, and the rate of decay of fluorescence in the tear film is recorded for 30 to 60 minutes. A biphasic response is obtained. There is an initial rapid decay as a result of reflex tearing, followed by a slower (physiological) decay after about 5 minutes. Tear volume can be calculated by extrapolation of the decay curve to zero time. Tear volume by this method averages about 7 μL, and tear turnover rate is between 13% and 16% per minute.[44, 71] This is a laboratory and not a clinical technique.

Tear Film Breakup Tests

Tear Breakup Time With Fluorescein

The tear film breakup time (BUT) measures the quality rather than quantity of tears. Usually performed by instilling fluorescein into the eye and observing the time required before the first dark spots of breakup areas are formed in the green tear film, it is an invasive procedure that in itself may cause disruption of the tear film (see Fig 8–12).[77]

The range of BUTs recorded with this technique is large. Normal patients are defined as those who show breakup in more than 10 seconds, many patients exceeding 60 seconds before the first breakup takes place.[54] Marginal dry patients are those with the tear BUT of 5 to 10 seconds. Patients with pathological dry eye have less than 5-second BUTs.[9, 58] This BUT is fairly reproducible.[55] To avoid problems, however, one should use liquid fluorescein, should not keep the patient's lids open during the test, and should have the patient maintain normal blinking at intervals when measurements are not being taken. Also, normal room humidity should be maintained throughout the test, which should be repeated several times.

Important for a stable tear film is a tear BUT that exceeds the normal interblink period. This is perhaps more important even than the actual tear BUT.[58]

Noninvasive Breakup Times

Because instillation of fluorescein into the conjunctival sac of itself can be disruptive to the tear film, techniques that do not have this requirement have been developed. The noninvasive breakup time (NIBUT) was first developed by Mengher et al.[69] In the technique a grid pattern is projected onto the anterior ocular surface, which is observed using a biomicroscope under low magnification. The first rupture of the tear film is seen when this grid pattern is disrupted. Normal values obtained with this technique average 40 seconds, with a range of 4 to 150 seconds; 85%

of the patients exceed 10-second BUTs. Dry eye patients, on the other hand, average 12 seconds, with a range of 2 to 20 seconds. A 10-second NIBUT is taken as the level of suspicion for dry eye.

Another form of NIBUT has been developed by Patel et al.[82] Similar to the Mengher et al.[69] technique, Patel et al.[82] used the keratometer mire image to observe tear film rupture. The tear film thinning time (TTT) measured by this technique has a normal value of 18 seconds, 10 seconds being the cutoff value for dry eyes.

Tear breakup time has been found to be the most valid predictive test in identifying those patients who are less likely to achieve success in contact lens wear because of dry eye.[99] The Schirmer test was found to have little predictive value.[40, 77, 99]

Tear breakup tests are discussed in more detail in Chapter 8.

Tear Evaporation

Several laboratory techniques have been used to measure the evaporation rate of tears from preocular or prelens surfaces. These techniques include resistance hygrometry,[103] pressure gradient evaporimetry,[104] and the relative humidity measurements within a goggle placed over the eyes.[89] Studies show a wide variation in evaporation rates between normal subjects and increased evaporation rates with contact lens wear and dry eye pathological conditions[90] (see Fig 8–23). In view of the experimental nature of these techniques, they are not applicable as clinical tests for dry eye.

Tear Film Structure

Relatively simple biomicroscopic techniques have been developed to observe the interference fringe patterns produced by the tear film on the preocular and prelens surfaces.[29, 31] Characteristic tear film patterns are seen as the result of the destructive interference taking place at the thin films that comprise the tear film. Unstable tear films are characterized by certain interference fringe patterns. Patients who show contaminated marmoreal patterns or colored fringe patterns are thought to be unsuitable for contact lens wear.[29] A detailed description of these techniques is found in Chapter 8 (see Figs 8–3 to 8–7).

Tear Fern Patterns

Samples of tears applied to a microscope plate and viewed under moderate magnification provide fernlike patterns for observation. The form of the fern pattern provides a means of tear assessment. The concept of this technique is similar to that of the Papanicolau smear test for cervical mucus.

Techniques vary in the method of collection of tears. Some workers[88] use a spatula to take a scraping of conjunctival mucus, whereas others[48, 75] use a microcapillary technique.

The technique provides a simple in-office procedure that could add valuable information on the quality of the tears. At this time, however, opinions differ on the interpretation of the fern patterns. Kogbe and Liotet[48] associate sparse ferning patterns with abnormal tear protein profiles, suggesting that the tear fern pattern is not an indicator of mucus inadequacy. Rolando et al.[88] also maintain that dense ferning patterns are indicators of normal tear profile, a sparse ferning being seen in patients with pathological dry eyes. Norn,[75] on the other hand, maintains that ferning is rarely seen in normal subjects and is more evident in diseases that produce larger amounts of mucus, such as allergic and infectious conjunctivitis. The criteria for normal tear ferning patterns must be defined before this technique can be used for diagnosis of dry eye.

Tear Osmolality

Gilbard[22] developed a technique of nanoliter osmometry in which the precise freezing point depression method is applied to determine the melting point of small tear samples. Normal values of tear osmolality are 300 to 310 mOsm/kg. Higher values are found in keratoconjunctivitis sicca (KCS) (329 mOsm/kg) and in contact lens wear (316 mOsm/kg).[19, 23] A comparison of the relative prediction value of various tests found the tear osmolality test to have the highest sensitivity (90%) and specificity (95%) compared with the lactoferrin assay technique (35% sensitivity, 70% specificity) and the Schirmer test (25% sensitivity, 90% specificity).[61] The technique is not applicable to in-office measurement of tear osmolality (see Fig 8–22), however.

Leukocyte Esterase Test

An application of the commercially available dip stick for detection of urinary infections has been developed for tear analysis.[76] The technique can be used to detect an associated ocular infection in dry eye, ocular surface disorders, and in contact lens wearers. The technique measures the presence of leukocyte esterase in tear samples in patients who are suspected of having an infection.

Lysozyme Test

A lysozyme agar diffusion test can be used to measure the amount of lysozyme in the tears. A decrease in the quantity of tears produces a subsequent decrease in lysozyme levels. The technique involves taking a tear sample by placing a small disc of filter paper (6-mm diameter) onto the lower conjunctival sac and allowing it to absorb tears. The disc is then placed on agarose gel plate containing *Micrococcus lysodeikticus,* and the zone of inhibited bacterial growth is measured.[8] Zone diameters less than the normal level of 21.5 mm indicate inhibition of tear production.[107] The technique is similar to the lactoferrin assay.

Lactoferrin Assay

Lactoferrin assay is a laboratory test that measures tear protein concentration using a lactoferrin immunodiffusion assay test (Lactoplate, Eagle Vision, Memphis, Tenn.). The procedure includes placing a filter paper circle onto the inferior conjunctiva to absorb tears. This disc is then placed on an immunoreactive plate for 3 days, and the size of the ring surrounding the disc is measured. The size of the ring indicates the amount of lactoferrin in the tear sample. The larger the ring, the greater the concentration of lactoferrin[42]; reduced diameters are measured in cases of dry eyes.[26]

A comparative evaluation of the lactoferrin assay technique (Lactoplate) indicated that lactoferrin measurements had the highest specificity among five tests evaluated for dry eye (i.e., Schirmer I test, Schirmer basal test, tear film BUT, and rose bengal staining).[41] Therefore, the test appears to be a valuable tool for early and accurate diagnosis of dry eye states.

Impression Cytology

The technique of removing ocular surface cells by pressing strips of cellulose acetate material onto the conjunctiva was described by Egbert et al.[16] Discs 6.2 mm in diameter are applied to the conjunctiva with a constant pressure from an ophthalmodynamometer. Specimens are then placed on glass slides, fixed, and stained to allow examination by light microscopy for goblet cell density and epithelial cell morphology (Figs 9–9 and 9–10).[16, 72] The technique has been used to study mucus and epithelial cells in KCS[65, 73] and to study goblet cell density in contact lens wearers and those taking oral contraceptives.[13] Goblet cell density is found to increase in contact lens wearers, but it decreases in those taking oral contraceptives, perhaps explaining lens intolerance in these patients.[13] As yet the technique has not been widely applied, but its relative ease of application makes it a potential in-office procedure.

Meibomian Gland Dysfunction

Korb and Henriquez[49] described a syndrome of meibomian gland dysfunction found in contact lens wearers in which

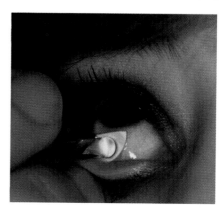

FIG 9–9.
Impression cytology procedure for measurement of dry eye. Sample collection is achieved by applying the Millipore filter paper against the bulbar conjunctiva and pressing with a glass rod for 2 seconds. This procedure is repeated three times over the same area. The filter paper is then attached to a microscope slide and fixed in 95% ethanol. The samples are then developed in a multiple-stage procedure involving staining with hematoxylin and development in saturated lithium carbonate. (Courtesy of C. Conner.)

minimal or transient symptoms of dryness, fluorescein staining of the cornea, and deficient or inadequate meibomian gland secretions occurred. Meibomian gland dysfunction is evidenced by cloudy or absent gland output on expression[40] and is found in problematic contact lens patients.[83] Meibomian gland assessment has been advocated as a standard procedure in contact lens patients with dry eye symptoms[83] and has been used to observe changes in gland morphology with age,[80] which can account for significant increases in tear film evaporation.[85] The technique is simple; the patient looks up, firm digital pressure is applied to the lower lid, and resulting gland secretions are observed with the biomicroscope. Secretions can be classified as clear (normal), cloudy (somewhat deficient), thick (toothpaste-like, deficient), or absent (inspissated, definitely deficient) (Fig 9–11). Meibomian gland deficiencies can often be overcome by the simple application of lid scrubs and warm compresses.[49]

Tear Prism Height

Biomicroscopic observation of the marginal tear strip or meniscus at the edge of the lower lid can reveal dry eye problems if the height is decreased. The technique is best carried out with a graticule in the eyepiece of the biomicroscope. A tear meniscus height of 0.3 mm is normal, with a regular and uniform tear prism along the lower lid margin. In dry eye patients the tear meniscus height is reduced, and the appearance of the tear prism may be irregular or scalloped.[101] Just more than half of the practitioners surveyed use 0.2 mm as a cutoff for dry eye,[38] and

A

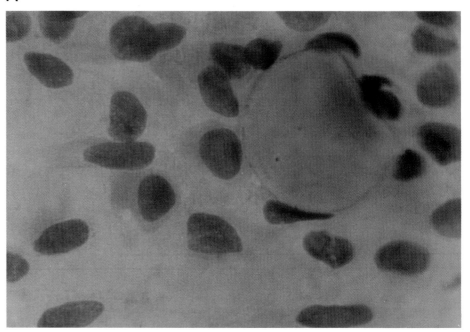

B

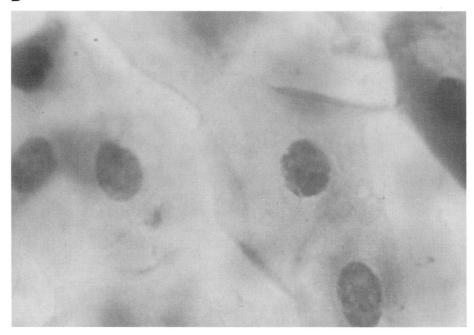

FIG 9–10.
Examples of the cell formations obtained by impression cytology from normal eyes **(A)** and dry eye patients **(B).** Goblet cells from a normal eye will stain red as illustrated in **A.** The high mucin content, rich in carbohydrates, causes the goblet cells to stain with periodic acid–Schiff reagent and appear red. In the dry eye, the absence of goblet cells and the prevalence of single cells rather than clusters are seen **(B).** (Courtesy of C. Conner.)

only 3% use 0.1 mm as a cutoff value.[38, 101] The technique can be carried out with or without the application of fluorescein to the tear film (Fig 9–12).[58]

Staining of the Cornea and Conjunctiva

Vital staining of the cornea is used by the majority of practitioners as an objective test for dry eye.[38] Almost 90% of practitioners use this staining technique, about one half using both rose bengal and fluorescein; fluorescein is used exclusively by about one third.

Fluorescein Dye

Fluorescein is an aniline dye that stains areas of epithelial cell loss where the cells are not devitalized. A small amount of sodium fluorescein 2% solution is instilled into the lower conjunctival sac. In a dry eye patient the inferior or interpalpebral portion of the cornea and conjunctiva

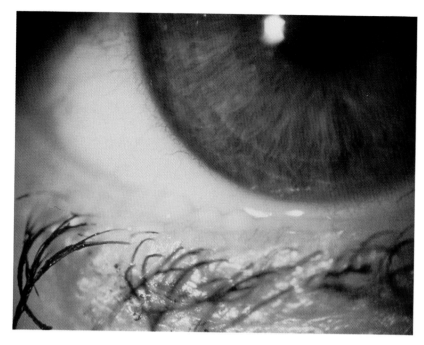

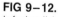

FIG 9-11.
Example of meibomian gland dysfunction in a patient wearing RGP lenses who complained of poor wettability. Expression of the lower meibomian glands revealed a marked degree of gland dysfunction, with a toothpaste-like residue being expelled from the glands. Lid scrubs, warm compresses, expression, and low doses of oral tetracycline resulted in sufficient regression to allow all-day wear of contact lenses. (Courtesy of Bausch & Lomb, Rochester, N.Y. and L. Jones.)

may stain with the dye. It is usually the area within the lid aperture that is most likely to stain. The degree of staining may vary from scattered spots to large areas of epithelial breakdown (Fig 9–13). Often when the patient is asked to gaze straight ahead, a line of staining is seen immediately below the upper lid.[58] Because tears are drawn from the precorneal tear film into the upper tear prism by surface tension, drying of the cornea occurs below the tear prism, resulting in this epithelial breakdown.

Rose Bengal

This aniline dye stains degenerated and dead epithelial cells, together with mucus strands and filaments. A drop of 1% rose bengal is instilled into the conjunctival sac. Because this solution may be irritative to the eye, a reduced volume may be instilled via a cotton-tip applica-

tor.[70] Using the green filter in the biomicroscope, one may view areas of corneal and conjunctival staining (Fig 9–14). Intense conjunctival staining in the temporal and nasal interpalpebral zone is commonly found in cases of dry eye. Diffuse corneal involvement may occur as the dry eye condition becomes more severe.[70] Corneal staining in the latter stages of these conditions is diagnostic and helps to differentiate them from ocular pemphigoid, keratitis medicamentosa, and blepharitis, where corneal staining occurs earlier.[70] Typically in KCS the inferior cornea and conjunctiva will exhibit a large amount of staining.

Rating systems have been developed to record staining patterns on the cornea and conjunctiva. Zuccaro[110] suggested a system in which 0 = no staining, 1 = less than one third of the cornea, 2 = one third to two thirds of the

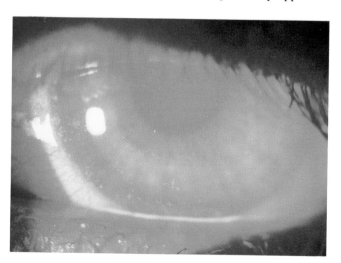

FIG 9-12.
Inferior lid tear prism height in a patient with dry eye. The tear prism height is reduced, and the appearance of the prism may be irregular or scalloped in these patients. (Courtesy of J. Dougal.)

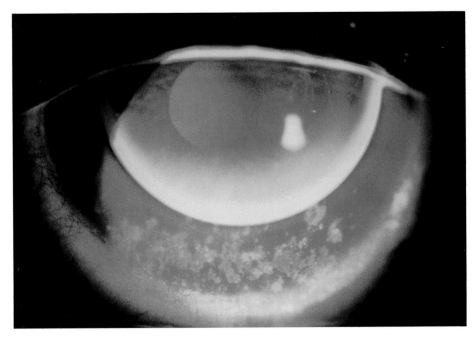

FIG 9–13.
Fluorescein staining of the inferior interpalpebral portion of the cornea in a dry eye patient wearing RGP contact lenses. (Courtesy of P. Caroline.)

cornea, 3 = two thirds to complete cornea stained, 4 = total cornea stain, and 5 = inferior conjunctival staining.

Alcian Blue Dye

Alcian blue dye may be used to specifically stain mucus and connective tissue so that mucus in the tear film, strands in the inferior fornix, and mucus fibrils from the goblet cells may be seen.[62]

Dry Eye Questionnaires

A patient's history may be highly significant in indicating the presence of a dry eye in contact lens wear from a series

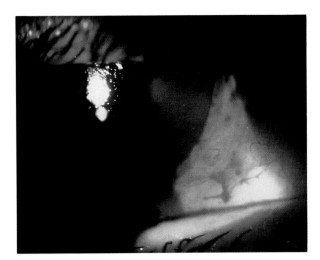

FIG 9–14.
Rose bengal staining of the inferior conjunctiva and cornea in a patient with dry eye. (Courtesy of G. Lowther.)

of questions concerning primary and secondary symptoms experienced.[58] This is a method used by the majority of practitioners in the detection of dry eye.[38] Often the patient answers a self-directed questionnaire before the contact lens fitting. This questionnaire seeks specific information on refractive error, ocular symptoms, current illnesses, medications, duration of present dry eye problems, and family history of similar problems. A number of questionnaires have been designed.[58, 66] The questionnaire designed by McMonnies[66] has received the widest validation (Table 9–3).[67, 68, 87] The questions from this questionnaire are encoded to allow for discriminant analysis.[67] In a group of dry eye patients compared with normal patients, the questionnaire was found to have 98% sensitivity and 97% specificity.

MANAGEMENT

Should a patient who is defined before contact lens fitting as borderline or marginally dry eyed be fitted with contact lenses? Patients with dry eye states have the potential for compromised ocular surfaces.[53] These patients suffer deficiencies of various ocular defense mechanisms such as tear volume and certain tear components (lysozyme, lactoferrin and β-lysin, the mucin network, cellular exfoliation, and subsurface immune secretions). If such individuals are fitted with contact lenses, the wear of the lenses may increase the risk of ocular infection. The risk is heightened if the patient is fitted with soft contact lenses that provide little tear exchange beneath their surfaces and produce a se-

TABLE 9–3.

Dry Eye Questionnaire*

Please answer the following by underlining the responses most appropriate to you: female/male. Age: less than 25 years, 25–45 years, more than 45 years. Currently wearing: no contact lenses, hard contact lenses/soft contact lenses.

1. Have you ever had drops prescribed or other treatment for dry eyes? Yes/No/Uncertain
2. Do you ever experience any of the following eye symptoms? (Please *underline* those that apply to you.) 1. Soreness 2. Scratchiness 3. Dryness 4. Grittiness 5. Burning
3. How often do your eyes have these symptoms? *(underline)* Never/Sometimes/Often/Constantly
4. Are your eyes *unusually* sensitive to cigarette smoke, smog, air conditioning, or central heating? Yes/No/Sometimes
5. Do your eyes easily become very red and irritated when swimming? Not applicable/Yes/No/Sometimes
6. Are your eyes dry and irritated the day after drinking alcohol? Not applicable/Yes/No/Sometimes
7. Do you take (please *underline*) antihistamine tablets or use antihistamine eyedrops, diuretics (fluid tablets), sleeping tablets, tranquilizers, oral contraceptives, medication for duodenal ulcer, digestive problems, high blood pressure, or ? (Write in any medication you are taking that is not listed.)
8. Do you suffer from arthritis? Yes/No/Uncertain
9. Do you experience dryness of chest or vagina? Never/Sometimes/Often/Constantly
10. Do you suffer from thyroid abnormality? Yes/No/Uncertain
11. Are you known to sleep with your eyes partly open? Yes/No/Sometimes
12. Do you have eye irritation as you wake from sleep? Yes/No/Sometimes

*From McMonnies CW: *J Am Optom Assoc* 1986; 57:512.

quested environment. The limited tear flow allows a greater buildup of lens deposits, already a problem in dry eye patients, and metabolic waste products. It also provides increased tear evaporation from the lens surface. (Dry eye patients have increased tear osmolarity and evaporation rates.[23, 90])

The pathogenesis of infection in patients with dry eye when fitted with contact lenses[53] is attributed to various mechanisms, including decreased tear flow beneath the lens, decreased tear components,[53] stagnation of the mucin network,[105] changes in surface cell exfoliation,[56] and the putative changes in the subsurface immune secretive system. Therefore, patients with dry eyes run a greater risk of bacterial conjunctivitis, blepharitis, and sterile corneal infiltrates when fitted with contact lenses. However, in many cases the demand for contact lenses is great enough for many clinicians to fit patients identified as marginally dry eyed with contact lenses. Correct identification of the patient who is potentially at risk because of a marginally dry eye condition can lead to a choice of correct lenses. Careful supervision of the patient and the implementation of various strategies minimize the potential for serious complications during lens wear.[20]

The management of dry eye is best achieved by a stepwise approach that identifies the minimum amount of therapy required to achieve satisfactory wear with lenses. Simpler treatment regimens will increase patient compliance and long-term success with lenses.[60]

Several strategies have been employed to enable the marginally dry eye patient to wear contact lenses (Fig 9–15); these include (1) patient selection, (2) patient education, (3) lens material selection, (4) environmental factors, (5) hot compresses and lid scrubs, (6) lubrication, and (7) punctal plugs.

Patient Selection

Proper patient selection depends on a comprehensive case history and prefitting evaluation involving prediction tests for dry eye.[9] Patient history is supplemented by a dry eye questionnaire.[66, 68] It is also important to determine whether the patient is taking any medications that may affect tear chemistry.[84]

Patient Education

The patient should be educated to have lower expectations in terms of wearing time and comfort than those of the normal contact lens patient. In addition, the need for scrupulous cleaning of lenses should be emphasized for those patients who have a greater predisposition to heavy deposits. Abrasive cleaners and surfactant cleaning agents must be used together for RGP lenses. Both soft and hard lenses require weekly or more frequent enzymatic cleaning. Patients with marginally dry eye conditions must clean their lenses immediately on removal from the eye to effectively remove surface deposits while they are still in the relatively hydrated state.[9] It is important to make clear to patients that their difficulty with lenses is not caused by failure of the contact lens material or by poor technical fitting but by the underlying dry eye problem.[12]

Because of the greater risk of serious complications, such as corneal ulcers, marginally dry eye patients should be advised of the possibilities of complications and instructed to return immediately for consultation if pain, redness, or photophobia develops during lens wear. The need for frequent after-care visits should be stressed to these patients. Because of the greater risk for complications, only daily wear lenses should be prescribed.

Lens Material Selection

Whether to prescribe rigid or hydrogel lens materials for marginally dry eye patients is a difficult choice. Both types of materials offer advantages and disadvantages. The ac-

Management Of Borderline Dry Eye

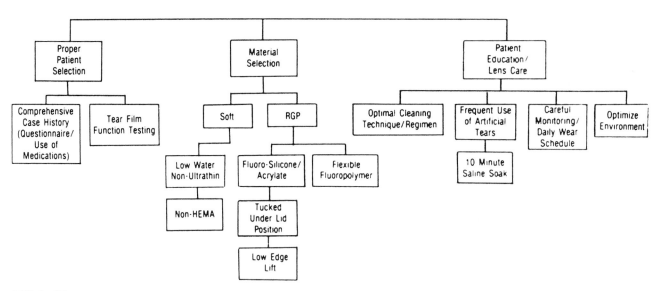

FIG 9–15.
Diagram of the management of borderline dry eye patients. Patient selection and education and the choice of lens material and care regimen are outlined. (From Bennett ES, Gordon JM: *Contact Lens Forum* 1989; 14(7):52. Used by permission.)

tual choice of the material will depend on the individual patient's needs.[12]

Rigid gas-permeable lenses have the advantage of not requiring hydration from the tear film. If lens deposits are anticipated as a major problem, low Dk, fluorinated materials are indicated. Rigid lens design in the potential dry eye patient is important. An interpalpebral or superior-positioning lens fit with minimum edge lift to minimize corneal dessication is preferred.[9] Therefore, an on-K or slightly flat-fitting base curve in combination with minimum center and edge thickness is desirable.

Hydrogel lens materials may be indicated for other patients. Generally, low water content, standard thickness lenses are preferred to those that are ultrathin.[9, 99] If one wishes to offset the problems of deposit formation on hydrogels, low water content, nonionic materials are preferred, and the use of disposable lenses is an option. To offset the tendency for corneal dessication beneath the hydrogel lens in the area of the lid aperture, Finnemore[20] advocates prism ballast incorporations into spherical lens designs to give greater lens thickness in this region. In some cases medium water content lenses may be indicated. Slightly increased center thicknesses of 0.1 to 0.12 mm in 55% water content materials have been found to be beneficial for patients with dry eye.[20] These lenses provide good oxygenation without suffering from the disadvantages of corneal dessication attendant on high water con-

tent lenses. For patients with pingueculae, soft contact lenses are preferred over rigid varieties.

Environmental Factors

Environmental factors may be controlled to enhance patient comfort during contact lens wear. Avoiding drafts and excessive air conditioning, sitting near hot air vents, and using a portable humidifier are advocated. The use of overspectacles for wear during windy or strong air current conditions can be beneficial.[9] In addition, patients performing close work for long periods should be encouraged in correct blinking habits.

Hot Compresses and Lid Scrubs

In cases where lipid deficiency is suspected as a cause of the dry eye condition, lid scrubs, hot compresses, and lid massage are an important part of the contact lens–wearing regimen.[49] This simple procedure may facilitate the successful wear of contact lenses. One should remember, however, that therapy must be ongoing to be effective.[12]

Lubrication

The lubrication of the anterior ocular surface and contact lens with an artificial tear preparation is the mainstay therapy for patients with marginally dry eyes.[4, 12, 52, 60] Artificial tear supplements should be prescribed for all contact lens dry eye cases (Table 9–4). The avoidance of preservatives, particularly benzalkonium chloride, is necessary in view of its tendency to affect corneal epithelium. It is found to increase corneal epithelial permeability by a factor of 3 over other preservatives in dry eye patients.[25] Frequent use of preservative solutions applied to a partially compromised ocular surface can result in irritation, lacrimation, hyperemia, photophobia, and corneal edema. [52] Therefore, preservative-free artificial tear preparations such as Refresh, Celluvisc, or Vit-A-Drops are preferred.[39] Hypotonic artificial tears such as Hypotears, Liquifilm, and Vit-A-Drops have the benefit of counteracting the hypertonicity of the tear film often found in dry eye states.[24]

Hypotears and Tears Naturale have adsorptive properties by virtue of their formulation with polymers, which increase the retention time of the solution and provide greater symptomatic relief for the patient.[52, 60] Polymers for this purpose include cellulose derivatives (carboxymethylcellulose, hydroxyethyl cellulose, and hydroxypropylmethol), dextrans, polyols (glycerine, polyethylene glycol, and polysorbate), polyvinyl alcohol, gelatin, and povidone. Solutions with these formulations are relatively innocous and can prolong the effects of the drops for up to 1½ hours after instillation.[52] Refresh has a preservative-free supplement containing polyvinyl alcohol–providone.

One percent carboxymethylcellulose, which is preservative-free, is also available as Celluvisc. These artificial tears are useful for patients who require drops more frequently than four to six times daily.[60]

Other tear solutions have been formulated with ingredients such as chondroitin sulfate and hyaluronic acid. In patients with moderate tear production deficiencies, tear solutions with polyvinyl alcohol or hyaluronic acid are preferred to those containing chondroitin sulfate.[57] The use of eye drops that contain physiological lipids (phospholipids, fatty acids, and triglycerides) normally found in the tear film has been shown to significantly increase tear BUT, improve Schirmer test results, and reduce complaints of "dry eye."[86] Polymers in several products claim mucomimetic properties, implying that the components mimic lacrimal surfactants that stabilize the tears. These claims are not usually substantiated by laboratory data.[39]

In addition to the use of tear supplements, soft lens wearers may benefit from a saline solution soak, lenses being removed at midday and rehydrated by soaking them in unpreserved saline solution for 15 minutes.[18]

The use of artificial tears can be of great benefit to the marginally dry eye patient wearing contact lenses, but overuse of the solutions is not recommended. If solutions are used more than ten times daily, this may lead to the development of medicamentosa, a form of keratitis associated with the destabilization of the tear film and consequent toxic effects on the epithelium resulting from the

TABLE 9–4.

Composition and Properties of Various Tear Substitutes*†

| Trade Name | Manufacturer | Composition | | Tonicity |
		Polymeric	Preservatives	
Celluvisc	Allergan Pharmaceuticals	CMC	None	Isotonic
Dakrina	Dakryon	PVAs, PVP	SORB, EDTA	Isotonic
Dwelle	Dakryon	PVAs, DEX	SORB, EDTA	Isotonic
Hypotears	IOLAB	PVA, PEG	BAC(h), EDTA	Hypotonic
Liquifilm	Allergan Pharmaceuticals	PVA	CHB	Hypotonic
Moisture Drops	Allergan Pharmaceuticals	HPMC	BAC(h), EDTA	Isotonic
Neo Tears	Barnes-Hind Pharmaceuticals	HEC, PVA	THIM	Isotonic
Nutra Tear	Dakryon	PVAs	BAC(l), EDTA	Isotonic
Refresh	Allergan Pharmaceuticals	PVA, PVP	None	Isotonic
Tears Naturale	Alcon Laboratories	DEX, HPMC	BAC(h), EDTA	Isotonic
Tears Naturale II	Alcon Laboratories	DEX, HPMC	PQUT, EDTA	Isotonic
Tears Plus	Allergan Pharmaceuticals	PVA, PVP	CHB	Isotonic
Vit-A-Drops	Vision Pharmaceuticals	PSB	None	Hypotonic

*From Holly FJ: *Contact Lens Forum* 1991; 16(4):19. Used by permission.
†BAC(h) = 0.01% benzalkonium chloride; BAC(l) = 0.004% benzalkonium chloride; CHB = chlorobutanol; CMC = carboxymethyl cellulose, sodium salt; DEX = dextran; EDTA = ethylenediamine tetracetic acid; HEC = hydroxyethyl cellulose; HPMC = hydroxypropyl cellulose; MC = methyl cellulose; PEG = polyethylene glycol; PQUT = Polyquat; PSB = polysorbate 80; PVA = polyvinyl alcohol; PVAs = synergistic mixture of two different PVAs; PVP = polyvinyl pyrrolidone; SORB = sorbic acid–sorbate.

compounds contained in the supplements. This level of use of artificial tear solutions is an indicator for other forms of therapy.[96]

Punctal Plugs

A form of tear preservation advocated for the contact lens–induced dry eye patient involves occlusion of the lid puncta by a temporary plug or a permanent surgical procedure.[15, 96] Some[52] advocate caution in applying this procedure to young patients because of the "waxing and waning" course of dry eye conditions. Punctal occlusion can lead to the development of epiphora, which is very disturbing to patients. For these reasons, occlusion using a temporary plug is advocated, at least for a period of time, to assess the efficacy of the technique before permanent measures are implemented.

Most advocates[15] suggest the use of collagen implants, which absorb after about 1 week, before the more permanent (but still reversible) silicone plugs are used. These plugs are 2 mm long and come in diameters of 0.2, 0.3, and 0.4 mm. The two larger sizes are more commonly used because the smaller ones can occasionally get lost in the punctum.[64] After the instillation of an anesthetic, the punctum is dilated and one or two of the medium- or large-size implants inserted. It is important that the implant gets well into the canaliculus so it is no longer

visible. This provides a good block and avoids any interaction with the contact lens or the anterior ocular surface.[96] Collagen plugs are usually left in the eye until they dissolve. During this time patients use artificial tear solutions in the normal manner.[15, 96] It is usual to carry out initial plugging only in the inferior punctum so that an assessment may be made of the potential benefits of the procedure in alleviating dry eye symptoms.

At the end of the period in which the collagen plugs hydrolize, an assessment can be made as to the benefits of the procedure. Those patients showing significant improvement in comfort may have permanent (silicone) plugs inserted into the inferior and, occasionally, superior puncta (Fig 9–16). Although more long term than the collagen plugs, silicone plugs can be removed if epiphora occurs. This is rare in dry eye syndromes.[106] The disadvantages of silicone plugs are that they may interfere with contact lens wear, irritate the anterior ocular surface, and may occasionally spontaneously extrude.[96] For these reasons more permanent occlusion by cautery[96] using thermal techniques or argon laser punctoplasty[60] may be undertaken. Punctal occlusion by these techniques in the contact lens patient are usually restricted to the inferior puncta, a procedure that never has to be reversed.[96]

Several systems have been developed to grade degrees of dry eye. Lemp[52] describes a system based on a Latin square diagram that takes the results of the Schirmer, rose

A
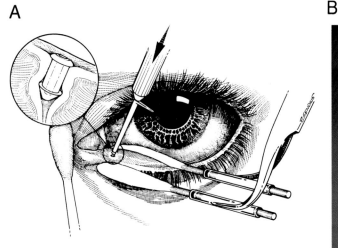

B
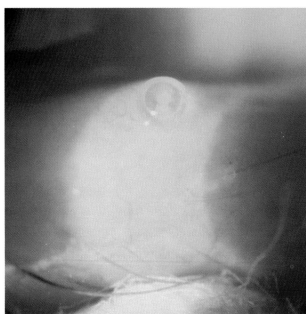

FIG 9–16.
Diagram of the installation procedure for the punctal plugs. **A,** after dilation of the inferior punctum, the plug is inserted with an applicator. The plug should be inserted until the dome rests on the surface of the lid margin *(insert).* The diagram shows the use of lid fixation forceps to prevent rolling of the lid during the insertion process. **B,** the domed end of a punctal plug in situ. (Courtesy of Eagle Vision, Memphis, Tenn.)

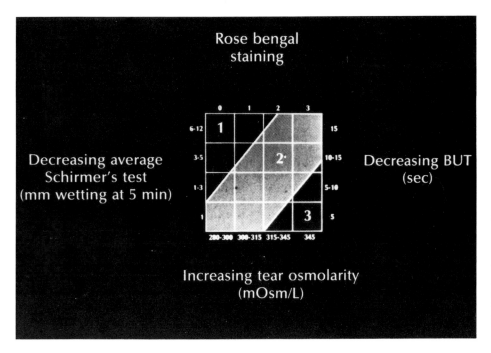

Rose bengal
staining

Decreasing average
Schirmer's test
(mm wetting at 5 min)

Decreasing BUT
(sec)

Increasing tear osmolarity
(mOsm/L)

FIG 9–17.
A Latin square diagram for grading dry eyes. Grade 1 is represented by the dark gray area *(upper left)*, grade 2 by the light gray area *(center)*, and grade 3 by the medium gray area *(lower right)* BUT = tear film breakup time. (From Lemp MA: *Int Ophthalmol Clin* 1987; 27:36. Used by permission.)

bengal staining, tear BUT, and tear osmolarity tests (Fig 9–17). Generally speaking, the borderline dry eye cases considered in this chapter would fall into the grade 1 category and would have a management system that includes artificial tears and the use of overnight lubricating ointments. The more rigorous treatment modalities, including frequent use of artificial tear solutions and ointments, sustained-release tear inserts, and mucolytic agents, are reserved for grade 2 dry eye conditions. Punctal occlusion, bandage lenses, estrogens therapy, and moisture chambers are prescribed in the grade 3 category.

CONCLUSION

The correct management of contact lens patients with marginally dry eye symptoms can provide great satisfaction for the clinician and facilitate the successful wear of contact lenses by these patients. A partnership between practitioner and patient provides the best chance for success. In this the patient must fully understand the potential limitations imposed on his or her contact lens wear by the dry eye condition and the need to rigorously maintain lens care.

REFERENCES

1. Andrasko G: Hydrogel dehydration in various environments. *Int Contact Lens Clin* 1983; 10:22–28.
2. Andres S, et al: Factors of precorneal tear film breakup time (BUT) and tolerance of contact lenses. *Int Contact Lens Clin* 1987; 14:103–107.
3. Arner RS: Corneal contact lens design by minimal corneal insult. *J Am Optom Assoc* 1969; 40:308–309.
4. Asbell P: How to make dry eyes wet. Paper presented at the Tenth International Contact Lens Conference, Atlantic City, NJ, 1989.
5. Barabas RJ: Juxtaposition staining. *Contacto* 1967; 11:3–5.
6. Barr JT: Optimizing gas permeable hard contact lenses. *Int Contact Lens Clin* 1984; 11:72.
7. Barr JT: Problem solving with rigid lenses. *Rev Optom* 1986; 123:58–65.
8. Belos P, Cherry PM, Miller DO: An improved method for measuring human tear lysozyme concentration. *Arch Ophthalmol* 1985; 103:31–33.
9. Bennett ES, Gordon JM: The borderline dry eye patient and contact lens wear. *Contact Lens Forum* 1989; 14(7):52–73.
10. Bennett ES, et al: DW investigation of aspheric posterior Boston IV lens design. *Contact Lens Forum* 1987; 12(4):65–69.
11. Bennett ES, Egan DJ: Rigid gas permeable lens problem solving. *J Am Optom Assoc* 1986; 57:504–511.
12. Campbell RC: Practical management of dry eye in contact lens wearers. *Contact Lens Update* 1989; 8:94–96.
13. Connor CG, Broadman DA: Decreased goblet cell density in contact lens patients taking oral contraceptives. *Invest Ophthalmol Vis Sci* 1990; 31(suppl):548.
14. Cotie B: How to manage 3 and 9 o'clock staining. *Contact Lens Forum* 1990; 15:42–43.
15. Dornic DI: Put in a plug for your dry eye patients. *Rev Optom* 1989; 126(8):49–51.
16. Egbert PR, Laubers S, Maurice DM: A simple conjunctival biopsy. *Am J Ophthalmol* 1977; 84:798–801.

17. Epstein AB, Donnenfeld ED: Ultrathin high water content lenses and epithelial fractures. *Contact Lens Forum* 1991; 16:32.

18. Epstein AB, Freedman JM: The two sides of dry eye syndrome. *Contact Lens Forum* 1985; 10(8):33–40.

19. Farris RL: Tear osmolarity variation in the dry eye. *Trans Am Ophthalmol Soc* 1986; 84:250–268.

20. Finnemore VM: Is the dry eye contact lens wearer at risk? Not usually. *Cornea* 1990; 9(suppl):51–53.

21. Franck C: Eye symptoms and signs in buildings with indoor climate problems (office-eye syndrome). *Acta Ophthalmol (Copenh)* 1986; 64:306–311.

22. Gilbard JP: Tear film osmolarity and keratoconjunctivitis sicca, in Holly FJ (ed): *The Preocular Tear Film in Health, Disease, and Contact Lens Wear.* Lubbock, Tex, Dry Eye Institute, 1986, p 127.

23. Gilbard JP, Farris RL, Santamaria J: Osmolarity of tear microvolumes in keratoconjunctivitis sicca. *Arch Ophthalmol* 1978; 96:677–681.

24. Gilbard JP, Kenyon KR: Tear diluents in treatment of KCS. *Ophthalmology* 1985; 92:646–650.

25. Gobbels M, Spitznas M: Influence of artificial tears on corneal epithelium in dry eye syndrome. *Graefes Arch Clin Exp Ophthalmol* 1989; 227:139–141.

26. Goren MB, Goren SB: Diagnostic tests in patients with symptoms of keratoconjunctivitis sicca. *Am J Ophthalmol* 1988; 106:570–574.

27. Graham R: Persistent nasal and temporal stippling. *Contacto* 1968; 12:20–21.

28. Grohe RM, Lebow KA: Vascularized limbal keratitis. *Int Contact Lens Clin* 1989; 16:197–207.

29. Guillon JP: Tear film structure on contact lenses, in Holly FJ (ed): *The Preocular Tear Film in Health, Disease, and Contact Lens Wear.* Lubbock, Tex, Dry Eye Institute, 1986, p 914.

30. Halberg G, Berens C: Standardized Schirmer tear test kit. *Am J Ophthalmol* 1961; 51:840–842.

31. Hamano H: The change of precorneal tear film by the application of contact lenses. *Contact Lens* 1981; 7:205–209.

32. Hamano H, et al: Tear secretion test (preliminary report). *J Contact Lens Soc* 1982; 24:103–107.

33. Henry VA, Bennett ES, Forrest JM: Clinical investigation of the Paraperm EW rigid gas permeable contact lens. *Am J Optom Physiol Opt* 1987; 64:313–320.

34. Herskowitz R, et al: Advantages of fluoropolymers. *Contact Lens Forum* 1988; 13(2):50–54.

35. Holden BA, Sweeney DF, Seger RG: Epithelial erosions caused by thin high water content lenses. *Clin Exp Optom* 1986; 69:103–107.

36. Holden T, et al: The effect of secondary curve liftoff on peripheral corneal desiccation. *Am J Optom Physiol Opt* 1987; 64:108P.

37. Holly FJ: Tear film physiology in contact lens wear: part 2. Contact lens tear film interactions. *Am J Optom Physiol Opt* 1981; 58:331–341.

38. Holly FJ: Diagnosis and treatment of dry eye syndrome. *Contact Lens Spectrum* 1989; 4(7):37–44.

39. Holly FJ: What is new in artificial tears? *Contact Lens Forum* 1991; 16(4):19–21.

40. Hom M, Silverman MW: Displacement technique and meibomian gland expression. *J Am Optom Assoc* 1987; 58:223–226.

41. Hu FR, et al: Tear lactoferrin in KCS. *Taiwan I Hsueh Hui Tsa Chih* 1989; 88:422–425.

42. Janssen PT, VanBijsterveld OP: A simple test for lacrimal gland function: A tear lactoferrin assay by radial immunodiffusion. *Graefes Arch Clin Exp Ophthalmol* 1983; 220:171–174.

43. Jones DH, Bennett ES, Davis LJ: How to manage peripheral corneal desiccation. *Contact Lens Spectrum* 1989; 4(5):63–66.

44. Jordan A, Baum JL: Basic tear flow: Does it exist? *Ophthalmology* 1980; 87:920–930.

45. Kline LN, DeLuca TJ: Effect of gel lens wear on the precorneal tear film. *Int Contact Lens Clin* 1975; 2:56–59.

46. Kline LN, DeLuca TJ: Pitting stain with soft contact lenses—hydrocurve thin series. *J Am Optom Assoc* 1977; 48:372–376.

47. Kline LN, Deluca TJ, Fishberg GM: Corneal staining relating to contact lens wear. *J Am Optom Assoc* 1979; 50:353–357.

48. Kogbe S, Liotet S: An interesting use of the study of tear ferning patterns in contactology. *Ophthalmologica* 1987; 194:150–153.

49. Korb DR, Henriquez AS: Meibomian gland dysfunction and contact lens intolerance. *J Am Optom Assoc* 1980; 51:243–251.

50. Korb DR, Korb JM: A new concept in contact lens design: Parts 1 and 2. *J Am Optom Assoc* 1970; 41:1–12.

51. Korb DR, Korb JM: A study of 3 and 9 o'clock staining after unilateral lens removal. *J Am Optom Assoc* 1970; 41:233–236.

52. Lemp MA: Management of the dry eye. *Int Ophthalmol Clin* 1987; 27:36–43.

53. Lemp MA: Is the dry eye contact lens wearer at risk. Yes? *Cornea* 1990; 9(suppl):48–50.

54. Lemp MA, Dohlmann CH, Holly FJ: Corneal desiccation despite normal tear volume. *Ann Ophthalmol* 1970; 2:258–261.

55. Lemp MA, Hamill JR: Factors affecting tear breakup in normal eyes. *Arch Ophthalmol* 1973; 89:88–94.

56. Lemp MA, et al: An in vivo study of corneal surface morphologic features in patients with keratoconjunctivitis sicca. *Am J Ophthalmol* 1984; 98:426–428.

57. Limberg MB, et al: Topical application of hyaluronic acid and chondroitin sulfate in the treatment of dry eyes. *Am J Ophthalmol* 1987; 103:194–197.

58. Lowther GE, Malinovsky V: Dry eye: A clinical overview. Fort Worth, Tex, Alcon Laboratories, 1988.

59. Lowther GE, Paramore JE: Clinical comparison of silcon resin lenses to PMMA, CAB and polycon lenses. *Int Contact Lens Clin* 1982; 9:106–118.

60. Lubniewski AJ, Nelson JD: Diagnosis and management of dry eye and ocular surface disorders. *Ophthalmol Clin* 1990; 3:575–593.

61. Lucca JA, Munez JN, Farris RL: A comparison of diagnostic tests for keratoconjunctivitis sicca: Lactoplate, Schirmer and tear osmolarity. *CLAO J* 1990; 16:109–112.

62. Lupelli L: A review of lacrimal function tests in relation to contact lens practice: part 1. *Contact Lens J* 1988; 16:4–17.

63. Mackie IA: Localized corneal drying in association with dellen, pterigia and related lesions. *Trans Ophthalmol Soc UK* 1971; 91:129–145.

64. Maguire LJ, Bartley GB: Complications associated with the newer size Freeman punctal plug. *Arch Ophthalmol* 1989; 107:961–962.

65. Marner K: "Snakelike" appearance of nuclear chromatin in conjunctival epithelial cells from patients with keratoconjunctivitis sicca. *Acta Ophthalmol (Copenh)* 1980; 58:849–853.

66. McMonnies CW: Key questions in dry eye history. *J Am Optom Assoc* 1986; 57:512–517.

67. McMonnies CW, Ho A: Patient history in screening for dry eye conditions. *J Am Optom Assoc* 1987; 58:296–301.

68. McMonnies CW, Ho A: Responses to the dry eye questionnaire from a normal population. *J Am Optom Assoc* 1987; 58:588–591.

69. Mengher LS, et al: Noninvasive assessment of tear film stability, in Holly FJ (ed): *Precocular Tear Film in Health, Disease, and Contact Lens Wear*. Lubbock, Tex, Dry Eye Institute, 1986, p 64.

70. Millodot M, O'Leary DJ: Corneal fragility and its relationship to sensitivity. *Acta Ophthalmol* 1981; 59:820–828.

71. Mishima S, et al: Determination of tear volume and tear flow. *Invest Ophthalmol Vis Sci* 1966; 5:264–276.

72. Nelson JD: Impression cytology. *Cornea* 1988; 7:71–81.

73. Nelson JD, Havener VR, Cameron JD: Cellulose acetate impressions of the ocular surface. *Arch Ophthalmol* 1983; 101:1869–1872.

74. Nelson PS: A short Schirmer test. *Optom Weekly* 1982; 73:568–569.

75. Norn M: Ferning in the conjunctival-cytologic preparations. *Acta Ophthalmol* 1987; 65:118–123.

76. Norn M: Tear stix tests for leucocyte-esterase, nitrate, haemoglobin and albumin in normals and in a clinical series. *Acta Ophthalmol (Copenh)* 1989; 67:192–198.

77. Norn MS: Desiccation of the precorneal film, part 1: Corneal wetting time. *Acta Ophthalmol* 1969; 47:865–880.

78. Osborn GN, Zantos SG: Corneal desiccation staining with thin high water content contact lenses. *CLAO J* 1988; 14:81–85.

79. Osborn GN, Zantos SG: Practitioner survey: Management of dry eye symptoms in soft lens wearers. *Contact Lens Spectrum* 1989; 4(9):23–26.

80. Pascucci SE, et al: An analysis of age related morphologic changes of human meibomian glands. *Invest Ophthalmol Vis Sci* 1988; 29(suppl):213.

81. Patel S: Constancy of the front surface desiccation times for IGEL 67 lenses in vivo. *Am J Optom Physiol Opt* 1987; 64:167–171.

82. Patel S, et al: Effects of fluorescein on tear breakup time and on tear thinning time. *Am J Optom Physiol Opt* 1985; 62:188–190.

83. Paugh JP, et al: Meibomian therapy in problematic contact lens wear. *Am J Optom Physiol Opt* 1990; 67:803–806.

84. Polak BC: Side effects of drugs and tear secretions. *Doc Ophthalmol* 1987; 67:115–117.

85. Refojo MF, et al: Tear evaporimeter for diagnosis and research, in Holly FJ (ed): *The Preocular Tear Film in Health, Disease, and Contact Lens Wear*. Lubbock, Tex, Dry Eye Institute, 1986, p 117.

86. Rieger G: Lipid-containing eye drops: A step closer to natural tears. *Ophthalmologica* 1990; 201:206–212.

87. Robboy M, Osborn G: The responses of marginal dry eye lens wearers to a dry eye survey. *Contact Lens J* 1989; 17:8–9.

88. Rolando M, Baldi F, Calabria GA: Tear mucus ferning test in keratoconjunctivitis sicca, in Holly FJ (ed): *The Preocular Tear Film in Health, Disease, and Contact Lens Wear*. Lubbock, Tex, Dry Eye Institute, 1986, p 203.

89. Rolando M, Refojo M: Tear evaporimeter for measuring water evaporation from the tear film under control conditions in humans. *Exp Eye Res* 1983; 36:25–33.

90. Rolando M, Refojo MF, Kenyon KR: Increased tear evaporation in eyes with keratoconjunctivitis sicca. *Arch Ophthalmol* 1983; 101:557–558.

91. Sarver MD, Nelson W: Peripheral corneal staining accompanying contact lens wear. *J Am Optom Assoc* 1969; 40:310–313.

92. Schnider C, et al: Unusual complications of RGP extended wear. *Am J Optom Physiol Opt* 1986; 63:35P.

93. Schnider CM: Rigid gas permeable extended wear. *Contact Lens Spectrum* 1990; 5(9):101–106.

94. Schnider CM, Terry RL, Holden BA: Clinical correlates of peripheral corneal desiccation. *Invest Ophthal Vis Sci* 1988; 29(suppl):336.

95. Sevigny J, Bennett ES: Troubleshooting with silicone acrylate lenses. *Rev Optom* 1985; 122(12):24–30.

96. Shenon P: Why you need to know about punctal occlusion. *Contact Lens Spectrum* 1990; 5(7):43–49.

97. Smiddy WE: Therapeutic contact lenses. *Ophthalmology* 1990; 97:291–295.

98. Solomon J: Causes and treatments of peripheral corneal desiccation. *Contact Lens Forum* 1986; 11(6):30–36.

99. Sorbara L, Talsky C: Contact lens wear in the dry eye patient: Predicting success and achieving it. *Can J Optom* 1989; 50:234–241.

100. Swarbrick HA, Holden BA: RGP lens binding: Significant and contributory factors. *Am J Optom Physiol Opt* 1987; 64:815–823.

101. Terry JE: Eye diseases of the elderly. *J Am Optom Assoc* 1984; 55:23–29.

102. Tomlinson A: Choice of materials—a material issue. *Contact Lens Spectrum* 1990; 5(9):27–36.

103. Tomlinson A, Cedarstaff TH: Tear evaporation from the human eye: Effects of contact lens wear. *J Br Contact Lens Assoc* 1982; 5:141–150.

104. Trees GR, Tomlinson A: Effect of artificial tear solutions

and saline on tear film evaporation. *Optom Vis Sci* 1990; 67:886–890.

105. Tseng SC, et al: Possible mechanism for the loss of goblet cells in mucin deficient disorders. *Ophthalmology* 1984; 91:545–552.

106. Tuberville AW, Frederick WR, Wood TO: Punctal occlusion in tear deficient syndromes. *Ophthalmology* 1982; 89:1170–1172.

107. VanBijsterveld OP: Diagnostic tests in the sicca syndrome. *Arch Ophthalmol* 1969; 82:10–14.

108. Zadnik K, Mutti DO: Inferior arcuate corneal staining in soft contact lens wearers. *Int Contact Lens Clin* 1985; 12:110–115.

109. Zantos SG, et al: Studies on corneal staining with thin hydrogel contact lenses. *J Br Contact Lens Assoc* 1986; 9:61–64.

110. Zuccaro VS: Rose bengal: A vital stain. *Contact Lens Forum* 1981; 6(10):39–43.

PART IV

Inflammation

Ocular Inflammation and Contact Lens Wear

Joel A. Silbert, O.D.

Inflammation represents a generalized reaction to cellular injury in which a variety of defensive and reparative events occur in adjacent tissues. Although the overall design of such mechanisms is protective, inflammatory responses often cause loss of function, and may in and of themselves create more damage, in addition to causing considerable discomfort for the patient.

Inflammation affecting the cornea and anterior segment may be caused by infectious microbes, mechanical trauma, and chemical toxicity, as well as from allergenic sources. In contact lens practice, examples of these might arise from extended wear ulcerative keratitis, corneal abrasion, thimerosal toxicity and hypersensitivity, and mast cell degranulation seen in giant papillary conjunctivitis.

When host tissues have had no prior exposure to the inciting inflammatory agent, the inflammatory response is considered "toxic." Toxic agents may produce local inflammatory responses without significant tissue damage (nonnecrotizing) or, in contrast, may produce profound tissue damage (necrotizing).[22] An example of the former might be a reaction to a drug or solution preservative, whereas the latter might be the corneal melting that occurs from necrotizing toxins and enzymes released in *Pseudomonas* corneal ulcers.

When host tissues have had prior exposure to an inflammatory agent, the response is likely to be one involving the acquired immune system. Acquired immunity is a response to repeated exposure to antigenic substances in which a larger and more effective defensive response is mounted. Acquired immunity may be noncellular or humoral, in which the immune defense system relies on various components in plasma, circulating antibodies, and the complement enzyme cascade. On the other hand, acquired immunity may be cellular, depending on the presence of macrophages and T lymphocytes.[1] Although the acquired immune system is inherently designed to be protective after an inflammatory stimulus, the immunological response may at times exceed normal bounds, giving rise to exaggerated hypersensitivity reactions.

Inflammatory reactions may vary in their intensity depending on the inherent nature of the inflammatory agent or stimulus, as well as the host tissue reaction. Both the stimulus quantity and contact time will determine the severity of the inflammatory response.

The classical signs of general inflammation described for centuries are quite apropos in any description of ocular inflammation, with or without the presence of a contact lens. "Tumor," or tissue swelling, results from increased capillary permeability, resulting in edematous tissue swelling. "Rubor" (hyperemia or redness) and "calor" (heat) both arise from increased vascular dilatation, as well as from internal immunological reactions. "Dolor" (pain) may be caused by stretched nerve endings in swollen tissues, as well as from irritated nerve fibers caused by release of certain inflammatory substances in the involved site. Pain associated with photophobia is often seen in corneal inflammation, abrasion, keratitis, and anterior uveitis. Tissue swelling and nerve fiber involvement are responsible primarily for loss of function accompanying inflammatory reactions.[40]

MECHANISMS OF INFLAMMATION

The mechanisms that come into play when an inflammatory stimulus occurs are both extraordinarily complex and elegant and could present the basis for several texts in and of themselves. As such, only an outline of some of the major components of the inflammatory response can be covered here. The host tissue involved in such a response contains substances that are responsible for identification and elimination of the inflammatory stimulus while at the same time providing mechanisms for tissue repair. Let us look at the mechanisms of inflammation and their sequelae.

Increased Capillary Permeability

During an inflammatory response, capillary permeability is increased, causing tight junctions between the capillary endothelial cells to be loosened. This increase in permeability arises from a number of mediators released from mast cells, basophils, macrophages, polymorphonuclear leukocytes, and platelets.[22] For example, when mast cells are ruptured during inflammatory, allergic, or traumatic events, granules of histamine and heparin are released in large numbers. If the mast cells are near blood vessels, their degranulation causes vasodilation and increased capillary permeability.[1] Leakage of plasma and proteins causes tissue edema, further compounded by leakage of neutrophils, lymphocytes, and macrophages into the damaged tissue.

Other agents that contribute to increased vascular permeability include bradykinins, leukokinins, kallikrein, globulin permeability factor, and prostaglandins.[22] Platelet-activating factors (PAFs) are gaining more recognition recently as powerful mediators of vascular permeability, including chemotaxis for neutrophils and induction of prostaglandin precursors.[34]

Neutrophils and macrophages play an important role in the phagocytosis and digestion of foreign organisms. This process is highly complex, triggered by a series of enzymatic reactions in the plasma, known as the complement cascade.

Complement Cascade

The complement cascade plays a critical function in inflammatory and immune reactions. After an antigen-antibody reaction, a series of cascading enzymatic reactions in the plasma involving nine plasma proteins (C1–C9) is responsible for chemotactic attraction of phagocytic polymorphonuclear leukocytes to the site of inflammation, the adherence of foreign microbes to the surface of these cells, vasodilation and increased capillary permeability, and cell lysis with release of tissue-damaging enzymes. In addition, further potentiation of mast cell degranulation occurs, releasing not only histamine and heparin but also serotonin, PAF, leukotrienes, and prostaglandins.[13]

The complement cascade also assists in the elimination of foreign organisms too large to be phagocytosed by neutrophils and macrophages. It does so by activating eosinophils, which proteolytically destroy the cell membranes of large microbes.[1] The complement system also acts to trigger the clotting system, as well as the production of plasmin and collagenase.

The classic complement system in the plasma is initiated by the binding of specific antibodies to foreign proteins, or antigens. Antibodies, which provide acquired immunity, are formed by plasma cells that develop from B lymphocytes.[1] An alternate complement-initiating pathway involving properdin- and endotoxin-activating factors has been discovered, and it further adds to the inflammatory response.[13]

Type I Hypersensitivity (Anaphylaxis)

Inflammatory events can also be part of the body's allergic response, particularly when mast cell degranulation later gives rise to newly formed inflammatory mediator substances.

In the body's immune system, specific antibodies form to counter foreign antigenic substances. This acquired immunity may be extremely beneficial, especially when harmful foreign antigens are present, as in the case of pathogenic microbes. The response itself may be harmful, however, if antibodies are produced to nonforeign antigens, as is the case in autoimmune states. In hypersensitivity or allergic states, allergens trigger an excessive immune response by binding with two adjacent immunoglobulin E (IgE) molecules present on the mast cell membrane. The primary response is an immediate or anaphylactic reaction occurring within seconds or minutes after exposure in which mast cell degranulation releases histamine, other biologically active vasoactive amines, and, of equal importance, longer-acting inflammatory substances created from phospholipids in the mast cell membranes (Figs 10–1 and 10–2).[1] Immediate allergic reactions to the presence of allergens such as pollen, dust, pet dander, and drugs are well-known examples of type I hypersensitivity reactions. Whereas the cornea and iris have no mast cells, the conjunctiva is rich with mast cells and vascular tissue.[2] It is thus no surprise that the conjunctiva is often the prime site of ocular anaphylaxis and sustained inflammatory reactions. Mast cell degranulation in type I hypersensitivity reactions also plays an important role in contact

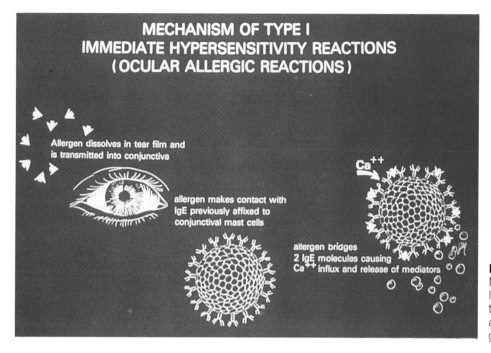

FIG 10–1.
Mechanism of type I (anaphylactic) hypersensitivity reactions. (Courtesy of Fisons Pharmaceuticals, Loughborough, England.)

lens–related papillary conjunctivitis (which is discussed in detail in Chapter 11).

The anaphylactic response in type I hypersensitivity reactions comes about from the release of preformed mediators contained in secretory granules within mast cells and basophils. These include histamine, heparin, serotonin, and chemotactic factors for phagocytic cells. The inflammatory component of type I allergy occurs when phospholipids in the mast cell membrane create arachidonic acid, a fatty acid precursor, which, in turn, gives rise to newly formed mediators such as prostaglandins, leukotrienes, thromboxane, and PAF.[1]

Prostaglandins

As noted, prostaglandins are a complex group of fatty acids formed as a result of membrane disturbances that release arachidonic acid. Prostaglandins are released from a

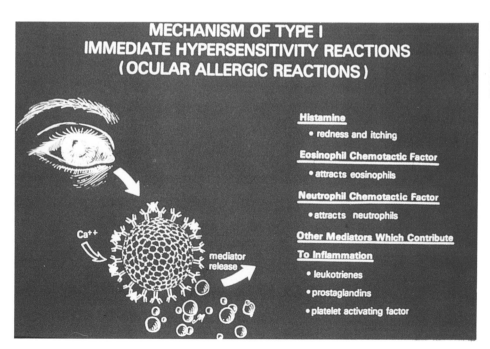

FIG 10–2.
Inflammatory mediators released in type I hypersensitivity reactions. (Courtesy of Fisons Pharmaceuticals, Loughborough, England.)

variety of tissues, including the eye, in response to primarily mechanical inflammatory stimuli and are synthesized as needed at the local tissue site.[22]

In the eye, the enzyme prostaglandin synthetase, now more commonly called cyclo-oxygenase, is present in practically all ocular tissues. The highest levels are in the conjunctiva,[5] which is not surprising given the large concentration of mast cell activity. Moderate levels are found in the iris and ciliary body, whereas low levels are present in the cornea and retina.

Prostaglandins are released into the anterior chamber primarily by mechanical irritation and are intimately involved with the inflammatory response to ocular irritation. This includes pupillary miosis (smooth muscle contraction), hyperemia, production of cells, flare and protein into the anterior chamber (breakdown of the blood-aqueous barrier), and consequent intraocular pressure elevation.[3, 36]

Although prostaglandins are released primarily as a response to mechanical irritation, they are also found in higher quantities in chemical injury (e.g., in mustard gas) and in neural stimulation (trigeminal nerve stimulation). High concentrations of prostaglandins are found in acute uveitis,[9] ocular trauma, cataract extraction, and other "traumatic" anterior segment surgery.[22]

PHARMACOLOGICAL INTERVENTION IN INFLAMMATORY PROCESSES

Pharmacological intervention in a variety of strategies can mitigate the inflammatory effects of increased capillary permeability, edema, the complement cascade, prostaglandin release, and anaphylaxis. For example, corticosteroids disrupt the production of arachidonic acid from the mast cell membrane phospholipids.[12] Nonsteroidal anti-inflammatory drugs (NSAIDs) such as aspirin, indomethacin, and indoxole inhibit cyclo-oxygenase, the enzyme required to convert already formed arachidonic acid into a precursor of prostaglandins.[43]

Although aspirin and salicylates are rarely used to control inflammation specifically within the eye, a number of NSAIDs have been under development for the control of ocular inflammation. Many have been found effective in combating inflammation and have been free of the more significant side effects encountered with corticosteroids, but most have a wide variety of adverse systemic reactions.[6] Considerable research is still needed before NSAIDs are widely used for the treatment of ocular inflammatory disease.

Corticosteroids are widely used for their nonspecific anti-inflammatory properties in the treatment of inflamma-

tion of the cornea and the anterior segment. Suppression of inflammation occurs regardless of whether the cause of inflammation is from infection, trauma, or allergy. As we have seen, inflammation occurs when there are changes in vascular permeability and resultant movement of white blood cells (WBCs) to the site of injury. The increase in vascular permeability resulting in edema is caused not only by type I hypersensitivity mediator release but also by prostaglandins, which can be inhibited by corticosteroids. Corticosteroids thus act on the inflamed site by inhibiting vasoactive mediators, WBC migration, and immune reactions.

Although corticosteroids can be highly effective in suppressing inflammation, these drugs do not affect the actual cause of the inflammatory stimulus. Nevertheless, prevention of the tissue damage caused by inflammation is very important in preserving vision. The judicious and conservative use of such palliative agents is essential not only in obtaining the desired effects but also in preventing complications and side effects known to be associated with their use. For example, because corticosteroids have an immunosuppressive role, bacterial, viral, and even fungal suprainfection can occur with prolonged usage.[6] In addition, prolonged corticosteroid therapy can cause an elevation in intraocular pressure in about one third of the population (steroid responders) who have a genetic predisposition to this effect with strong topical corticosteroids.[35]

For the topical treatment of ocular inflammation, the clinician will make use of prednisolone, dexamethasone, fluorometholone, or medrysone, which are typically available in solution, suspension, and ointment forms. Fluorometholone and medrysone are less potent anti-inflammatory agents and rarely cause intraocular pressure elevation.[35]

Topical corticosteroid therapy is preferred when ocular inflammation affecting the anterior segment is treated. Treatment typically comprises one drop every 2 hours for the first 24 to 48 hours, with gradual tapering as the inflammatory signs and symptoms abate. Systemic therapy is indicated for more severe and nonresponsive anterior uveitis, severe allergic states, and posterior segment inflammation.

Nonsteroidal drugs used to treat the immediate allergic or anaphylactic aspects of inflammatory disease include the ocular decongestants or vasoconstrictors and the antihistamines. Drugs that suppress both the immediate and long-term allergic effects are typified by sodium cromolyn, which inhibits mast cell degranulation in the presence of an allergen. The use of cold compresses should not be overlooked as a useful adjunct therapy to enhance vasoconstriction, free of side effects, in allergic and inflammatory states.

CORNEAL INFILTRATION

Corneal infiltrates are aggregates of neutrophils, macrophages, and lymphocytes that chemotactically migrate into the site of tissue involvement as one of the effects of the inflammatory response. These will be observed in the cornea and limbus as intraepithelial, subepithelial, or stromal infiltrates. Vasodilation, increased vascular permeability, and corneal edema allow for WBC migration from the limbal vasculature along the corneal lamellae to the site of tissue insult.[4]

White blood cells can also be recruited from chemotactic substances in the tears, which may originate from limbal transudation and the conjunctival lymphatics.[33] Thus, infiltrates may reach a site through intracorneal and external migration. Additional sources of infiltrate induction may come from inflammatory stimuli such as toxicity and hypersensitivity, viruses,[29] and bacterial exotoxins and endotoxins.[44]

Infiltrates may be observed in a wide variety of presenting symptoms ranging from a single focus in a white and quiet eye (with intact epithelium) to single or multiple foci in an inflamed, hyperemic eye (with or without epithelial defect).[19] They may vary in appearance as small, translucent, focal spheroids in the anterior cornea to large, diffuse, "snowball" opacities in the central stroma (Figs 10–3 and 10–4).[18] Contact lens–induced infiltrates are typically found within 2 mm of the limbus and can be overlooked, especially in an asymptomatic patient, if the clinician does not do a detailed biomicroscopic examination of the superior limbus.

Limbal and marginal corneal infiltrates often develop as a response to staphylococcal exotoxins associated with chronic blepharitis. Such marginal infiltrates are sterile and may be associated with inferior punctate staining of the cornea and conjunctival inflammation. Both of these signs are caused by the presence of α, β, γ, and δ toxins, exfoliative toxin, and leukocidin, which are toxic to both cornea and conjunctiva.[25] The infiltrates may represent neutrophilic clouding of the cornea in these marginal areas or more likely represent an immune hypersensitivity reaction to staphylococcal toxins. Grayish white, ovoid marginal ulcers that typically have a clear zone separating them from the limbus may develop (Fig 10–5).[25]

An even more severe inflammatory reaction may be observed in patients with phlyctenulosis. Large, gelatinous limbal nodules associated with an inflammatory pannus may develop as an immune response to chronic staphylococcal toxins. These may progress into clear cornea and may produce episodes of considerable discomfort as peripheral corneal scarring, thinning, and neovascularization progress (Fig 10–6). Both marginal ulcers and phlyctenules respond to corticosteroids. However, control or elimination depends in good measure on effective lid hygiene to reduce the presence of staphylococcal toxins.[37]

When infiltrates are observed in a contact lens–wearing patient, lens wear should be temporarily discontinued until the infiltrates have resolved. If the patient is asymptomatic, this may be a difficult task for the practitioner. However, patient education as to the importance of eliminating signs of inflammation, however slight, is usually effective, and the patient may return to lens wear as the infiltrate resolves. If, on the other hand, the patient is symptomatic, it is important to rule out infective keratitis. Should epithelial staining be present with a zone of underlying infiltration, corneal infection should be assumed and immediate institution of therapy begun. In the absence of infection, however, symptoms will gradually disappear with lens discontinuance, typically before resolution of the infiltrates themselves. Close monitoring of the patient during this period is recommended. Infiltrates observed in an extended wear hydrogel lens patient are at higher risk, because they may represent inflammatory prodromes to potential infection. Once infiltrates have completely resolved, daily wear with fresh lenses can be reinstituted and the patient followed for several weeks before resumption of extended wear. Disposable or frequent-replacement lenses are preferred if the patient is to be refitted on an extended wear basis. However, the lens fit should also be carefully reassessed. Should infiltrates return under condi-

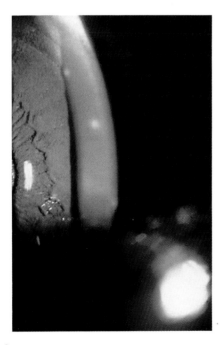

FIG 10–3.
Focal, subepithelial corneal infiltrate (with intact epithelium) typically observed in allergic and viral inflammations.

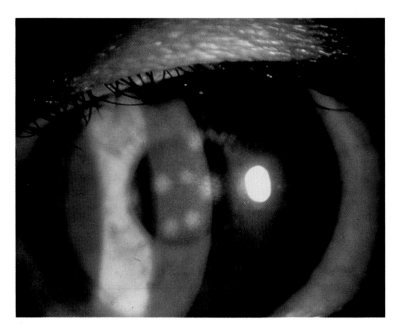

FIG 10–4.
Diffuse, "snowball" infiltrative opacities in the central corneal stroma, observed as an inflammatory response to thimerosal.

tions of extended wear, the patient should permanently discontinue using this modality and instead use either daily wear hydrogel or rigid gas-permeable (RGP) lenses.

INFLAMMATORY CONSEQUENCES OF INFECTION

Infection is certainly a prime stimulus for inflammation. Although the presence of corneal infiltrates may signal an inflammatory reaction, it does not necessarily signify in-

fection. For a confirmed diagnosis of infection, the clinician must use a constellation of signs, symptoms, and clinical intuition, along with laboratory tests, to identify the causative organism.

In contact lens wear, the cornea is exposed not only to microorganisms naturally resident in the tears and on the lids but also to contaminants on lenses, in contact lens cases, and in solutions. Mechanical trauma associated with lens wear, as well as from the physiologically compromising effects of hypoxia, as, for example, in extended wear, accounts for the majority of infections in contact lens users.[39]

The corneal epithelium serves a protective function

FIG 10–5.
Marginal "ulcers" are ovoid, sterile infiltrative aggregations representing an immune hypersensitivity reaction to staphylococcal toxins. (Courtesy of J. Josephson and from Bennett ES, Weissman BA: *Clinical Contact Lens Practice*. Philadelphia, JB Lippincott Co, 1991. Used by permission.)

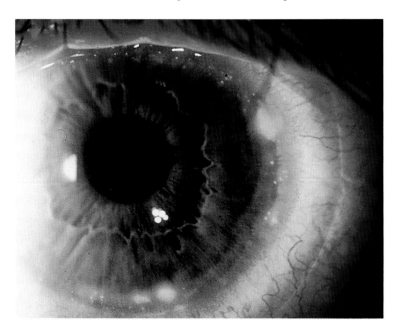

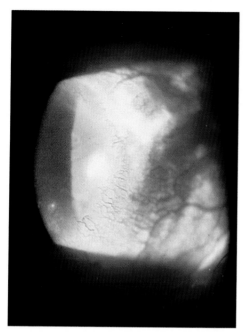

FIG 10-6.
Phlyctenule with associated inflammatory pannus.

against infection, as does the precorneal tear film, which contains numerous antibacterial substances (the immunoglobulins, lysozyme, lactoferrin, ceruloplasmin, lymphocytes, and complement, to name a few). Despite these excellent defensive mechanisms, an epithelial defect may allow opportunistic microbes in the tears, on the corneal epithelium, or adherent to contact lenses to invade the stroma, establishing an infection.

The presence of an epithelial defect or ulceration in association with underlying diffuse cellular infiltration and an anterior chamber reaction are strong clinical evidence for infection. The clinician's suspicion will be further heightened in the presence of pain, photophobia, hyperemia, mucopurulent discharge of the lids, or exudate on the ulcerated corneal surface, as well as in the presence of decreased vision. Because many of these signs are nonspecific, smears and cultures are required to make an appropriate identification of the causative pathogen.[23]

The inflammatory consequences of microbial infection may range from mild focal ulceration with minimal tissue damage to stromal abscess with ring ulcer, hypopyon, and even perforation (Figs 10-7 and 10-8). The severity of the inflammatory process depends not only on the virulence of the pathogen but also on the condition of the host defenses.

Inflammation is worsened in bacterial infections because of release of damaging toxins. Actively replicating bacteria release exotoxins, whereas endotoxins are released by some bacteria only after microbial death, causing ring infiltrates and postinfective tissue damage.[32] Enzymes released by infectious bacteria can also cause considerable tissue damage. These include collagenases, coagulases, proteases, nucleases, lipases, elastase, fibrinolysins, and hemolysins.[23] A virulent strain of *Pseudomonas*, for example, elicits a necrotizing enzyme, proteoglycanase, which can rapidly cause stromal destruction with descemetocele.[7]

The reader is encouraged to read Chapter 12 for further discussion of the diagnosis and management of ulcerative keratitis and its inflammatory consequences.

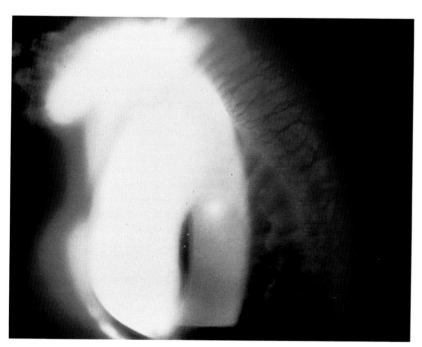

FIG 10-7.
Focal corneal ulcer caused by *Staphylococcus aureus*. Note intense sectoral injection, limited tissue damage, and generally clear cornea.

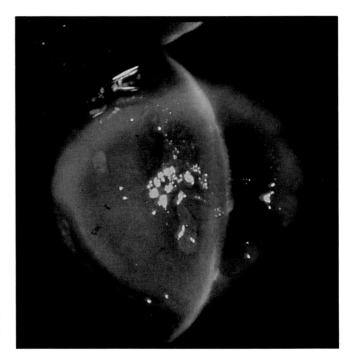

FIG 10–8.
Necrotizing corneal ulcer with diffuse tissue damage, including loss of corneal transparency, stromal abcess, and ring ulcer.

CORNEAL NEOVASCULARIZATION

The development of corneal neovascularization, particularly in a contact lens wearer, is a complex event. Although significant vascular incursion is not frequently encountered with today's more oxygen transmissive hydrogel lenses, any new vessel growth represents an adverse response. Hypoxia, trauma from damaged lenses, vascular compression from tight-fitting lenses, and solution sensitivity all are potential causes of vascularization.[26] In most cases, a vasostimulatory or angiogenic factor is released by existing blood vessels, which directly stimulates the development of new vascular endothelial cells, fibroblasts, pericytes, and smooth muscle cells.[21] Although it is unclear how hypoxia exerts its common vasostimulatory effect on the limbal plexus, it is believed that the vasostimulatory and inflammatory effects of prostaglandins are directly involved in these mechanisms.[8]

A recent model of contact lens–induced vascularization has been proposed by Efron,[10] who describes a sequence of events: initially, contact lens wear creates hypoxia, corneal edema, and stromal softening. Subsequent epithelial microtrauma from the effects of the contact lens releases enzymes, which, in turn, are chemotactic for inflammatory cells. When the cells reach the site of epithelial injury, they release angiogenic factors, which induce new vessel growth directed toward the site of injury.

The incidence of vascularization among wearers of rigid corneal lenses is quite low,[21] whereas the neovascu-lar response to hydrogel extended wear has shown incidence rates of 9%[42] and 17%,[41] respectively. In extended wear, factors such as the use of large lenses spanning the limbus, hypoxia, overwear, and reduced lens movement are factors playing a role in the formation of corneal vascularization.

Most contact lens–related neovascularization is superficial and limited to a zone 2 mm from the limbus, although in the presence of a strong stimulus vessels can extend beyond this zone, as well as trigger stromal invasion (Figs 10–9 and 10–10). Baseline examination of the corneolimbal area in any contact lens wearer is desirable to document the appearance of the normal limbal vasculature. This is best accomplished by marginal retroillumination using a slit-lamp biomicroscope.[27] After contact lens wear, the clinician should document with drawings or photography the extent of neovascular penetration beyond the normally translucent limbal transition zone. Vessels that demonstrate spikes or branches leaving a looped arcade should be closely monitored on subsequent visits.

When vascularization is observed, attempts should be made to remove the offending stimulus whenever possible. The use of thinner lenses is advantageous for both the benefits of less edge trauma and increased oxygen transmissibility. Increasing lens movement and using preservative-free solutions are also helpful changes. To prevent further vascularization when it is observed in an extended wear user, the clinician should change the wearing modality to daily wear. If vascularization is observed in a daily wear user, further restriction on wearing time is encouraged if

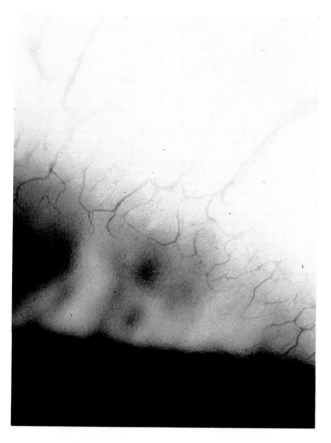

FIG 10–9.
Early superficial vascularization associated with hydrogel lens wear. (From Bennett ES, Weissman BA: *Clinical Contact Lens Practice.* Philadelphia, JB Lippincott Co, 1991. Used by permission.)

the cause cannot be identified or rectified. Any patient with documented neovascularization needs to be closely monitored on an ongoing basis.

ACUTE RED EYE SYNDROME

An inflammatory response observed in some extended wear hydrogel lens wearers has been termed the acute red eye, or ARE, syndrome.[11] The affected, lens-wearing patient is typically awakened in the very early hours of the morning with extreme unilateral pain, bulbar and limbal injection, pronounced photophobia, and lacrimation. Epithelial staining is usually absent. However, subepithelial or anterior stromal infiltrates are present within a few millimeters of the limbus (Figs 10–11 and 10–12).

The ARE syndrome is usually caused by a tightly adherent extended wear soft lens.[17] It can also come about from a number of other etiologies, including inflammatory toxic effects from trapped postlens debris,[28] mechanical irritation from poor lens design,[46] irritative response from acute hypoxia or lens deposits,[24] thinning and dehydration of the tear film during sleep,[24] and hypersensitivity or tox-

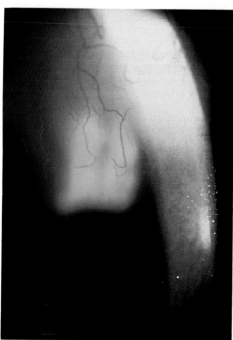

FIG 10–10.
Pronounced corneal neovascularization associated with long-term wear of hydrogel extended wear lenses.

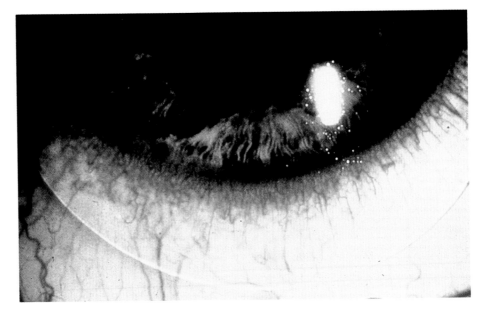

FIG 10–11.
Adherent extended wear hydrogel lens observed in the acute red eye (ARE) syndrome. Note the perilimbal injection or flush. (From Bennett ES, Weissman BA: *Clinical Contact Lens Practice.* Philadelphia, JB Lippincott Co, 1991. Used by permission.)

icity to solution preservatives, especially when used with high water content extended wear hydrogels.[16, 20]

The inflammatory reaction of the ARE syndrome in an acutely distressed patient necessitates a careful differential diagnosis on the part of the clinician, because the potential for infective keratitis in such a patient is also high. Although ARE syndrome typically manifests inflammatory infiltrates, there is no staining or ulceration. Epithelial defects with underlying infiltration require a presumption of infection and necessitate rapid and aggressive intervention.

This syndrome typically resolves with lens removal, with infiltrates clearing within a few weeks. Topical corticosteroids may reduce the inflammatory response, but their

use in an eye suffering from acute extended wear hypoxia carries too much risk and may actually facilitate microbial infection.[40] Although some believe that therapeutic management is not warranted with the ARE syndrome,[15] I believe that an eye experiencing acute hypoxic inflammation under conditions of extended wear is particularly susceptible to infection, especially in light of bacterial proliferation on surfaces of biofilm-coated hydrogels. As such, I treat ARE syndrome with broad-spectrum aminoglycoside antibiotics (gentamicin or tobramycin) during the initial 24 to 48 hours after an ARE episode to protect the eye, along with the quieting afforded by lens removal.

Lens wear should not be resumed until all inflamma-

FIG 10–12.
Anterior stromal infiltrates seen in ARE syndrome.

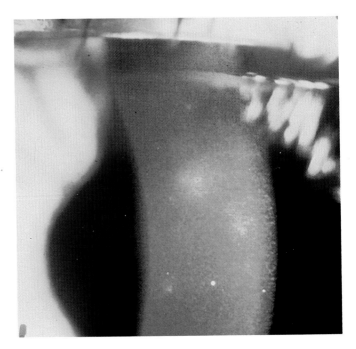

tory signs have disappeared. Daily wear, as well as the use of fresh lenses, should be encouraged. The incidence of the ARE syndrome can be greatly reduced, although not eliminated, with the use of disposable extended wear lenses worn on a weekly replacement schedule.[14] Because the ARE syndrome does have a propensity to recur in certain individuals, extended wear should be discontinued if this is observed, with future use of hydrogels strictly on a daily wear basis, or the patient refitted with gas-permeable lenses.

HYPERSENSITIVITY AND TOXICITY TO PRESERVATIVES

As noted previously, an inflammatory agent is considered toxic if there has been no prior exposure of the host tissue and where there is rapid injury to tissue. Toxic reactions may occur from exposure to chemicals used in contact lens solutions. The most common toxic effects are seen with benzalkonium chloride (BAK) and chlorhexidine.

Sensitivity reactions occur after there has been prior exposure to an inflammatory or allergic agent and occurs when the immune system detects that the offensive agent is not the same as the host. An allergic and often inflammatory reaction occurs as a defensive response to the reintroduced agent. The most commonly observed sensitivity reaction is caused by thimerosal.

Benzalkonium Chloride

Benzalkonium chloride is a bactericidal quaternary ammonium salt used as a preservative in ocular solutions because of its high effectivity against both gram-positive and gram-negative organisms. It is quickly adsorbed onto hydrogel lenses, reaching toxic levels rapidly.[30] This effect may be observed (and once seen never forgotten) by the clinician who inadvertently rinses a hydrogel lens with BAK-preserved irrigating solution rather than with hydrogel saline solution. An almost instantaneous red eye with diffuse epithelial punctate stippling will often be observed (Fig 10–13). This toxic effect is so rapid as to eliminate an immunological or allergic cause. As such, BAK is used only in solutions designed for polymethylmethacrylate hard lenses. It is not used in any hydrogel lens solutions, nor should it be used with RGP lenses, because BAK also binds to deposits on siloxanes and reduces RGP lens wettability.

Other quaternary ammonium chemicals with molecules large enough to prevent penetration into the hydrogel polymer have been developed for soft lens use, thus pre-

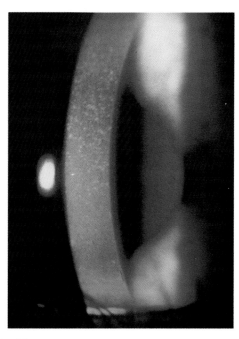

FIG 10–13.
Diffuse epithelial punctate staining observed as an immediate toxic effect to benzalkonium chloride adsorption on to a hydrogel lens. (From Bennett ES, Weissman BA: *Clinical Contact Lens Practice.* Philadelphia, JB Lippincott Co, 1991. Used by permission.)

venting gradual leaching of the agent and prolonged chemical insult.

Chlorhexidine

Chlorhexidine digluconate is a bactericidal preservative also effective against gram-positive and gram-negative organisms, with the exception of *Serratia*.[30] It binds strongly to hydrogel polymers and then leaches to complex with proteins in the tears. Tear protein complexing can reduce the preservative's antimicrobial effectivity. In addition, chlorhexidine is known to bind to mucins on lens surfaces, creating a more hydrophobic surface and contributing to ocular discomfort. It is typically combined with thimerosal in contact lens solutions because of chlorhexidine's weak action against fungi and *Serratia*.[30]

Although animal studies show little toxicity associated with direct application of chlorhexidine to the cornea, chlorhexidine does demonstrate toxicity in humans, causing punctate staining and hyperemia,[30] as well as localized limbal chemosis (Fig 10–14).

In toxic reactions, lens wear should be temporarily withdrawn to allow the cornea to heal. Topical corticosteroids are often helpful in reducing the inflammatory effects of toxic reactions. Lenses should be thoroughly purged of the offending agent before being reused. Because this is

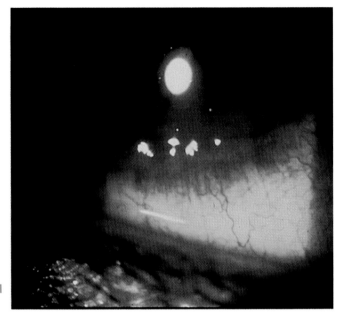

FIG 10–14.
Chlorhexidine toxicity leading to localized, chemosis limbal and hyperemia.

difficult, it is often wise to replace the lenses whenever possible.

Thimerosal

Thimerosal is a bacteriostatic mercurial compound used against a wide range of microbes in contact lens care solutions. Direct application of thimerosal to rabbit corneas in concentrations 200 times more concentrated than that used in contact lens solutions does not show corneal toxic effects. However, with hydrogel lenses, the chemical is adsorbed and slowly released, and repeated application produces sensitivity reactions.

Historically, thimerosal has been widely used as a preservative in numerous contact lens–related solutions and often is combined with other less effective preservatives. The incidence of hypersensitivity reactions associated with thimerosal has been reported as high as 40%.[30] Typically patients have used it for at least 3 months, after which signs and symptoms begin to manifest. Ocular reactions can include diffuse conjunctival redness and edema, discomfort, and anterior stromal infiltrates (Figs 10–4 and 10–15).[31, 45]

Because the sensitivity response to long-term thimerosal usage is similar to other sensitivity reactions, it is often a clinical challenge to differentiate thimerosal reactions from a wide variety of clinical entities. Because staining, folliculosis, and lymphadenopathy are typically not present in thimerosal reactions, viral, chlamydial, herpetic, and staphylococcal etiologies can usually be excluded. The

FIG 10–15.
Thimerosal hypersensitivity often leads to diffuse bulbar and palpebral (seen here) conjunctival hyperemia. (From Bennett ES, Weissman BA: *Clinical Contact Lens Practice.* Philadelphia, JB Lippincott Co, 1991. Used by permission.)

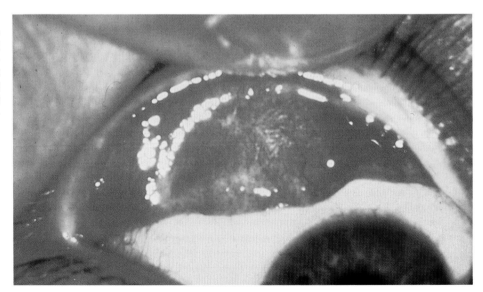

history is very important, and patients must be questioned in depth regarding products used in their care systems. Patients demonstrating positive ocular findings in thimerosal sensitivity reactions have also been shown to have delayed hypersensitivity reactions to thimerosal-containing solutions used in challenge tests with chemically soaked lenses, occlusive dermal patch testing, and intradermal injections.[31]

Today, thimerosal use is very low, because most practitioners have educated their patients and are using thimerosal-free preparations. Nevertheless, thimerosal-containing solutions are still sold, and the patient looking for "bargains" in lens care solutions is still likely to switch products and inadvertently begin using thimerosal-containing ones.

When thimerosal hypersensitivity is diagnosed, lens wear should be temporarily discontinued and lenses replaced with new ones. The patient must scrupulously avoid contact with mercurials in the future. Corticosteroids may be used to mitigate the sensitivity response only if the clinician can reasonably exclude bacterial, chlamydial, and herpetic causes.

Toxic and hypersensitivity reactions are described in more detail in Chapter 6.

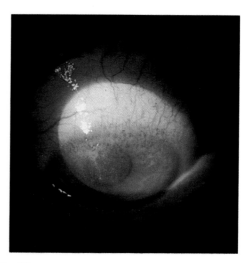

FIG 10–16.
Contact lens–induced superior limbic keratoconjunctivitis (CLKC). Note superior corneal staining and vascularization. (From Bennett ES, Weissman BA: *Clinical Contact Lens Practice.* Philadelphia, JB Lippincott Co, 1991. Used by permission.)

A detailed description of the etiology, symptoms, course, and management of CLKC is included in Chapter 6.

CONTACT LENS–INDUCED SUPERIOR LIMBIC KERATOCONJUNCTIVITIS

An inflammatory syndrome of soft contact lens use in which thimerosal is often implicated as the etiological agent is that of contact lens–induced superior limbic keratoconjunctivitis, or CLKC. Although often mimicking the appearance of true superior limbic keratoconjunctivitis (SLK), CLKC is not associated with thyroid disease, nor does it have a predilection for middle-aged women. The clinical signs of CLKC encompass:

1. Intense injection of the superior bulbar conjunctiva
2. Punctate staining of the superior limbus and cornea
3. Epithelial and subepithelial opacities
4. Superior corneal vascularization
5. Fine papillary hypertrophy of the superior tarsus

Whereas true SLK rarely affects vision,[38] the corneal changes seen with CLKC can reduce visual acuity because the inflammatory events may encroach into the pupillary zone. The corneal changes often start at the superior limbus and progress centrally in a V-shaped wedge, with its apex toward the pupil (Figs 10–16 to 10–18).

CONCLUSION

This chapter has reviewed the mechanisms of ocular inflammation, with particular attention to the anterior seg-

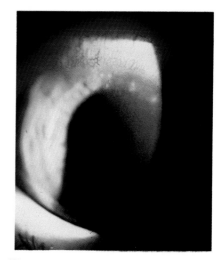

FIG 10–17.
Contact lens–induced superior limbic keratoconjunctivitis showing intense superior conjunctival hyperemia, vascularization, staining, and infiltrative response encroaching into the visual axis. (From Bennett ES, Weissman BA: *Clinical Contact Lens Practice.* Philadelphia, JB Lippincott Co, 1991. Used by permission.)

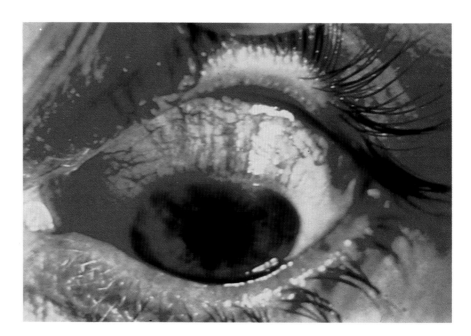

FIG 10–18.
True superior limbic keratoconjunctivitis (non–contact lens related) observed in a middle-aged woman with concurrent thyroid disease. Note similar appearance to CLKC.

ment and contact lens wear. Inflammatory reactions may arise, as we have seen, from a variety of mechanical, infectious, toxic, and allergic etiologies. A complex series of events occurs during any inflammatory reaction, and our knowledge is still incomplete with regard to a full understanding of the biochemical and cellular interrelationships at play during these events.

The clinical consequences of inflammation have been described, along with examples of specific inflammatory conditions and syndromes affecting the contact lens–wearing patient. The clinician must be alert to identify the presenting signs and symptoms of inflammation, to differentiate between the many possible causes in a contact lens–wearing population, and to act promptly to suppress the sequelae of inflammatory responses.

REFERENCES

1. Allansmith MR: Immunology of the external ocular tissues. *J Am Optom Assoc* 1990; 61:S16–S22.
2. Allansmith MR, Greiner JV, Baird RS: Number of inflammatory cells in the normal conjunctiva. *Am J Ophthalmol* 1978; 86:250–259.
3. Ambache N, Kavanaugh L, Whiting J: Effect of mechanical stimulation on rabbits' eyes: Release of active substance in anterior chamber perfusates. *J Physiol* 1965; 176:378.
4. Basu PK, Minta JO: Chemotactic migration of leukocytes through corneal layers: An in vitro study. *Can J Ophthalmol* 1976; 11:235.
5. Bhattacherjee P, Eakins KE: Inhibition of the PG-synthetase systems in ocular tissues by indomethacin. *Br J Pharmacol* 1973; 15:209.
6. Bartlett JD: Pharmacology of allergic eye disease. *J Am Optom Assoc* 1990; 61:S23–S31.
7. Brown SI, Bloomfield SE, Wai-Fong IT: The cornea-destroying enzyme of *Pseudomonas aeruginosa*. *Invest Ophthalmol* 1974; 11:174.
8. Cooper CA, Bergamini MVW, Leopold IH: Use of flurbiprofen to inhibit corneal neovascularization. *Arch Ophthalmol* 1980; 98:1102.
9. Eakins KE, Whitelocke RF, Bennett A, et al: Prostaglandin-like activity in ocular inflammation. *Br Med J* 1972; 3:452.
10. Efron N: Vascular response of the cornea to contact lens wear. *J Am Optom Assoc* 1987; 58:836–846.
11. Fichman S, Baker VV, Horton HR: Iatrogenic red eyes in soft lens wearers. *Int Contact Lens Clin* 1978; 15:202–209.
12. Flower RJ, Blackwell GJ: Anti-inflammatory steroids induce biosynthesis of a phospholipase A2 inhibitor which prevents prostaglandin generation. *Nature* 1979; 278:456.
13. Foster CS: Basic ocular immunology, in Kaufman HE, Barron BA, McDonald MB, et al (eds): *The Cornea*. New York, Churchill Livingstone, 1988, pp 101–102.
14. Grant T, Chong MS, Holden BA: Which is best for the eye: Daily wear, 2 nights, or 6 nights? *Am J Optom Physiol Opt* 1988; 65:S40.
15. Grant T, Terry R, Holden BA: Extended wear of hydrogel lenses, in Harris MG (ed): *Problems in Optometry: Contact Lenses and Ocular Disease*. Philadelphia, JB Lippincott Co, 1990, p 609.
16. Holden BA, Vannas A, Nilsson K, et al: Epithelial and endothelial effects from the extended wear of contact lenses. *Curr Eye Res* 1985; 4:739–742.
17. Holden BA, Zantos SG: The ocular response to continuous wear of contact lenses. *Optician* 1979; 177:50–56.
18. Josephson JE, Caffrey BE: Infiltrative keratitis in hydrogel lens wearers. *Int Contact Lens Clin* 1979; 6:223–242.

19. Josephson JE, Zantos S, Caffery BE, et al: Differentiation of corneal complications observed in contact lens wearers. *J Am Optom Assoc* 1988; 59:679–685.

20. Kotow M, Grant T, Holden BA: Avoiding ocular complications during hydrogel extended wear. *Int Contact Lens Clin* 1987; 14:95–99.

21. Larke JR: *The Eye in Contact Lens Wear*. Stoneham, Mass, Butterworths, 1985, p 54.

22. Leopold IH, Gaster RN: Ocular inflammation and anti-inflammatory drugs, in Kaufman HE, Barron BA, McDonald MB, et al (eds): *The Cornea*. New York, Churchill Livingstone, 1988, p 67.

23. Liesegang TJ: Bacterial and fungal keratitis, in Kaufman HE, Barron BA, McDonald MB, et al (eds): *The Cornea*. New York, Churchill Livingstone, 1988, p 217.

24. Mandell RB: *Contact Lens Practice*, ed 4. Springfield, Ill, Charles C Thomas, Publisher, 1989, p 699.

25. Mannis MJ: Bacterial conjunctivitis, in Kaufman HE, Barron BA, McDonald MB, et al (eds): *The Cornea*. New York, Churchill Livingstone, 1988, p 193.

26. McMonnies CW: Risk factors in the etiology of contact lens–induced vascularization. *Int Contact Lens Clin* 1984; 11:286–293.

27. McMonnies CW, Chapman-Davies A, Holden BA: The vascular response to contact lens wear. *Am J Optom Physiol Opt* 1982; 59:795–799.

28. Mertz GW, Holden BA: Clinical implications of extended wear research. *Can J Optom* 1981; 43:203–205.

29. Meyers RL, Pettit TH: Chemotaxis of polymorphonuclear leukocytes in corneal inflammation: Tissue injury in herpes simplex virus infection. *Invest Ophthalmol* 1974; 13:187.

30. Morgan JF: Problems associated with current care systems, in Stein HA, Slatt BJ, Stein RM (eds) *Fitting Guide for Rigid and Soft Contact Lenses: A Practical Approach*. St Louis, CV Mosby Co, 1990, pp 435–440.

31. Mondino BJ, Groden LR: Conjunctival hyperemia and corneal infiltrates with chemically disinfected soft contact lenses. *Arch Ophthalmol* 1980; 98:1767–1770.

32. Mondino BJ, Rabin BS, Kessler E, et al: Corneal rings with gram negative bacteria. *Arch Ophthalmol* 1977; 95:2222.

33. Pfortner T, DeAldama EB, Korbenfeld P, et al: Immunological action of the precorneal tear film with the use of contact lenses. *Int Contact Lens Clin* 1977; 4:65.

34. Rosenbaum JT, Boney RS, Samples JR, et al: Synthesis of platelet activating factor by ocular tissue from inflamed eyes. *Arch Ophthalmol* 1991; 109:410–413.

35. Schlaegel TF: Nonspecific treatment of uveitis, in Duane TD (ed): *Clinical Ophthalmology*. Philadelphia, Harper & Row, Publishers, 1986, vol 4, chapter 43, p 3.

36. Silbert JA: Prostaglandins and the ocular inflammatory response. *Rev Optom* 1978; 115(3):53–54.

37. Silbert JA: Contact lens related pathology: part I. *Rev Optom* 1984; 121(4):104–112.

38. Silbert JA: Contact lens related pathology: part II. *Rev Optom* 1984; 121(7):51–60.

39. Silbert JA: Microbial infection in contact lens patients, in Harris MG (ed): *Problems in Optometry: Contact Lenses and Ocular Disease*. Philadelphia, JB Lippincott Co, 1990, pp 572–573.

40. Silbert JA: Contact lens-related inflammatory reactions, in Bennett ES, Weissman BA (eds): *Clinical Contact Lens Practice*. Philadelphia, JB Lippincott Co, 1991.

41. Spoor TC, Hartel WC, Wynn P, et al: Complication of continuous-wear soft contact lenses in a nonreferral population. *Arch Ophthalmol* 1984; 102:1312–1313.

42. Stark WJ, Martin NF: Extended wear soft contact lenses for myopic correction. *Arch Ophthalmol* 1981; 99:1683.

43. Vane JR: Inhibition of prostaglandin synthesis as a mechanism of action for aspirin-like drugs. *Nature* 1971; 231:232.

44. Ward PA, Lepow IH, Neuman LJ: Bacterial factors chemotactic for polymorphonuclear leukocytes. *Am J Pathol* 1968; 52:725.

45. Wilson LA, McNath J, Reutschel R: Delayed hypersensitivity to thimerosal in soft lens wearers. *Ophthalmology* 1981; 88:804–809.

46. Weissman BA: An introduction to extended wear contact lenses. *J Am Optom Assoc* 1982; 53:183–186.

Giant Papillary Conjunctivitis

Carolyn G. Begley, O.D., M.S.

Giant papillary conjunctivitis (GPC) is a relatively new disease, which was not fully described until the 1970s. It is usually associated with contact lens wear,[6, 36, 45, 47] but it has also been known to occur in conjunction with ocular prostheses,[61, 62] an extruded scleral buckle,[50] cyanoacrylate adhesive,[36] and nylon sutures.[49, 63] It affects primarily the upper tarsal conjunctiva, where it causes hyperemia, excess mucus, and the formation of giant papillae (Fig 11–1). Patients with GPC also experience itching, foreign body sensation, and eventually contact lens intolerance.[6]

In 1970, Kennedy[33] provided what is probably the earliest report of a GPC-like condition. In a case report of a patient suffering from a polymethylmethacrylate (PMMA)–induced overwear corneal abrasion, he noted that the upper tarsus demonstrated vascularized papillary elevations. Spring,[60] in 1974, more fully described an allergic-like reaction of the upper lid in a population of 176 soft contact lens wearers. Seventy-six of these patients displayed large tarsal papillae with discomfort and excessive mucous formation.

In 1977, Allansmith et al.[6] published a landmark paper describing papillary changes on the upper tarsal conjunctiva of 58 hard and soft contact lens wearers. They also dubbed the disorder GPC and outlined the typical clinical signs and symptoms. The disease was compared to vernal conjunctivitis, and an allergic etiology was suggested.

Giant papillary conjunctivitis still occurs relatively frequently in the contact lens–wearing population, with recent estimates of the incidence varying from 4.23% to 15%.[36, 57] However, despite its regular appearance in clinical practice, the disease remains poorly understood by practioners and researchers alike. The following chapter outlines controversial aspects of the disease and current methods of diagnosis and treatment.

THE CAUSE OF GIANT PAPILLARY CONJUNCTIVITIS: AN OPEN QUESTION

Despite the best efforts of many researchers, the etiology of GPC remains unclear. As clinicians we routinely treat patients with GPC while lacking a clear grasp of the disease we are managing. It has been labeled both an allergic reaction of various types and a pure response to mechanical trauma of the upper lid.

Evidence for an Allergic Reaction

In 1977, Allansmith et al.[6] proposed that GPC represents an allergic reaction based largely on biopsy specimens of numerous papillae from patients with GPC. They noted that the papillae exhibited an atypical cellular profile, including mast cells, eosinophils, and basophils in the conjunctival epithelium and eosinophils and basophils in the substantia propria.[5] Normal palpebral conjunctiva, on the other hand, contained no eosinophils and few other inflammatory cells.[4] Allansmith et al.[3] also compared GPC to vernal conjunctivitis, which is a very similar but clinically more severe allergic disorder. Biopsy specimens of papillae from patients with GPC and vernal conjunctivitis showed analogous profiles, but the numbers of inflammatory cells were greatly increased in vernal conjunctivitis and included an infiltrate of plasma cells in the epithelium. Both diseases also exhibited a high number of partially or fully degranulated mast cells in the epithelium.[30]

Cutaneous Basophilic Hypersensitivity

The cellular infiltrate evident in both GPC and vernal conjunctivitis, including the unusual presence of basophils, led Allansmith et al.[3, 6] to suggest that the two diseases

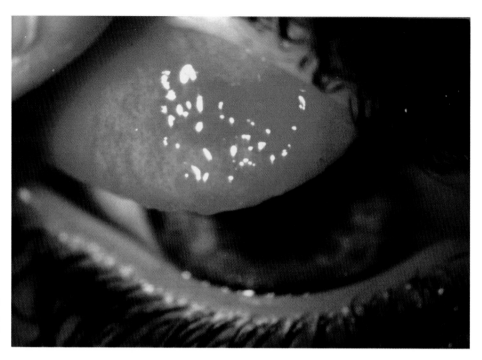

FIG 11–1.
Upper tarsus of giant papillary conjunctivitis (GPC) patient. Note nasal orientation of papillae.

may at least partially represent a delayed hypersensitivity reaction of the cutaneous basophilic type. Cutaneous basophilic hypersensitivity refers to a basophil-rich skin reaction, with a delayed time course that may be mediated in part by sensitized T lymphocytes and by antibodies.[19, 29] An animal model has been established for cutaneous basophilic hypersensitivity of the upper tarsal plate by Hann et al.,[28] who obtained a GPC-like reaction in guinea pig eyelids after injection of various antigens.

The appropriateness, however, of categorizing GPC as a cutaneous basophilic hypersensitivity reaction is uncertain. In this cutaneous reaction, basophils constitute almost half of the inflammatory cells present,[19, 53] but GPC patients show less than 5% basophils in the epithelium and substantia propria of the upper tarsal conjunctiva.[5] The low percentage of basophils in GPC and vernal conjunctivitis[42] may actually better reflect the classic tuberculin type of delayed hypersensitivity reaction, in which variable numbers of basophils[53] can also be present.

IgE-Mediated Immediate Hypersensitivity

There is evidence that an IgE-mediated immediate hypersensitivity reaction (type 1, anaphylactic) may be involved in the etiology of GPC.[8, 15] This type of hypersensitivity reaction is stimulated by an antigen (foreign substance) that causes the proliferation of specific IgE antibodies. As Figure 11–2 indicates, the antigen-specific IgE molecules attach to the membrane of locally circulating mast cells. Subsequent exposure to the antigen sets off a chain reaction, ultimately causing degranulation of the mast cell and release of vasoactive and chemical mediators of inflamma-

tion, including histamine, serotonin, leukotrienes, prostaglandins, and platelet-activating factor, and eosinophil and neutrophil chemotactic factors. In addition, other substances that affect tissue damage and repair, such as β-glucoronidase, amylosidase, β-hexaminidase, chymase, tryptase, and heparin, may be released, depending on the type of mast cell.[52, 53] Mast cell degranulation has far-reaching consequences, causing edema, hyperemia, and itching.

The large number of degranulated mast cells found in the conjunctival epithelium of GPC patients[30] support the involvement of IgE-mediated mechanisms in GPC. Tear tryptase levels are also increased in GPC patients over normals,[12] reflecting heightened mast cell degranulation (see Fig 11–2). In addition, IgE levels in the tears are significantly elevated in GPC patients, implying an increased local synthesis of these antibodies in the conjunctival tissue.[8, 15] However, Abelson et al.[1] failed to demonstrate histamine in the tears of GPC patients, whereas patients with hay fever and vernal conjunctivitis had increased levels of tear histamine.

Association With Atopy

Reports on the connection of GPC with other allergies are varied. Allansmith et al.[6] found no connection between atopy and GPC. Henriquez et al.[30] also described a GPC patient who had normal skin test reactions to airborne allergens, no hay fever, no asthma, no eczema, and no allergic rhinitis. Other authors, however, have noted an increase in the incidence of allergies in GPC patients,[8, 47] which tends to substantiate an IgE-mediated mechanism

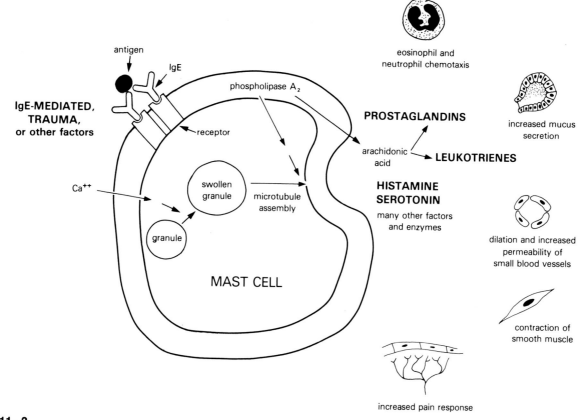

FIG 11–2.
Mast cell degranulation. (Adapted from Sell S: *Immunology, Immunopathology, and Immunity*, ed 4. New York, Elsevier North-Holland, 1987, p 478; and Smolin G, O'Connor RG: *Ocular Immunology*, ed 2. Boston, Little, Brown & Co, 1986.)

for the disease. Buckley,[11] for example, noted high levels of serum IgE, indicative of atopy, in his population of GPC patients.

The association of GPC with seasonal allergies has been pointed out by several authors. Begley et al.[9] found that the onset of GPC was seasonal in a population of 68 patients in southern Indiana. As Figure 11–3 indicates, the number of cases peaked in the spring and early fall, corresponding with spring and fall allergy seasons in the midwestern United States. The GPC patients in this study reported significantly more overall allergies than did a control group. Molinari[47] also found that allergies were a risk factor for GPC in his study of 20 patients with the disease. In addition, Soni and Hathcoat[57] noted an increase in the numbers of GPC patients in March compared with February, and Smolin and O'Connor[56] commented that atopic patients with GPC demonstrated an increase in symptoms during the spring pollen season.

Proposed Antigens

Contact lens deposits or associated materials are probably still the strongest contender for the antigen triggering GPC. It is evident to most clinicians that as the symptoms and signs of the disease increase, they are accompanied by

an increase in mucus and lens deposits (see Fig 11–8). In their earlier studies, Allansmith et al.[6] pointed to an unknown factor in the contact lens deposits as providing the stimulus. Proteins, adsorbed to the surface of the contact lens, or adherent bacteria[22] were suggested as the antigenic

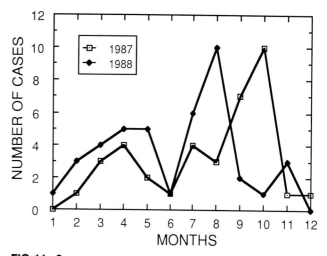

FIG 11–3.
Seasonal occurrence of GPC. (From Begley CG, Riggle A, Tuel JA: *Optom Vis Sci* 1990; 67:192. Used by permission.)

culprit. However, scanning electron microscopy[23, 24] and immunohistochemical staining[27] demonstrated no difference between deposits on the contact lenses of patients with or without GPC. In addition, as Reynolds[49] noted, the deposits on the lens may be the result rather than the cause of the condition.

The plastic in the contact lens has also been suggested as an antigenic stimulus for GPC.[49] However, replacement of a deposited lens with a new lens of the same type provides, at least, temporary relief for most symptomatic GPC patients (see discussion of treatment). It is not therefore likely that the plastic itself serves as the antigenic stimulus, although its potential for surface irregularities may provide increased trauma to the palpebral conjunctiva.

Evidence for Mechanical Trauma

Mechanical trauma has also been proposed as a cause for GPC.[49] This body of evidence is derived largely from GPC associated not with contact lens wear but with plastics that obviously abrade the upper lid. For example, GPC occurs fairly frequently in patients wearing plastic ocular prostheses.[61, 62] Frequent polishing or smoothing of the prosthesis often provides symptomatic relief in these patients. Giant papillary conjunctivitis has also been reported to occur in conjunction with an extruded scleral buckle,[50] bulging cyanoacrylate adhesive used to patch a corneal perforation,[13] and protruding nylon sutures.[49, 63] In each of these cases, removing or smoothing the plastic irregularity relieved the symptoms and signs of GPC. Similarly, in patients who had contracted GPC after cataract surgery, Reynolds[49] noted that the causative nylon suture end projected "little more than the diameter of the suture itself—a mere 22 microns." He hypothesized that analogous small defects on the surface of a contact lens could irritate the tarsal conjunctiva.

Dunn et al.[18] made another interesting observation in a GPC patient who had never worn contact lenses but had hardened corneal deposits resulting from an earlier accident. These deposits apparently caused a severe focal case of GPC through mechanical abrasion of the superior tarsal conjunctiva. Debridement of the cornea, with subsequent smoothing of the surface, produced a resolution of the GPC. This case report suggests that even in the absence of plastics (contact lenses, sutures, prostheses, etc.), long-term trauma alone can produce GPC.

The large numbers of degranulated mast cells present in the epithelium and substantia propria of GPC patients could also implicate trauma in the etiology of the disease, along with an IgE-mediated hypersensitivity reaction. As Figure 11–2 indicates, a number of factors are known to cause mast cell degranulation, including trauma.[32, 53,58] In a study involving eye rubbing in rats, Greiner et al.[26] found that the conjunctival epithelium was disrupted and 50% of the mast cells were degranulated. They presumed that trauma caused this effect on mast cells and also found a 2,300% increase in neutrophils in the first 4 hours.

Another palpebral change investigated by Greiner et al.[25] involved the excessive mucus discharge found in GPC patients. They found that both asymptomatic contact lens wearers and patients with GPC demonstrated increased numbers of vesicles containing mucus in nongoblet epithelial cells. The group hypothesized that these vesicles are responsible for the excess mucus often noted clinically even in asymptomatic contact lens wearers and likely represent a response to upper lid trauma. In addition, Ehlers et al.[20] found increased levels of neutrophil chemotactic factor, which is released by traumatized conjunctiva, in both GPC patients and asymptomatic contact lens wearers. The GPC patients showed almost 15 times the normal level of neutrophil chemotactic factor, again supporting the concept that the etiology of GPC involves trauma.

DIAGNOSIS

Giant papillary conjunctivitis is diagnosed largely by upper lid changes, although the symptoms are also very characteristic of the disease. Lid eversion, therefore, should be performed routinely on all contact lens patients to establish the baseline lid appearance and to note any changes in the upper tarsal conjunctiva. A preexisting drawing of both everted upper lids on standard clinic forms is helpful so that the examiner can quickly sketch in upper lid findings for a particular patient.

Traditionally the first step in diagnosing pathological changes in the upper tarsal conjunctiva is to learn to differentiate between papillae and follicles. Papillae occur in allergic diseases, such as GPC and vernal conjunctivitis, and are usually described as conjunctival elevations with a vascular tuft in the center (Fig 11–4, arrow). Follicles, on the other hand, are hallmarks of viral or chlamydial infections of the conjunctiva. Follicles have whitish centers, with vessels around the outside of the elevation. Unfortunately, papillae and follicles can be hard to distinguish because inflamed or scarred papillae can effectively mimic follicles. In fact, papillae with whitish centers are relatively common in the latter stages of GPC (see Fig 11–7,E and G). The centers of these papillae are presumably filled with inflammatory cells or scar tissue, masking the central tuft of

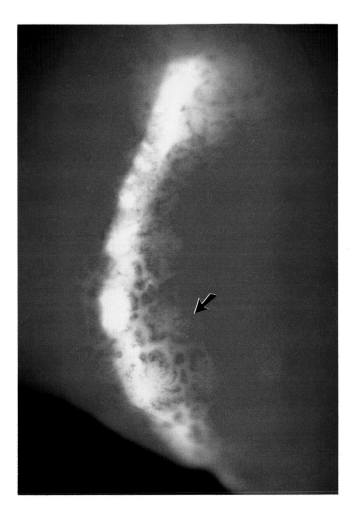

FIG 11–4.
Papilla *(arrow)* in GPC patient. Note central vascular tuft.

vessels. Despite the potential difficulty in differentiating the two types of conjunctival elevations, however, the categories are often clinically useful when they are considered in association with other signs and symptoms.

The upper tarsal conjunctiva on normal (non-GPC) lids can be classified into three basic categories (Fig 11–5), according to Allansmith.[2] Only the tarsal plate is graded, because the junctional conjunctiva may contain large papillae or concretions even in normals. About 14% of people have satin or smooth lids (see Fig 11–5,a). This type is more common in older persons with somewhat flaccid lids and may be less likely to progress to GPC than other lid types. A large percentage (about 85%) of normal lids demonstrate small but uniformly sized "micropapillae" approximately 0.3 mm or less (see Fig 11–5,b). This lid type is often labeled as uniform papillary or uniform cobblestone appearance. The third classification, nonuniform papillary or nonuniform cobblestone appearance, occurs in less than 1% of the population (see Fig 11–5,c). The upper tarsal conjunctiva of these lids contains some larger "macropapillae" approximately 0.5 mm in diameter, which

contribute to the nonuniform appearance of the lids. In this author's experience, these individuals often report numerous allergies, and Allansmith[2] believes that they are at a greater risk of developing GPC.

Patients with GPC exhibit a range of lid types, including the uniform cobblestone (see Fig 11–5,b) and nonuniform cobblestone (Fig 11–5,c) found in normals. Although this is confusing to the beginner, one must remember that the giant papillae take a while to develop, so that intermediate stages may mimic "normal" lids. One constant feature seen in symptomatic GPC, however, is hyperemia of the upper lid. A useful technique is to compare the papillae and injection of the upper lid with that of the lower lid. This essentially uses the lower lid as a rough baseline for the amount of hyperemia and size of papillae usual for that patient. As Figure 11–6 indicates, a symptomatic patient with GPC will almost always demonstrate increased hyperemia of the upper lid compared with the lower.

The most severe lid manifestation in GPC is the giant papillary appearance in which the papillae reach 1 mm or

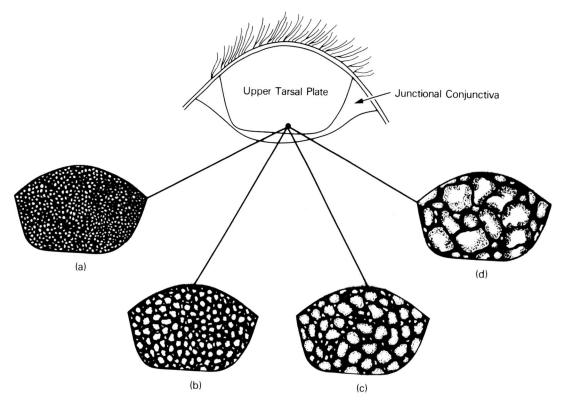

FIG 11–5.
Diagrammatic representation of upper tarsal types. Smooth or satin *(a)*, uniform papillary or cobblestone *(b)*, nonuniform papillary or cobblestone *(c)*, and giant papillary appearance *(d)*.

more in diameter (see Fig 11–5,d). The giant papillae often become ulcerated and contain adherent mucus strands. Papillae are easier to visualize if sodium fluorescein is instilled. The dye pools around the base of the papillae and serves to outline its circumference (Figs 11–7,B, D, F, and H). Fluorescein also stains mucus strands and the tips of large papillae. These features can be clinically graded on a 0 to 4+ scale, based on the amount of mucus, erythema, and the presence of fluorescein staining of the tops of the papillae.[6]

Another characteristic that may be important in management of the patient is the distribution of giant papillae on the upper lid. Allansmith et al.[6] recommend dividing the conjunctival surface of the upper eyelid into zones of equal size to note the location of the papillae. She[2] notes that hydrogel lens wearers with GPC often show more giant papillae in the superior tarsal area and less near the lash margin, whereas hard lens wearers tend to have large papillae closer to the lash margin.[34] The distribution of the papillae can certainly be uneven, as in Figure 11–1, where the papillae assume a nasal orientation. Simply sketching the location of the large papillae is recommended. In this way the size and location of the papillae can be followed over time.

Giant papillary conjunctivitis is usually diagnosed and categorized by stages 1 to 4 from the landmark 1977 paper of Allansmith et al.[6] Table 11–1 outlines the signs and symptoms of the disease. Stage 1 (see Figs 11–7,A and B) is largely preclinical and relatively asymptomatic. According to Allansmith et al.,[6] patients in stage 1 can be diagnosed by symptoms only, reporting an increase in mucus discharge on awakening and mild itching. These symptoms are very mild and do not often bring the patient to his or her eye care practioner at this point. One common exception to this rule, however, is the patient who has had GPC in the past and is very aware of the early symptoms of the disease. These patients, in my experience, demonstrate no papillary changes but do show a slight increase in hyperemia of the upper tarsal conjunctiva.

It is also relatively uncommon for patients to seek out medical help in stage 2 GPC. These individuals are more often detected on routine follow-ups and may divulge their symptoms on questioning. In this stage, the patient begins to notice lens discomfort later in the day and may report increased blurring because of lens deposits toward the end of the wearing time. The upper lid changes may be somewhat minimal in stage 2 and often consist of a few larger papillae interspersed with smaller, "normally sized" papil-

A

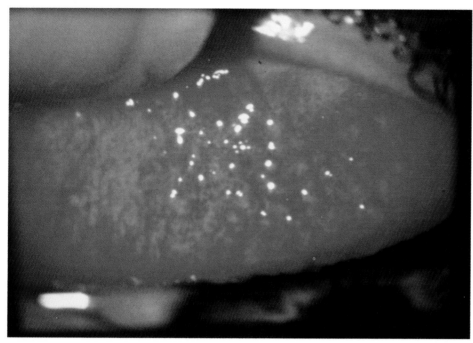

B

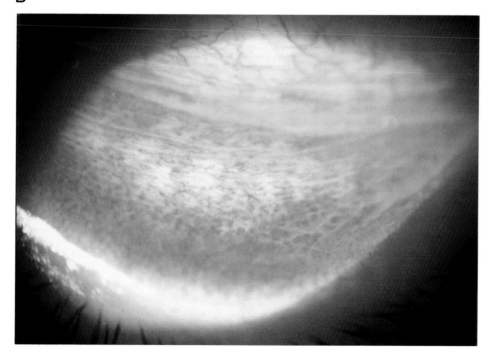

FIG 11–6.
A, upper tarsus of GPC patient. Note hyperemia. **B,** lower lid of same patient. (Yellow liquid is sodium fluorescein.)

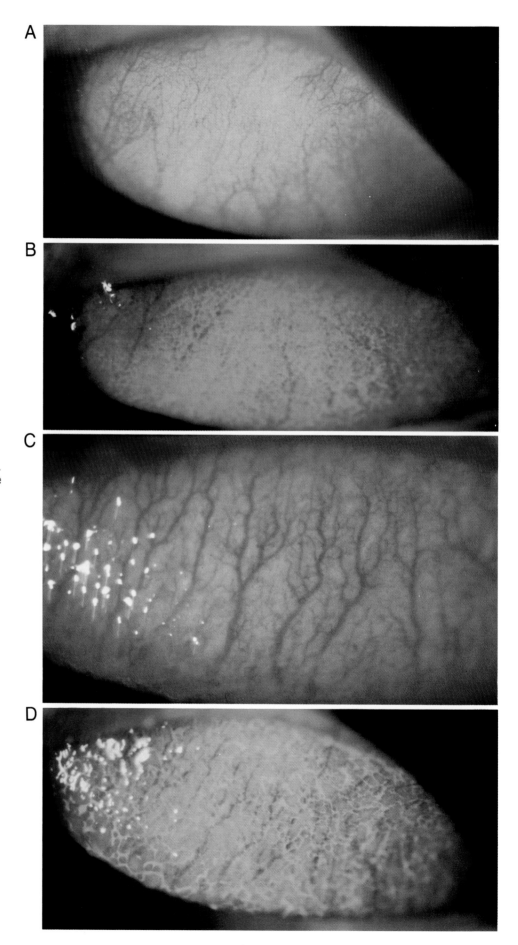

FIG 11–7.
Upper tarses in GPC.
Stage 1 (**A** and **B**), stage
2 (**C** and **D**), *Continued.*

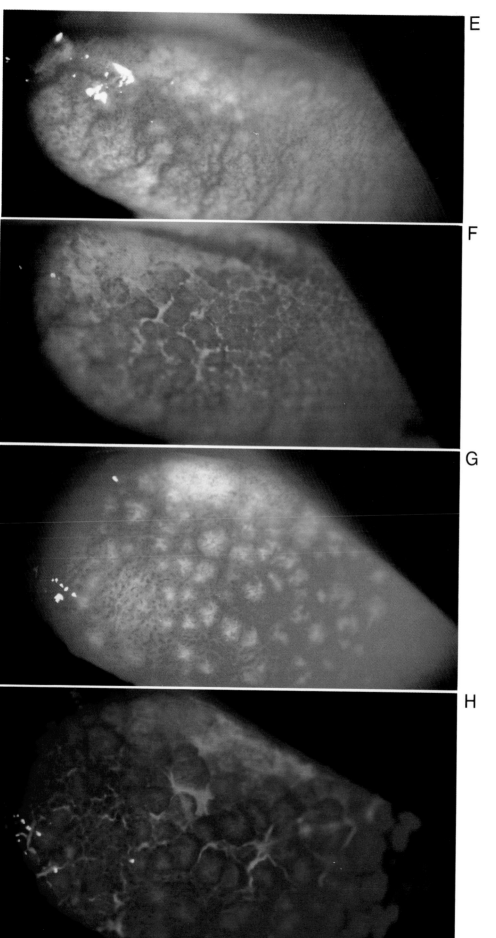

E

F

G

H

FIG 11–7 (cont.).
Stage 3 (**E** and **F**), and
Stage 4 (**G** and **H**). Instillation of sodium fluorescein (**B, D, F,** and **H**) delineates papillae for easy visualization.

TABLE 11–1.

Signs and Symptoms of Giant Papillary Conjunctivitis*

Stage	Symptoms	Signs
1	Mild itching Slight increase in mucus in A.M.	No signs or slight hyperemia of upper lid
2	Itching Increased mucus in A.M. Lens awareness and blurring of vision late in day	Enlargement of some papillae on upper tarsal plate Mucus strands over papillae Slight to moderate hyperemia of upper lid Mild coating of contact lens Rare punctate staining superiorly
3	Moderate to severe itching, especially on lens removal Moderate to severe mucus Increased lens awareness, often forcing a reduction in lens wear Moderate blurring of vision with lens Occasional decentering of lens	Increased size of papillae, with some giant papillae (>1 mm) present Heavy sheets and strands of mucus Upper lid hyperemic and edematous Moderate coating of contact lens, which may occasionally decenter superotemporally with blink May have superior punctate staining
4	Severe itching Severe mucus; eyelids may be stuck together in A.M. Discomfort forces an extreme reduction or discontinuation of lens wear Moderate to severe blurring of vision with contact lens Frequent decentering of lens	Giant papillae (>1 mm); some flattened on top (mushroom shaped); tips may stain with fluorescein Heavy sheets and strands of mucus Upper lid hyperemic and edematous Severe coating of contact lens, which often decenters frequently with blink May show superior punctate staining or infiltrates

*Adapted from Allansmith MR, Korb DR, Greiner JV, et al: *Am J Ophthalmol* 1977; 83:697–708.

lae (see Figs 11–7,C and D). The lid is usually graded as having a nonuniform cobblestone appearance and frequently shows an increased hyperemia of the palpebral conjunctiva.

Patients with stage 3 and 4 GPC are clearly symptomatic. In stage 3 the itching and mucus discharge have increased, and lens wear is less comfortable. The patient is often forced to remove the lens earlier in the day than usual and may conclude that his or her contact lens is "old" and needs replacement. Patients also begin to report that the lens moves around excessively or may decenter (Fig 11–8,A) under the upper lid. This presumably occurs because of the lens sticking to the mucus-laden giant papillae. On examination, the patient with stage 3 GPC demonstrates some giant papillae on the superior tarsus (see Figs 11–7,E and F). The upper lid is also hyperemic and edematous, and the contact lens usually shows moderate deposits. In addition, it is not uncommon for patients with stage 3 and 4 GPC to demonstrate superficial punctate staining or infiltrates in the superior cornea.[6, 10] One reported case of GPC also showed a diffuse limbitis, limbal nodules, and Tranta's dots reminiscent of the limbal form of vernal conjunctivitis.[44]

In stage 4 GPC, the symptoms usually worsen to the point that contact lens wear becomes minimal because of discomfort. Patients report a foreign body sensation and blurry vision because of excessive mucus and contact lens deposits (Fig 11–8,B). The lens also decenters frequently (see Fig 11–8,A) and may fold up and lodge under the upper lid. The extremely hyperemic upper tarsus demonstrates numerous giant papillae (see Figs 11–7,G and H), which may be mushroom shaped with flat apices. The tips of the papillae often stain with sodium fluorescein in this stage, presumably because of mechanical abrasion. The giant papillae on the upper lid may cause enough edema to result in a unilateral or asymmetrical ptosis.[54]

Table 11–1, however, does not reflect all clinical manifestations of GPC. It is not uncommon to find that the signs and symptoms of a given stage of GPC do not match.[1] For instance, a patient with upper lid changes consistent with stage 2 GPC may complain of symptoms best categorized as stage 3 or 4. Conversely, patients with stage 4 giant papillae on the upper tarsus may complain minimally. The mismatch between signs and symptoms in some patients may reflect individual tolerances to discomfort or pain.

A

B

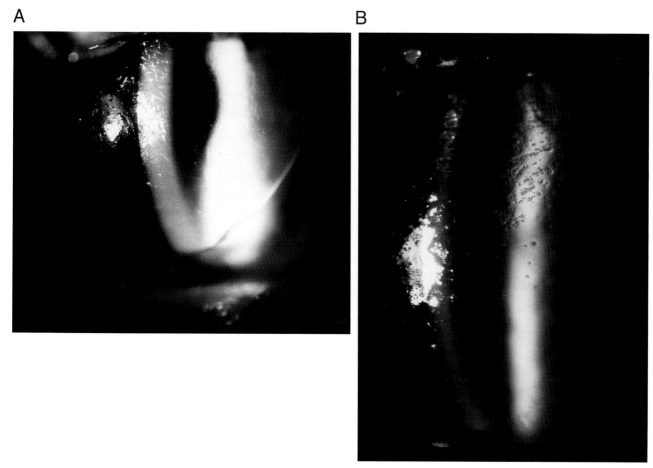

FIG 11–8.
A, decentered lens with heavy protein and mineral deposits. **B,** heavy deposits in stage 4 GPC.

Another important point in staging GPC is the hyperemia of the upper tarsal conjunctiva. Hyperemia is an important sign and often correlates better with symptoms than the size or number of papillae. For instance, a symptomatic patient with stage 4 GPC may demonstrate numerous large papillae on an extremely hyperemic and edematous upper tarsus. If the patient quits wearing contact lenses for 1 or 2 weeks, the symptoms of mucus and itching will virtually disappear. Examination of the upper lid will most likely reveal that the papillae are still large and numerous, but the hyperemia and mucus production have greatly decreased in conjunction with the symptoms. The palpebral conjunctiva may even appear pale at this point, but several more weeks may be required to significantly reduce the size of the papillae.

TREATMENT

Historically the treatment of GPC can be grouped into four general categories: (1) alteration in lens solutions or clean-

ers, (2) cessation of lens wear or replacement, (3) change of lens type or parameters, and (4) application of pharmaceutical agents. A discussion of this confusing array of recommended treatments follows, and these are then summarized for a practical approach at managing the disease. The wide variety of treatment modalities in common usage probably reflects the lack of understanding of the etiology of the disease.

Alteration in Lens Solutions or Cleaners

Relatively asymptomatic patients who demonstrate less severe GPC (stage 1 or 2) are often easily managed by enhanced cleaning efforts.[21, 51, 55] It is well known that heavy contact lenses deposits often parallel an increase in the symptoms of GPC patients, whereas cleaner lenses often result in fewer symptoms. More frequent enzyme cleaning, as often as two to three times per week, helps to reduce protein deposits and improve comfort. This applies to both soft[21, 51] and hard[35] contact lenses, although rigid gas-permeable (RGP) and PMMA lenses can simply be polished repeatedly. Some patients also need to be reinstructed in the use of a daily surfactant cleaner. It is important to mechanically rub both sides of the lens repeatedly with the cleaner for approximately 30 seconds to ensure maximum cleaning efficacy. Many clinicians also recommend using nonpreserved contact lens solutions for GPC patients[21, 46, 47, 51] because of the link between GPC and other allergies.[9, 47] Changing from chemical disinfection methods to heat or hydrogen peroxide has been suggested.

Cessation of Lens Wear or Replacement

Patients demonstrating stage 3 or 4 GPC are usually symptomatic and report discomfort with lens wear. Their lenses are often so heavily deposited that excessive cleaning and enzyming does not improve the condition of the lenses or the symptoms of the patient. At this point the practitioner may choose to discontinue lens wear, although this is not popular with many patients. Withdrawal of contact lens wear was identified early on as an effective treatment for GPC, because patients with even the most severe cases cease showing symptoms within 5 days to 2 weeks of lens removal.[6, 64] Hyperemia and excess mucus disappear quickly, whereas the giant papillae slowly become less elevated over several weeks.

Short-term withdrawal of lens wear is a useful management technique that may yield better patient cooperation than long-term discontinuation of wear. Symptomatic patients in stage 3 and 4 GPC may be asked to stop wearing their old deposited lenses for about 1 week while new lenses are ordered. This approach allows the excess ocular mucus and hyperemia to subside, along with most symptoms. Then, when new lenses are dispensed, the patient will be a better judge of increased discomfort or worsening of symptoms.

As an alternative to protracted withdrawal from contact lens wear, many practitioners opt for simply replacing the deposited contact lens with a new lens of the same type. It is well documented that a new, clean lens will improve GPC symptoms,[21, 64] at least for a while, especially if combined with a decreased wearing time. If the patient is currently on an extended wear schedule, a switch to daily wear is beneficial.

Lens Type or Parameter Changes

Traditional Soft Contact Lenses

Clinicians have also reported success with changing the lens design, polymer, or both.[21, 46, 47, 51, 55] Studies indicate that a smaller-diameter lens (13.5 or 13.8 mm) may contact and abrade the upper lid less, thereby reducing the patient's symptoms.[47] The debate over choosing the best soft contact lens polymer type has been more inconclusive.

In two separate clinical studies, Schussel and Farkas[51] and Farkas et al.[21] refit GPC patients with crofilcon A (CSI; Sola/Barnes-Hind Pharmaceuticals, Sunnyvale, Calif.). lenses. They claimed that the smooth, thin edge design of the CSI lens, along with its reported ability to deposit less, yielded amelioration of GPC symptoms and signs. However, other reports indicate that the CSI lens actually deposits more than polymers, which do not contain methyl methacrylate.[39] In addition, the thin, tapered edge of the CSI lens may actually tend to curl up and abrade the upper lid, especially when the lens becomes dry with heavy deposits. Smith[55] reported little success refitting his GPC patients with CSI lenses, preferring instead a tetrafilcon A material. In a study by Molinari,[47] another 20 GPC patients who had been wearing CSI-151 lenses were successfully refit with Hydrocurve (Barnes-Hind Pharmaceuticals) lenses (13.5 diameter).

The conflicting results of these clinical studies probably reflect the difficulty in constructing adequate controls for studies involving GPC patients. The disease is most often asymmetrical, so the patient's other eye cannot usually serve as a reliable control. In addition, simply ceasing lens wear or replacing the lens produces an improvement in symptoms. Therefore, it is difficult to draw clear conclusions about the "best" soft lens type for treating GPC.

Rigid Gas-Permeable Lenses

Clear-cut success can be achieved, however, by switching soft lens patients to RGP lenses. Although GPC does occur in RGP wearers, its incidence is much lower than with soft lenses. Rigid gas-permeable lenses also have the added benefit that they can be polished rather than replaced to remove heavy protein deposits. This may be more cost effective for the patient than frequent replacement of soft lenses. Despite the increased rate of success, the material and design of the RGP lens are still important for GPC patients. An interpalpebral fit, which does not position high under the upper lid, is often successful in reducing the signs and symptoms of GPC.[40] In addition, a recent study by Douglas et al.[17] indicates that GPC patients should be fit with a lower Dk material. They found that lower Dk value RGP lenses were correlated with a decreased incidence of GPC than higher Dk lenses.

Programmed Replacement or Disposable Lenses

A more recent lens treatment for GPC involves frequent replacement with disposable soft contact lenses. Clean lenses are correlated with fewer symptoms, so that daily wear with frequent replacement presents an attractive option for some patients. Lenses can be replaced on a 1-week, 2-week, or 1-month schedule, depending on the severity of the GPC. In general, patients with stage 3 or 4

GPC should begin on a 1-week schedule of daily wear. It may still be necessary to enzymatically clean the lenses midweek, and, of course, the lenses should still be disinfected nightly. When the mucus production and symptoms have begun to decrease, the replacement schedule may be gradually extended to 2 weeks and then to 1 month. Patients should still be warned, however, that if the symptoms of GPC start to increase, they should return to the clinic immediately. At this time the practitioner may want to drop the replacement schedule to 1 week until the symptoms and signs of GPC disappear.

This approach to managing GPC has been quite successful, although it tends to be more expensive for the patient. In a retrospective study comparing disposable contact lens wearers to controls wearing traditional soft lenses, Marshall et al.[42] found a lower incidence of GPC in the disposable lens wearers. This occurred despite the fact that many of the disposable lens wearers were on a frequent replacement schedule because of past episodes of GPC. In a separate study, Hamburg et al.[27] found that GPC patients wearing disposable lenses demonstrated significant subjective and objective improvements and that none became intolerant to the lenses on a 1- to 2-week schedule.

Pharmaceutical Agents

Mast Cell Stabilizers

One of the most widely used pharmaceutical treatments for GPC is cromolyn sodium or disodium cromoglycate, which is commercially available in a 4% ophthalmic solution (Opticrom). Opticrom is approved by the Food and Drug Administration (FDA) for treatment of GPC, as well as vernal keratitis, conjunctivitis, keratoconjunctivitis, and allergic keratoconjunctivitis. Cromolyn sodium acts to stabilize the mast cell membrane, thereby preventing degranulation and inhibiting the release of vasoactive and chemical mediators (see Fig 11–2). Stabilization of the membrane probably occurs by preventing an allergically induced influx of calcium ions[59] and by inhibiting intracellular cyclic adenosine monophosphate phosphodiesterase.[39]

Despite the extensive usage of cromolyn sodium, researchers have not overwhelmingly documented its effectiveness in treating GPC. Donshik et al.,[16] in a study evaluating several treatments for GPC, found a trend toward improvement but no significant difference between GPC patients medicated with 2% cromolyn and a group managed with contact lens parameter changes. Meisler et al.[43] reported that the symptoms and signs of five GPC patients wearing ocular prostheses or soft contact lenses improved greatly with the application of 2% or 4% cromolyn. Allansmith[2] recommends using ophthalmic cromolyn to treat early GPC, with the understanding that severe GPC cannot be treated with cromolyn.

In any case, cromolyn sodium is extensively used to treat GPC, often in conjunction with other methods.[2, 17, 21] In milder cases of GPC (stage 1 or 2), Opticrom drops can be instilled four times daily while lens wear is decreased to 8 or 10 hours. This allows lens wear during the working day, which accommodates the needs of most patients. It is preferable to instill the drops when lenses are removed, because in the United States, the FDA has not approved Opticrom usage with soft lenses. This prohibition is largely because of the presence of the preservative benzalkonium chloride (BAK), which is known to bind with soft lens polymers.[14] However, a recent Japanese study[31] found no binding of BAK in 56 soft lenses exposed to a commercial disodium cromoglycate solution four times daily.

Cromolyn management of patients with stage 3 or 4 GPC depends largely on the symptoms and mucous discharge exhibited by the patient. If the patient's symptoms are such that he or she is uncomfortable wearing even new soft lenses, a short-term withdrawal of lens wear is advisable. During this time, which usually encompasses about 1 week, Opticrom drops can be instilled up to six times daily. Symptoms and mucous discharge will usually decrease greatly, and new disposable or traditional soft lenses can be dispensed to the patient. The patient may then be started on a wearing schedule of 6 to 8 hours/day, instilling Opticrom four times daily. After a 2-week period, if no exacerbation of symptoms or signs are noted, the wearing schedule can be increased to 8 to 10 hours, with the drop instillation remaining at four times daily. (This schedule will require that the drops be instilled more frequently when the lenses are removed.) In 3 to 4 weeks, if the patient still shows improvement, the wearing time may be increased to 12 to 14 hours, with drop instillation decreased to two times daily. The patient may continue using Opticrom two times/day indefinitely to help prevent a recurrence of GPC.

Clinically, cromolyn sodium is effective in reducing the hyperemia and edema of the upper tarsal plate, but it seems to have little immediate effect in diminishing the diameter of the papillae. However, as noted previously, many of the acute symptoms of GPC, such as itching, discomfort, and mucus discharge, are more closely related to upper lid edema and hyperemia than to actual papillary diameter. It is also important for the clinician to realize that cromolyn sodium may require 1 or 2 days to begin to take effect. Application of Opticrom will stabilize the intact mast cells, but it will not affect the vasoactive and chemical mediators released by mast cells that have already degranulated. Therefore, it may be a few days before the effect of cromolyn treatment is felt by the patient. Cromolyn sodium is actually a preventive treatment, stabilizing the mast cell in advance of the stimulus for degranulation.[7]

Anti-inflammatory Agents

Another pharmaceutical approach to treating GPC involves the use of corticosteroidal and nonsteroidal anti-inflammatory drugs. These drugs are designed to decrease the inflammatory response once it has occurred rather than to prevent it. Corticosteroids suppress the formation of both prostaglandins and leukotrienes (see Fig 11–2),[53] as well as decrease the inflammatory response by other means. These drugs effectively improve the symptoms and signs of GPC, but it is difficult to justify their use with a contact lens–related disease such as GPC because of the numerous undesirable side effects. Also, GPC patients will improve if they simply stop wearing their lenses. Therefore, treatment with currently available corticosteroids is not recommended.[2] However, a newly developed corticosteroidal "soft drug" may show promise for GPC treatment in the future. Loteprednol etabonate, an analog of prednisolone, is rapidly transformed to an inactive metabolite in the anterior chamber, so that it apparently does not cause an increase in intraocular pressure. In a GPC study involving 37 patients, loteprednol etabonate significantly reduced the primary ocular signs of GPC when compared with a placebo.[37]

A nonsteroidal anti-inflammatory drug, suprofen, has also been used in the treatment of GPC. Nonsteroidal anti-inflammatory drugs inhibit prostaglandin synthesis (see Fig 11–2), and suprofen was effective as a topical ophthalmic drop in reducing papillary size and mucous discharge.[64] However, 48% of the patients tested reported ocular side effects, such as burning or stinging. Therefore, topical suprofen drops may not be a practical treatment for GPC in the formulation used.

Vitamin A Drops

Another treatment that has been proposed for GPC involves the use of vitamin A drops (Vit-A-Drops). Although the mechanism of action is unknown, Molinari and Rengstorff[48] found that Vit-A-Drops instilled four times daily caused a resolution of GPC signs and symptoms in one patient. Five weeks after running out of drops, the same patient developed the disease again. The authors concluded that Vit-A-Drops effectively treated GPC, perhaps by improving the quality of the tear film.

TREATMENT SUMMARY AND RECOMMENDATIONS

The previous discussions outline the confusing array of treatment possibilities for GPC patients. To simplify management techniques, I have prepared Table 11–2 for easy reference. Although Table 11–2 does not include all possible treatments for GPC, it does reflect the successful management techniques used in our clinic and by many practitioners.

Patients with stage 1 GPC have no clinical signs and are therefore difficult to identify. As Table 11–2 indicates, if diagnosed, these patients are often adequately managed by increasing the frequency of enzyme cleaning and changing to unpreserved solutions or hydrogen peroxide disinfection. Stage 2 GPC is slightly more severe and may, in addition, require replacement of the patient's lens or perhaps a change to a different-diameter soft lens. Opticrom may also be instilled two to four times daily when the contact lenses are removed.

Stage 3 and 4 GPC are managed similarly. As Table 11–2 suggests, it may be helpful to switch these patients to disposables or RGP lenses, although a smaller-diameter soft lens may be appropriate for stage 3. If the patient is extremely uncomfortable because of itching and mucus, a temporary withdrawal of lens wear may help the inflammation subside before new lenses are worn. As previously mentioned, the patient can be advised to wear glasses for approximately 1 week while the lenses are ordered (even if the lenses are in stock). During this time, Opticrom drops should be instilled four to six times daily. When the new lenses are dispensed, it is probably a good idea to keep the wearing time at about 6 to 8 hours during the first 2 weeks. The wearing time can gradually be increased as the patient's progress is monitored.

TABLE 11–2.

Summary of Recommended Treatments for Giant Papillary Conjunctivitis*

Stage of GPC	Frequent Enzyming	Temporary Withdrawal of Lens Wear	Replacement of Original Lens	Smaller-Diameter Soft Lens	Disposables	RGP	Opticrom
1	+	–	–	–	–	–	(+ or –)
2	+	–	(+ or –)	(+ or –)	–	–	+
3	+	(+ or –)	–	(+ or	+ or	+)	+
4	+	+	–	–	(+ or	+)	+

*GPC = giant papillary conjunctivitis; RGP = rigid gas-permeable.

Table 11–2 does not, however, directly deal with the problem of recurrent GPC episodes. It is significant that many patients seen with relatively mild GPC (stage 1 or 2) have had the disease in the past. They tend to come in more quickly the second or third time around when they first begin to notice increased itching or mucous discharge. If the patient has had several recurrences, it is probably wise to switch to RGP or disposable lenses, even if the present episode is fairly mild.

It is also important to monitor for GPC carefully after the first episode. Because the disease frequently recurs, regular checkups, at least every 6 months, will help to catch problems early. At these follow-ups, lid signs, as well as the deposits on the contact lenses, should be monitored. If the patient is not already wearing disposable or RGP lenses, lenses should be replaced frequently at the first sign of deposit buildup. In addition, it may be wise for the recurrent patient to continue using Opticrom drops twice daily indefinitely. This is especially important during allergy season when the incidence of GPC is known to increase.[9]

Probably the most important management technique for GPC, as with many other diseases, is patient education. Patients need to understand the natural course of the disease, so that they will return quickly at the first sign of increased mucus in the morning, itching, or lens displacement under the upper lid. The patient can be treated more easily at these early stages and tends to blame the physician less for not producing a "cure."

REFERENCES

1. Abelson MB, Baird RS, Allansmith MR: Tear: Histamine levels in vernal conjunctivitis and other ocular inflammations, *Ophthalmology (Rochester)* 1980; 87:812–814.
2. Allansmith MR: Pathology and treatment of giant papillary conjunctivitis, The U.S. perspective. *Clin Ther* 1987; 9:443–450.
3. Allansmith MR, Baird RS, Greiner JV: Vernal conjunctivitis and contact lens–associated giant papillary conjunctivitis compared and contrasted. *Am J Ophthalmol* 1979; 87:544–555.
4. Allansmith MR, Greiner JV, Baird RS: Number of inflammatory cells in the normal conjunctiva. *Am J Ophthalmol* 1978; 86:250.
5. Allansmith MR, Korb DR, Greiner JV: Giant papillary conjunctivitis induced by hard or soft contact lens wear: Quantitative histology. *Trans Am Acad Ophthalmol Otolaryngol* 1978; 85:766.
6. Allansmith MR, Korb DR, Greiner JV, et al: Giant papillary conjunctivitis in contact lens wearers. *Am J Ophthalmol* 1977; 83:697–708.
7. Allansmith MR, Ross RN: Ocular allergy and mast cell stabilizers. *Surv Ophthalmol* 1986; 30:229–244.
8. Barishak Y, Aavaro A, Samra Z, et al: An immunological study of papillary conjunctivitis due to contact lenses. *Curr Eye Res* 1984; 3:1161–1168.
9. Begley CB, Riggle A, Tuel JA: Association of giant papillary conjunctivitis with seasonal allergies. *Optom Vis Sci* 1990; 67:192–195.
10. Benvenuto PB: Giant papillary conjunctivitis with resultant keratitis. *South J Optom* 1979; 8:43–44.
11. Buckley RJ: Pathology and treatment of giant papillary conjunctivitis: II. The British perspective. *Clin Ther* 1987; 9:451–457.
12. Butrus SI, Laby DM, Zacharia JS, et al: Tryptase in tears: A marker for mast cell activation in giant papillary conjunctivitis (GPC). *Inv Ophthalmol Vis Sci* 1991; 32(4):740.
13. Carlson AN, Wilhelmus KA: Giant papillary conjunctivitis associated with cyanoacrylate glue. *Am J Ophthalmol* 1987; 104:437–438.
14. Chapman JM, Cheeks L, Green K: Interactions of benzalkonium chloride with soft and hard contact lenses. *Arch Ophthalmol* 1990; 108:244–246.
15. Donshik PC, Ballow M: Tear immunoglobulins in giant papillary conjunctivitis induced by contact lenses. *Am J Ophthalmol* 1983; 96:460–466.
16. Donshik PC, Ballow M, Luistro A, et al: Treatment of contact lens-induced giant papillary conjunctivitis. *CLAO J* 1984; 10:346–350.
17. Douglas JP, Lowder CY, Lazorik R, et al: Giant papillary conjunctivitis associated with rigid gas permeable contact lenses. *CLAO J* 1991; 14:143–147.
18. Dunn JP, Weismann BA, Mondino BJ, et al: Giant papillary conjunctivitis associated with elevated corneal deposits. *Cornea* 1990; 9:357–358.
19. Dvorak HF, Dvorak AA: Cutaneous basophil hypersensitivity, in L. Brent, EJ Holborow (eds): *Progress in Immunology II.* New York, Elsevier North-Holland, 1974, vol 3.
20. Ehlers WH, Fishman JB, Donshik PC, et al: Neutrophil chemotactic factors derived from conjunctival epithelial cells: Preliminary biochemical characterization. *CLAO J* 1991; 17:65–68.
21. Farkas P, Kassalow TW, Farkas B: Clinical management and control of giant papillary conjunctivitis secondary to contact lens wear. *J Am Optom Assoc* 1986; 57:197–200.
22. Fowler SA, Greiner JV, Allansmith MR: Attachment of bacteria to soft contact lenses. *Arch Ophthalmol* 1979; 97:659–660.
23. Fowler SA, Greiner JV, Allansmith MR: Soft contact lenses from patients with giant papillary conjunctivitis. *Am J Ophthalmol* 1979; 88:1056–1061.
24. Fowler SA, Korb DR, Finnemore VM, et al: Surface deposits on worn hard contact lenses. *Arch Ophthalmol* 1984; 102:757–759.
25. Greiner JV, Kenyon KR, Henriquez AS, et al: Mucus secretory vesicles in conjunctival epithelial cells of wearers of contact lenses. *Arch Ophthalmol* 1980; 98:1843–1846.
26. Greiner JV, Peace DG, Baird RS, et al: Effects of eye rubbing on the conjunctiva as a model of ocular inflammation. *Am J Ophthalmol* 1985; 100:45–50.
27. Hamburg TR, O'Brien TP, Kracher GP, et al: Management

of giant papillary conjunctivitis (GPC) using soft contact lenses. *Inv Ophthalmol Vis Sci* 1991; 32(suppl):739.

28. Hann LE, Cornell-Bell AH, Marten-Ellis C, et al: Conjunctival basophil hypersensitivity lesions in guinea pigs, *Inv Ophthalmol Vis Sci* 1986; 27:1255–1259.

29. Haynes JD, Rosenstein RW, Askenase PW: A newly described activity of guinea pig IgG1 antibodies: Transfer of cutaneous basophil reactions. *J Immunol* 1978; 120:886–893.

30. Henriquez AS, Kenyon KR, Allansmith MR: Mast cell ultrastructure. *Arch Ophthalmol* 1981; 99:1266–1272.

31. Iwaske W, Kosaka Y, Mosmoe T, et al: Absorption of topical disodium cromoglycate and its preservatives by soft contact lenses. *CLAO J* 1988; 14:155–158.

32. Kaliner M: Asthma and mast cell activation. *J Allergy Clin Immunol* 1989; 83:510–520.

33. Kennedy JR: A mechanism of corneal abrasion. *Am J Optom* 1970; 47:564–569.

34. Korb DR, Allansmith MR, Greiner JV, et al: Biomicroscopy of papillae associated with hard contact lens wearing. *Ophthalmology* 1981; 88:1132–1136.

35. Korb DR, Greiner JV, Finnemore VM, et al: Treatment of contact lenses with papain. Increase in wearing time of keratoconic patients with papillary conjunctivitis. *Arch Ophthalmol* 1983; 101:48–50.

36. Kowtow M, Holden BA, Grant T: The value of regular replacement of low water content contact lenses for extended wear. *J Am Optom Assoc* 1987; 58:461–464.

37. Laibovitz RA, Ghormley NR, Insler MS: Treatment of giant papillary conjunctivitis with loteprednol etabonate: A novel corticosteroid. *Inv Ophthalmol Vis Sci* 1991; 32(suppl):734.

38. Lavin N, Rachelefsky GC, Kaplan SA: An action of disodium cromolglycate: Inhibition of cyclic 3′,5′-adenosine monophosphate phosphodiesterase. *J Allergy Clin Immunol* 1976; 57:80–88.

39. Levy B: Calcium deposits on glyceryl methyl methacrylate and hydroxyethyl methacrylate contact lenses. *Am J Optom Physiol Opt* 1984; 61:605–607.

40. Mackie IA, Wright P: Giant papillary conjunctivitis (secondary vernal) in association with contact lens wear. *Trans Ophthalmol Soc UK* 98:3-9, 1978.

41. Maggi E, Biswas P, Del Prete G, et al: Accumulation of Th-2-like helper T cells in the conjunctiva of patients with vernal conjunctivitis. *J Immunol* 1991; 146:1169–1174.

42. Marshall EC, Begley CG, Nyugen CHD: Frequency of complications among wearers of disposable and conventional soft contact lenses. *Int Contact Lens Clin* 1992 (in press).

43. Meisler DM, Berzins UJ, Krachmer JH, et al: Cromolyn treatment of giant papillary conjunctivitis. *Arch Ophthalmol* 1982; 100:1608–1610.

44. Meisler DM, Zaret CR, Stock EL: Trantas dots and limbal inflammation associated with soft contact lens wear. *Am J Ophthalmol* 1980; 89:66–69.

45. Modino BJ, Salamon SM, Zaidman GW: Allergic and toxic reactions in soft contact lens wearers. *Surv Ophthalmol* 1982; 26:337–344.

46. Molinari JF: A case report: A procedure for the clinical management of giant papillary conjunctivitis in a patient wearing contact lenses. *Aust J Optom* 1980; 63:288–290.

47. Molinari JF: The clinical management of giant papillary conjunctivitis. *Am J Optom Physiol Opt* 1981; 58:886–890.

48. Molinari JF, Rengstorff R: Management of soft lens–induced GPC with vitamin A aqueous drops. *Contact Lens J* 1988; 16:169–170.

49. Reynolds RMP: Giant papillary conjunctivitis: A mechanical aetiology. *Aust J Optom* 1978; 61:320–323.

50. Robin JB, Regis-Pacheco LF, May WN, et al: Giant papillary conjunctivitis associated with an extruded scleral buckle. *Arch Opthalmol* 1987; 105:619.

51. Schussel AB, Farkas B: Giant papillary conjunctivitis. *Rev Optom* 1983; 81:2.

52. Seldin DC, Austen KF: Mast cell subclasses and growth dependence, in Schrader JW (ed): *Lymphokines: A Forum for Immunoregulatory Cell Products.* New York, Academic Press, 1988, vol 15.

53. Sell S: *Immunology, Immunopathology, and Immunity,* ed 4. New York, Elsevier North-Holland, 1987, p 478.

54. Sheldon L, Biedner B, Geltman C, et al: Giant papillary conjunctivitis and ptosis in a contact lens wearer. *J Pediatr Ophthalmol Strabismus* 1979; 16:136–137.

55. Smith RN: Managing GPC with tetrafilicon, A: A retrospective study of 122 patients. *Contact Lens Spectrum* 1988; 5:57–59.

56. Smolin G, O'Connor RG: *Ocular Immunology,* ed 2. Boston, Little, Brown & Co, 1986.

57. Soni PS, Hathcoat G.: Complications reported with hydrogel extended wear contact lenses. *Am J Optom Physiol Opt* 1988; 65:545–551.

58. Soter NA: Experimental studies of the mast cell in the inflammatory response in human skin, in Suran A, Gery I, Nussenblatt RB (eds): *Immunology of the Eye. Workshop III.* 1980. Information Retrieval, Washington DC.

59. Spataro AC, Bosmann HB: Mechanism of action of DSC: Mast cell calcium ion influx after a histamine-releasing stimulus. *Biochem Pharmacol* 1976; 25:505–510.

60. Spring TF: Reaction to hydrophilic lenses. *Med J Aust* 1974; 1:499–500.

61. Srinivasan BK, Jakobiec FA, Iwamato T, et al: Giant papillary conjunctivitis with ocular prostheses. *Arch Ophthalmol* 1979; 97:892–895.

62. Sugar A, Meyer RF: Giant papillary conjunctivitis after keratoplasty. *Am J Ophthalmol* 1981; 91:239–242.

63. Wille H, Molgaard I: Giant papillary conjunctivitis in connection with corneoscleral supramid (nylon) suture knots. *Acta Ophthalmol (Copenh)* 1984; 62:75–83.

64. Wood TS, Stewart RH, Bowman RW, et al: Suprofen treatment of contact lens–associated giant papillary conjunctivitis. *Ophthalmology* 1988; 95:822–826.

PART V

Infection

Corneal Infection Secondary to Contact Lens Wear

Barry A. Weissman, O.D., Ph.D.

Bartly J. Mondino, M.D.

Contact lens wear is associated with a great variety of potential physiological complications, although the number of patients suffering severe compromise of the ocular tissues is quite small. These complications include changes in the lids such as giant papillary conjunctivitis, changes in the bulbar conjunctiva such as hyperemia (from solution sensitivity for example), and corneal changes.

The surface of the cornea, its epithelial layer, is most affected by the presence of a contact lens, probably because of its proximity. Minor epithelial erosions, called *superficial punctate staining* (SPS), are commonly seen (Figs 12–1 and 12–2) and may be related to drying, allergic and toxic effects of solutions, mechanical problems with a lens surface or edge, or a host of other potential insults.

A contact lens forms a potential barrier to oxygen supply. Acute hypoxia induces metabolic changes in the epithelium, resulting in decreased glycogen stores, sensitivity, and adhesion. Epithelial edema may be seen as microcysts, microcystic edema, circular corneal clouding, and edematous corneal formations. Hypoxia may also be associated with vascularization of the cornea, stromal swelling, and changes in endothelial morphology.

The most severe complication of contact lens wear, however, is direct microbial infection. It is probably the least well understood but fortunately one of the less commonly encountered complications of contact lens wear.

DEFINITION

Claes Dohlman,[21] in his Friedenwald lecture, defined a corneal ulceration as an "epithelial defect which has become complicated by the disappearance of some underlying stromal substance, usually following infection, chemical burns, trauma or desiccation." Corneal ulceration is a nonspecific diagnosis; it implies *excavation of the corneal tissues* and an associated *inflammatory response* (keratitis) but does not provide information as to etiology. Corneal ulceration may be caused by sterile (i.e., Mooren's ulcer) or infectious (bacterial, viral, fungal, or protozoan) etiologies. Common corneal ulcers include those initiated by trauma or *herpes* and those secondary to staphylococcal blepharitis, whereas direct bacterial or fungal invasion of the intact cornea is relatively rare in healthy individuals.

Keratitis is inflammation of the cornea. Here too the etiology may be infectious or noninfectious. Noninfectious causes of keratitis include tear film abnormalities, exposure, immunological reactions (perhaps to topical or systemic medications or solutions), denervation, dystrophies, and photic, mechanical, and chemical injuries. Clinical signs of keratitis include corneal edema and infiltrates. Corneal infiltrates are transient, discrete collections of whitish material observed in the normally transparent corneal tissues (Table 12–1); these are usually presumed to be leukocytes that have migrated into the cornea from the

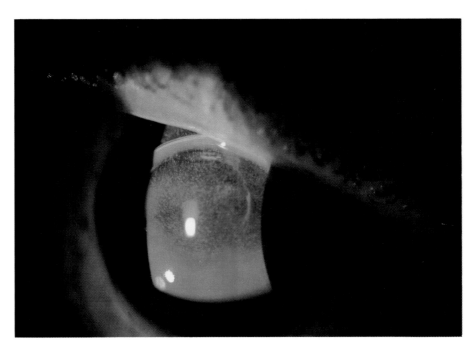

FIG 12–1.
Severe superficial punctate staining (SPS) in an aphakic patient with diabetes, demonstrating increased epithelial fragility. A rigid gas-permeable contact lens has been worn on a daily wear basis for several years, the patient is asymptomatic, and this staining problem is chronic and not responsive to any treatment.

limbal vasculature or through the tears in response to a chemotactic factor released from damaged local tissues. The inflammatory cells include polymorphonuclear leukocytes (PMNs), macrophages, and lymphocytes. These changes are usually seen just underneath the epithelium (Figs 12–3 and 12–4). Occasionally an infectious agent itself forms all or part of the infiltrate, as in fungal infection. Conjunctival edema and injection often accompany severe keratitis, as does an anterior chamber reaction seen as flare and cells in the aqueous humor. Hypopyon may be associated with severe inflammation of the anterior seg-

ment. Subjective symptoms include pain, photophobia, and decreased vision because of involvement of the corneal visual axis and cells in the aqueous humor. Patients with mild keratitis, however, may have minimal subjective symptoms. Neovascularization, scarring, and corneal thinning may result after episodes of acute or chronic keratitis.

Stein et al.[91] provide additional clinical help distinguishing between sterile infiltrates and corneal infection associated with contact lens wear. This group studied 50 patients with corneal infiltrates associated with contact lens wear to determine which clinical signs and symptoms are

FIG 12–2.
Slight SPS under a hydrogel contact lens in a patient with chronic mild dry eye; presumably this is associated with dehydration through the lens.

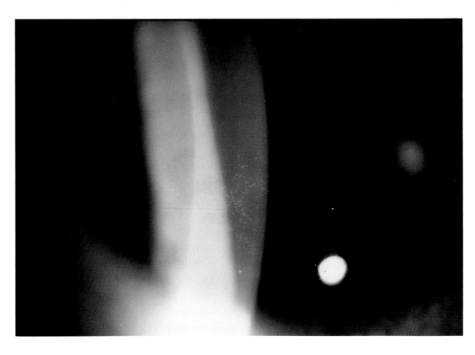

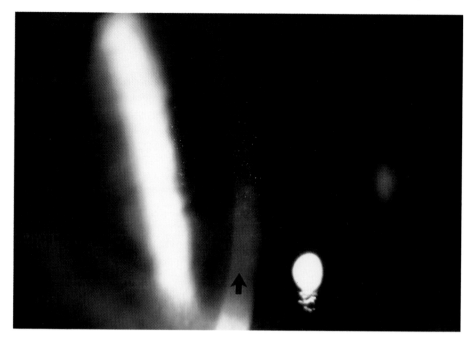

FIG 12–3.
Multiple subepithelial infiltrates *(arrow)* seen in the inferior cornea of an asymptomatic myopic patient wearing hydrogel extended wear lenses (2-week wear with chemical cleaning and disinfection). These lesions do not stain. Extended wear was discontinued.

important in predicting the results of microbial culture. In the presence of *corneal infiltrates* after *contact lens wear*, positive cultures were statistically associated with *increased pain, discharge, epithelial staining,* and *anterior chamber reactions*. Lesions that did not yield positive cultures were usually smaller, multiple, and without substantial pain, epithelial stain, or anterior chamber reaction. It is important to note, however, that clinicians diagnose microbial keratitis based on appearance. Large studies of corneal infection always include substantial numbers of patients who clinically appear to have microbial keratitis and

respond to treatment but also have negative cultures for any of a number of reasons, including previous antibiotic therapy and sampling error (see later discussion). Considering the risk and benefit of treating a sterile infiltrate vs. not treating an infectious keratitis, it is probably better to overrefer rather than underrefer and overtreat rather than undertreat.

Some have suggested as a diagnostic feature that small and peripheral corneal "ulcers" tend to be "sterile" (catarrhal ulcers, which are usually a relatively benign and self-limited entity commonly associated with *Staphylococ-*

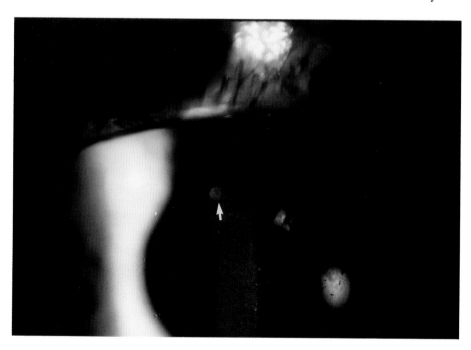

FIG 12–4.
Single infiltrate *(arrow)* seen in the cornea of a patient who wore daily wear hydrogel lenses and developed giant papillary conjunctivitis. This lesion did not stain.

TABLE 12–1.

Common Etiologies of Corneal Infiltrates

Infection
  Herpes
  Chlamydia
  Adenovirus
  Bacterial, fungal, and protozoan corneal infection or ulcer*
Hypersensitivity
  Solution sensitivity (e.g., thimerosal)
  Acute red eye syndrome (contact lens overwear?)
Mixed
  Staphylococcus aureus marginal infiltrate

*Topics of this chapter.

cus aureus lid infections), whereas large and central ulcers should be considered infectious. On the contrary, with contact lens wear, we believe that it is important to emphasize that size and location are not major distinguishing features. All infections may begin as small infiltrates or epithelial defects.[46] Mondino et al.[65] found that only 23 of 40 clinically diagnosed corneal infections associated with contact lens wear were central ulcers, and the remainder were peripheral.

HISTORICAL PERSPECTIVES

Contact lens–associated corneal infection was a relatively rare event until the introduction of extended wear. Only 14 cases of "lost" or "blinded" eyes could be documented in 1966 from almost 50,000 polymethylmethacrylate (PMMA) contact lens–wearing patients seen by a large group of ophthalmologists during a single year.[20] Eight of these patients had clear defects in their lens care by history. Several case reports in the late 1970s suggested there might be more infections with the use of hydrogel contact lenses,[33, 55] but Ruben[80] concluded (from his experience at Moorfield's Eye Hospital in England) that, although the rate of infection with hydrogels might be somewhat greater than that found with PMMA lenses, the overall incidence was low when hygiene and lens care were good.

Wilson et al.[102] then documented eight corneal ulcers in seven patients using hydrogel contact lenses with home-made saline solution for a care solution. This group identified the same bacterial serotypes of *Pseudomonas* in the corneal ulcers as in the contact lens care systems used by four of seven patients. It is important to note that all of these patients used homemade saline inappropriately as a wetting agent, eye drop, or bath after thermal disinfection of their contact lenses. Nontheless, in this important study, Wilson et al.[102] clearly linked microbial contamination of care solutions with microbial infection of the cornea.

Cooper and Constable[19] also reported eight cases of infective keratitis in wearers of soft contact lenses. One was wearing a lens continually for therapeutic reasons, and three were using their lenses daily or intermittently, but four of these patients appeared to have no predisposing factors except that they were using their lenses for "continuous" or "extended" wear. Cooper and Constable's[19] report thus introduced the modern concerns regarding infection in extended contact lens wear.

RISK FACTORS

In general, the process of infection is believed to depend on the mechanical and humoral or cellular defense mechanisms of the host, on the one hand, and the inoculum size, pathogenicity, and virulence of the microorganisms, on the other.

To defend the globe, the blinking action of the lid and flow of tears over the anterior segment of the eye mechanically remove microorganisms. Tears contain several antibacterial substances such as lysozyme, lactoferrin, and mucus that may envelope microorganisms. Tears also contain immunoglobulins, especially secretory IgA, which can trap and coat microorganisms, suppress adhesion, and, after binding to the surface antigen of the microorganism, result in lysis and enhanced phagocytosis through compliment activation. The epithelium itself poses a formidable mechanical barrier to most microbes[47]; only *Corynebacterium diphtheriae*, *Neisseria gonorrhoeae*, and *Haemophilus aegyptius* (Koch-Weeks bacillus) are able to invade the intact corneal epithelium.

In any infection, specific risk factors are believed to encourage the disease process. Several specific concerns have been raised with regard to contact lens wear, discussion of which follows.

Extended Wear Lenses

The definition of the term extended wear derives from the concept that contact lens wear can be extended through one or multiple sleep cycles before cleaning (and "disinfection"); this concept should be distinguished from "continuous" wear, which means that the lens is never removed for routine cleaning.

Patients as opposed to clinicians probably began the extension of contact lens wear. Anecdotal reports of the rare patient napping or sleeping with PMMA contact lenses still on the eye, perhaps parked on the sclera, were common 30 years ago. Soon after hydrogel contact lenses were introduced for the correction of refractive error, ophthalmologists were using these devices as bandage lenses to treat diseases of the anterior segment, and the lenses were often worn continuously.[9] Complications were common but disasters were few. Dohlman et al.[22] found that 11 of 278 patients so treated developed corneal infiltrates, 4 of which were definite infections that resulted in permanent damage to the eyes. These authors nonetheless concluded that the advantages of using therapeutic soft lenses on a continuous basis far outweighed their risks.

The Permalens (perfilcon A) was developed about 1970 by deCarle in England. This lens appears to be the first produced solely for extended wear and was originally fitted very small in diameter and steep in relation to the corneal curvature. The Food and Drug Administration (FDA) approved two contact lenses for aphakic extended wear use in this country in June 1979: Permalens (Cooper-Vision, San Jose, Calif.) and Hydrocurve (Barnes-Hind Pharmaceuticals, Sunnyvale, Calif.). Other materials and designs, for both aphakic and phakic (original FDA approval in January 1981) patients, followed over the next several years.[38]

Early clinical reports of the American experience suggested that this form of contact lens wear was a total success[10, 88, 89]; complications appeared, but rates were similar to those encountered with daily wear lenses, and benefits in patient satisfaction, both with myopes and aphakes, were substantial.[38]

In England, Hirji and Larke[40, 56] performed a clinical trial and also found that continual wearing of a soft contact lens (Sauflon 85) for 20 weeks was innocuous for 20 subjects. Although they monitored several corneal functions, they found only a decrease in corneal sensitivity and an increase in lens deposits; no significant corneal swelling or other complications were noted.

Yet trouble was brewing for extended wear lenses; Cooper and Constable's[19] report from Perth, Australia, was perhaps the first indication that something might be amiss. Zantos and Holden,[103] also in Australia, reported on a study of 35 patients who wore a variety of contact lenses on a continuous wear basis for up to 2 years. Multiple physiological complications were observed in this study, including corneal edema, neovascularization, microcysts, acute red eye syndrome (12/35), and infection. Three patients had small marginal ulcers, and one developed multiple small central epithelial lesions, which later coalesced into a large central ulcer. Every patient attempting continuous wear experienced some difficulty resulting in an interruption of lens wear.

Another report detailed the disasterous experience (multiple episodes of severe keratitis) of patients in both West Germany and Japan fitted with early silicone elastomer lenses for extended wear.[79]

As extended wear proliferated through North America in the early 1980s, the original glowing reports faded, and the reality predicted by the observations of Cooper and Constable[19] and Zantos and Holden[103] became clear. Several reports in the early 1980s gave strong evidence that extended wear was associated with a higher rate of corneal infection in both aphakic and phakic patients.[1, 30, 39, 81, 97]

For example, Mondino et al.[65] studied 40 patients with corneal infection associated with contact lens wear over 21 months. Eleven of these patients wore lenses intended for daily wear, and all were found to be noncompliant with good contact lens care, including eight reporting occasionally sleeping with their lenses in place. Twenty-nine patients used extended wear hydrogels (wearing their lenses from 3 days to 30 months), and 12 were believed to be compliant with the then-current lens care guidelines. Of the noncompliant 17, the most common problem was microbial contamination of their care systems. This study highlights the conclusion that must be reached from the literature just reviewed: Risk factors for corneal infection during contact lens wear include (1) sleeping with contact lenses on the eyes and (2) noncompliance with contact lens care and hygiene.

Because about 10% of the total population of the United States and a substantial number of Europeans and Asians wear contact lenses, often for extended wear, it is not surprising that many now believe contact lens–related microbial keratitis has the potential of becoming an important public health problem. About 30% of all corneal ulcers recently treated at three centers were found to be related to contact lens wear: 196 of 658 between October 1982 and June 1986 at the Bascon-Palmer Eye Institute (Florida)[54]; 60 of 191 between July 1983 and December 1984 at the Wills Eye Hospital (Pennsylvania)[24]; and 136 of 397 between June 1982 and December 1985 at the Massachusetts Eye and Ear Infirmary.[83] Extended wear of hydrogel contact lenses was associated with the majority of these infections at all centers.

These concerns led the Contact Lens Institute (CLI), an organization of the senior administrators of the major contact lens manufacturers in the United States, to sponsor a major epidemiological study of corneal infection and contact lens wear. This study confirmed that extended wear of hydrogel contact lenses significantly increases the risk of corneal infection[82] and will be discussed further later on.

Oxygen

Polse and Mandell[77] proposed that there was a "critical oxygen tension" (COT) for the anterior corneal surface, below which corneal metabolism would be compromised. By use of a goggle through which they passed gases of specified oxygen concentrations and observation of subsequent corneal swelling, they suggested that the COT was 11 to

19 mm Hg. Normal oxygen tension is found by multiplying the percentage of oxygen in the air (21%) by the barometric pressure (760 mm Hg at sea level) and is therefore about 155 mm Hg, so Polse and Mandell's[77] COT represents about 2% of the oxygen tension at sea level. Later human goggle studies, with better controls and additional subjects, increased the COT to 40 to 70 mm Hg (5%–10% oxygen).[43, 60] Others have looked at alternative corneal functions to define the COT. Millodot and O'Leary[62] found that there was a depression in human corneal sensitivity if the anterior oxygen tension was less than 60 mm Hg. In rabbits, Uniacke et al.[94] found epithelial glycogen was mobilized when the anterior oxygen tension was less than 40 mm Hg, Hamano et al.[37] found an increase in the production of lactate and a decrease in epithelial mitosis if the oxygen tension was less than 100 mm Hg, and Masters[61] found changes in the epithelial mitochondria redox state at less than 75 mm Hg.

Holden and Mertz[42] used contact lenses of known oxygen transmissibilities (Dk/L) to determine the "critical Dk/L" and found they could preclude human corneal swelling by using lenses with Dk/L values of 24×10^{-11} (cm $\times$ mL O_2)/(sec $\times$ mL $\times$ mm Hg) under daily wear conditions and 87×10^{-11} (cm $\times$ mL O_2)/(sec $\times$ mL $\times$ mm Hg) for extended wear conditions; presumably both of these situations allow for an oxygen tension under the lenses of 40 to 70 mm Hg or more. The concept of the COT level for the cornea is described in more detail in Chapter 1.

It is attractive to suggest that hypoxia at the corneal surface results in compromise of the epithelium, which then secondarily becomes less able to resist microbial infection. Although hypoxia causes all sorts of metabolic problems for the cornea resulting in multiple changes in the epithelium, stroma, and endothelium,[44] the link between these problems and infection per se has yet to be firmly established.[96] It is also clear, however, that all extended wear of contact lenses, from a wear schedule of 28 nights to only 4 nights in a row, cause ocular complications; no severe infections were encountered in one study, but epithelial microcysts, red eye syndrome, superficial punctate keratitis (SPK), and other changes occurred at similar rates across several wearing schedules.[51]

Compliance

Another risk factor that has been identified is that of noncompliance with contact lens care techniques.

Mondino et al.[65] provide a definition of compliance with regard to contact lens wear. A compliant patient (1) washes his or her hands before any contact lens manipulations, (2) appropriately uses an FDA-approved contact lens care system in a manner in agreement with both the manufacturer's published guidelines and good hygiene, (3) adheres to recommended contact lens–wearing schedule for either daily or extended wear, and (4) is found to have no microbial contamination of his or her contact lens solutions and cases.

Wilson et al.[102] established the link between poor contact lens care and hygiene and corneal infection by demonstrating the same serotype of *Pseudomonas* in corneal ulcers and the contact lens care systems of their patients. Others have since verified these results.[24, 65]

Both Collins and Carney[18] and Chun and Weissman[14] studied compliance in contact lens wear. They found that 40% to 70% of normal patients were noncompliant by history. This is quite a worrisome figure.

Several authors have also studied microbial contamination of contact lens solutions and cases. Pitts and Krachmer[75] cultured the contact lens cases and conjunctiva of 29 patients and found that 10 (34%) had contaminated cases despite use of heat disinfection. Donzis et al.[26] cultured all elements of the contact lens care systems of 100 asymptomatic contact lens users, including 38 rigid lens users and 62 hydrogel users (50 for daily wear and 12 for extended wear). More than 50% of these patients had microbial contamination in some element of their care system, and microbes found by culture included potential pathogens such as *Pseudomonas, Staphylococcus, Serratia, Bacillus,* and *Acanthamoeba.*

Campbell and Caroline[12] believe that even patients who use care regimens compliantly may not be able to eliminate microbes from their care systems. They suggest that care systems that are effective in the laboratory may become ineffective in the home environment because the bacteria encountered are more resistant through the development of bacterial biofilm. Thirty-nine of 45 patients studied used their disinfection techniques correctly, but 29% of the patients using heat disinfection, 50% of those using peroxide disinfection, and 75% of those using chemical disinfection were found to have bacteria culturable from their contact lens cases.

It is clear from a large collection of research that microbes can adhere to contact lens surfaces, most likely by formation of biofilms, and this raises the issue of the lens acting as a vector, transferring pathogenic agents from the contaminated case or solutions directly to the ocular surface. Because *Pseudomonas* appears to be responsible for one half to two thirds of culture-positive corneal infections in contact lens wearers,[23, 54, 65] several subtypes of this particular microorganism have been studied as to their ability to attach to corneas, as well as new and worn, rigid and hydrogel, high and low water content, ionic and nonionic contact lenses. The exact role of bacterial adherence in the pathogenesis of corneal infection, however, has yet to be clearly described. Baum and Panjwani[5] recently reviewed this topic.

Despite frequent noncompliance across all forms of contact lens wear, suggested by history and documented by contamination of care systems, however, the incidence figures suggest that infection is rare, at least until lenses are used for extended wear.

Diabetes

Diabetes has been suggested as a risk factor for corneal infection, specifically when contact lenses are used for extended wear. Eichenbaum et al.[30] studied 235 aphakic patients and were the first to suggest that diabetics using contact lenses for extended wear were at specific risk. One hundred patients wore hydrogel contact lenses for extended wear, and all three patients who were diabetic developed infections. A fourth patient, who concomitantly had cancer of the colon, also developed a corneal infection. None of 135 patients wearing spectacles, including 8 diabetics, developed corneal infections.

It is known that diabetic patients have metabolic abnormalities that place them at greater systemic risk for microbial infections. Millodot and O'Leary[63] also determined that both contact lens wear and diabetes (see Fig 12–1) increase the fragility of the corneal epithelial layer.

Epithelial Trauma

It is very likely that epithelial trauma that occurs during contact lens wear plays a role in subsequent infection. As noted earlier, the intact corneal epithelium is known to present a substantial barrier to infection. Experimentally, bacterial inoculation of a linear abrasion is effective in producing a corneal ulcer.[78, 93] Stern et al.[92] clearly showed that *Pseudomonas* tends to adhere to injured or exposed basal epithelial cells rather than to an intact epithelial surface or even exposed corneal stroma. And even without direct mechanical abrasion, an electron microscopy study of primate corneal epithelia after use of excessively thick hydrogels for daily or extended wear showed epithelial thinning (loss of superficial cells and flattening of the remaining ones), edema, and degenerative cytoplasmic changes.[8]

Adams et al.[1] found that five of six patients with corneal infections associated with extended wear of hydrogel lenses reported recent manipulations of their lenses, and they speculated that this may have resulted in epithelial defects that predisposed these patients to the infectious process. Mondino et al.,[65] however, could not support this particular contention in their series.

There is no doubt that minor epithelial erosion is a common occurrence in any contact lens practice (see Fig 12–2). What is not clear, however, is why such lesions appear to be clinically relatively innocuous when the lenses are used on a daily wear basis and whether the role of such lesions changes during extended wear.

Corticosteroid Use

Topical corticosteroids are generally recognized as a predisposing factor for corneal microbial infection.[49] These pharmaceuticals suppress immunological defense mechanisms and inflammatory reactions and by doing so may mask the severity of an infection.

Chalupa et al.[13] found that early inappropriate corticosteroid therapy was implicated as a major factor contributing to the severity of corneal infection after contact lens wear in their series.

Therapeutic Contact Lenses

The literature is consistent in reporting the clinical impression that the therapeutic use of hydrogel lenses as bandages presents an increased risk for infection. Diseases often managed with hydrogel bandage lenses include symptomatic relief of filamentary keratitis or bullous keratopathy, persistent nonhealing epithelial defects, the covering of exposed sutures (e.g., after keratoplasty), neurotrophic or exposure keratitis, keratitis sicca, and ocular pemphigoid; all of these situations involve disruption of the epithelial surface barrier. Many of these patients are elderly, some have diabetes, and frequently they may be using topical corticosteroids. This combination of known risk factors places these patients at particular risk, and it is not surprising that infection has been found to be a major concern in this group of patients.[23, 50]

For example, 6 corneal ulcers (both bacterial and fungal by culture) developed in 38 eyes treated with therapeutic hydrogel contact lenses for severe epithelial diseases, including Stevens-Johnson and Sjögren syndromes, ocular pemphigoid, neurotrophic keratis, herpes simplex keratitis, and ocular burns.[11] The authors[11] believe several factors contributed to these infections, including concurrent dry eye, use of antibiotics and corticosteroids, and the contamination of a bottle of sodium chloride drops in one case.

Smoking

A recent CLI study of corneal infection associated with contact lens wear investigated a number of potential risk factors, including age, sex, and race of the contact lens user, the age of the contact lens and type of fit (initial or replacement), length of time since last professional evaluation, and type of clinician seen. The only factor of these that appeared to have some statistical relation to corneal infection was smoking,[82] which was significant statistically for extended wear use of contact lenses and almost significant for daily wear use of lenses as well. The mechanism is unclear in this instance.

Other Risk Factors

Some have suggested additional risk factors, such as travel and warm weather,[13] but these have not been verified.

INCIDENCE

From the introductory discussion of this chapter it is easy to see that the first difficulty in arriving at an incidence is clearly defining the problem we wish to study: corneal ulcers, keratitis, or corneal infection. Clearly we are primarily interested here in understanding the specific issue of corneal microbial infection as described earlier.

Second, it is difficult to determine the frequency of this event because occurrence is relatively rare—so rare that many of the initial studies of extended wear contact lenses (as detailed earlier) did not encounter this complication at all.

One of the first modern reports attempting to give an incidence for corneal infection with extended wear of contact lenses was that of Salz and Schlanger.[81] They followed 100 aphakic eyes (70 patients) using hydrogel lenses for extended wear for 3 months to 7 years, and 5 peripheral or paracentral ulcers occurred. Eichenbaum et al.[30] similarly studied a group of 100 aphakic eyes wearing extended wear hydrogel lenses and found 4 infections in 1 year. Spoor et al.[87] studied 120 aphakic eyes wearing hydrogel lenses for extended wear and reported 4.3% incidence of infection over 3 years. (They also agreed with the earlier conclusion that diabetics were particularly at risk.)

Weissman et al.[95] reviewed the experience with corneal infection associated with contact lens wear at one major university hospital and concluded that the risk of infection was increased six times with extended wear compared with daily wear.

Chalupa et al.[13] presented their 2-year experience caring for a large population (estimated at 35,000–40,000) of contact lens wearers in Gothenburg, Sweden. Their study of 55 corneal infections suggested an incidence rate of about 1 in 15,000 for daily wear and 1 in 3,000 for extended wear of hydrogel lenses. Holden et al.[41] summa-

rized these data and their own: "The best estimate we can make is that in Western Australia in 1977, in Sweden in 1981–82, and in the US currently [1986], about 1 in every 100 patients will have a peripheral corneal erosion (ulcer) that heals without complications and about 1 in 1,000–5,000 will have a serious infection that adversely affects vision."

A large survey of the members of the American Optometric Association's Contact Lens Section, a self-selected body of practitioners with an expressed interest in contact lens care, was undertaken, and the results, from 440 respondees, suggested that corneal infection occurred at a rate of about 0.5% for daily wear and 3% for extended wear over 2-year blocks of time from 1980 to 1985.[98]

MacRae[59] summarized several years (1980–1988) of experience collected from the FDA-controlled studies of new contact lenses. These data involved 22,584 patients; there were 158 serious adverse reactions and 32 "corneal ulcers" reported. From these data MacRae[59] calculated an infection rate of 1 in 2,000 (number of events/patient-years) for daily wear, and 1 in 500 for cosmetic, and 1 in 200 for aphakic extended wear.

Finally, the long-awaited CLI studies of corneal infection with both daily and extended cosmetic hydrogel wear were published in the *New England Journal of Medicine* in September 1989. These two companion studies first estimated the relative risk of infection among the two groups with a case-control study and then secondly attempted to estimate the incidence of ulcerative keratitis among the groups. The first study found 86 patients with corneal infections and matched them with controls.[82] The authors found that either daily or extended wear hydrogel lenses used under closed-eye (extended wear) conditions resulted in a statistically significant increased risk of infection (9 times for daily wear lenses and 10 to 15 times for extended wear–approved lenses). And they noted that the risk increased with every night of additional lens wear.

The second CLI study surveyed all practicing ophthalmologists in a five-state area in New England to identify all new cases of corneal infection with contact lens wear over 4 months.[76] The denominator of the fraction was estimated from a telephone survey of 4,178 households in this same area. The annual incidence of corneal infection was found to be 20.9 out of 10,000 for extended wear and 4.1 out of 10,000 for daily wear.

This large collection of data is summarized in Table 12–2 and suggests that the incidence of corneal infection with contact lens wear is quite low but that extended wear, particularly for the correction of aphakia, substantially increases this risk.

TABLE 12–2.

Estimated Incidence of Corneal Infection Associated With Modes of Contact Lens Wear (1966–1989)*

	Estimated Incidence/10,000 Patient-yr		
Study (yr)	Cosmetic Daily Wear	Cosmetic Extended Wear	Aphakic Extended Wear
Dixon et al.[20] (1966)	2	—	—
Eichenbaum et al.[82] (1982)	—	—	400
Spoor et al.[87] (1984)	—	—	143
Holden et al.[41] (1986)	—	7–100	—
Chalupa et al.[13] (1987)	1	3	—
Weissman et al.[98] (1987)	25	150	—
MacRae[59] (1988)	5	20	50
CLI (1989)[76]	4	21	—
Means	7	45	198

*Note that compliance and type of contact lens are not considered in this table.

MICROORGANISMS

Human beings exist in a veritable soup of microbiological life: bacteria, fungi, viruses, and others. Some forms of these microorganisms are symbiotic, aiding us in the digestion of our food, producing vitamins as by-products of their own development, and so forth. Others ignore human life and are invisible to our existence. Yet other microbes are potentially pathogenic, in other words, capable of inducing human disease if given the appropriate opportunity.

Discussion of many of the specific groups of microorganisms associated with corneal infection follows.

Bacteria

Bacteria are usually grouped according to their shape (rod or cocci) and reaction to Gram, Giemsa, or other staining (negative or positive).

The corneal lesions (i.e., "ulcers") associated with gram-positive bacteria are usually smaller and relatively less purulent compared with those associated with gram-negative bacteria. Gram-positive bacteria, both *Staphylococcus epidermidis* and *S. aureus,* are very common contaminants of the normal lid. *Staphylococcus aureus* is often the cause of conjunctivitis and blepharitis and is associated with marginal infiltrates and corneal phlyctenules.[64] Both *Staphylococcus* species have also been frequently cultured from corneal ulcers associated with contact lens wear. *Streptococcus pneumoniae* (Fig 12–5) and *Streptococcus pyogenes* are the two *Streptococcus* species most often found in association with ocular disease, especially corneal ulcers. Both are also gram positive, as is *Bacillus,* a rare bacteria that can cause corneal infection and severe endophthalmitis. (*Bacillus cereus,* in particular, has emerged as a potentially virulent intraocular pathogen.) Several contact lens–associated corneal infections have been associated with *Bacillus* by culture.[24, 71, 100] *Bacillus* has also been found in the contact lens care systems of about 5% of asymptomatic patients[26] and forms spores resistant to heat and many forms of chemical disinfectants. (Heat of 121° C for 15 minutes or 5 hours of exposure to

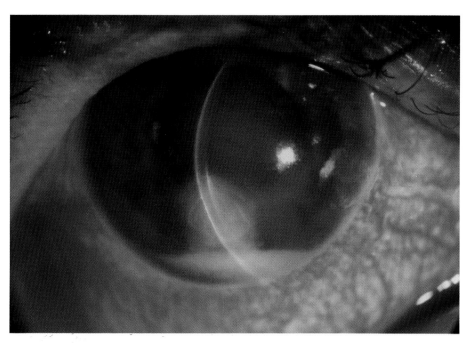

FIG 12–5.
Moderate corneal infection found to be caused by *Streptococcus pneumonia* (gram-positive cocci) by culture. Note corneal ulcer with minimal suppuration but hypopyon in the anterior chamber.

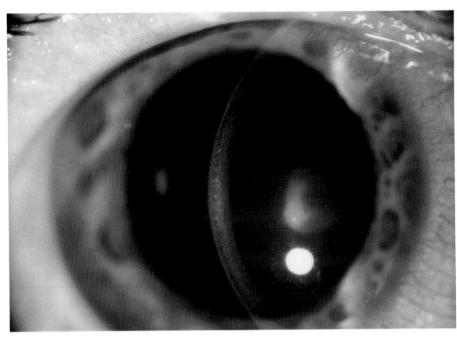

FIG 12-6.
Early (mild) corneal infection associated with *Pseudomonas aeruginosa* (gram-negative rod) by culture.

3% hydrogen peroxide, however, may eliminate viable forms of this bacteria.[24])

Pseudomonas (principally *Pseudomonas aeruginosa*) is a gram-negative, rod-shaped bacterium capable of producing devastating corneal infections. *Pseudomonas* is a ubiquitous microorganism, distributed widely in soil, water, plants, the mammalian gut, and sewage. This is a very virulent and aggressive agent in the cornea, liberating endotoxin and proteolytic enzymes that result in a rapidly progressive corneal ulcer, characterized by melting and purulence. *Pseudomonas* infections often manifest with large epithelial defects, dense anterior stromal infiltration, and mucoid material clinging to the lesion (Figs 12-6 and 12-7). Exotoxin is heat resistant and may not be eliminated from care systems even after thermal disinfection has killed all viable bacteria. It also has been known to cause corneal ring infiltrates.[6] Although *Pseudomonas* may injure host tissue through release of its own factors, in some instances, corneal damage from lysosomal enzymes released by stimulated host PMNs may be more important than the direct damage from the bacterial infection.

Capable of using many different organic compounds

FIG 12-7.
Advanced corneal infection caused by *P. aeruginosa* (by culture). Note severe epithelial defect, stromal melting, and mucoid material clinging to the lesion.

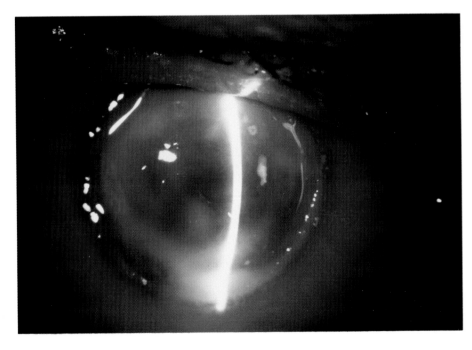

(including atmospheric carbon dioxide) as sources for carbon and energy, *Pseudomonas* is known to be able to contaminate distilled water, saline, fluorescein solutions, eye cosmetics, and the like. *Pseudomonas aeruginosa* is often found in and around sinks, faucets, bedpans, and other moist areas but rarely causes systemic infections in healthy individuals. It is, however, a major pathogen causing pneumonia in myelosuppressed patients undergoing cancer therapy, is a common cause of sepsis in burn patients, and is the most common cause of death in cases of cystic fibrosis.

Serratia marcescens is another gram-negative rod that also is capable of liberating endotoxin, but corneal infections appear not to be quite as devastating as those associated with *Pseudomonas*. *Serratia* has been found to become resistant to certain preservatives often used in contact lens care systems, such as benzalkonium chloride and chlorhexidine.[31]

Several other bacteria have also been rarely cultured from both contact lens care systems and corneal infections. *Propionibacterium acnes* is an example of a gram-positive bacteria occasionally cultured from corneal infections after contact lens wear. Similarly, gram-negative organisms occasionally found by culture include *Klebsiella, Proteus,* and *Moraxella;* the latter is more associated with angular blepharitis or corneal ulcers in alcoholic and debilitated patients.

Historically, Jones has advocated initiating antibiotic treatment of bacterial keratitis based on Gram's stain results, whereas Baum suggested a broad-spectrum "shotgun" approach based initially on clinical appearance.[4] Cultures should be acquired before initial medical therapy, and delay in care should not be tolerated. Initial therapy should be broad-spectrum antibiotics. Presumed bacterial infections are usually treated with first-generation cephalosporin and aminoglycosides (e.g., gentamicin and tobramycin) and often in fortified form. Treatment is then modified based on culture and sensitivity results and clinical course.

Fungi

Although fungal invasion of soft contact lenses has been noted in several studies, associated corneal infection has been very rare. Wilson and Ahearn[101] reported 11 instances of fungal contamination of hydrogel contact lenses from 450 patients using extended wear lenses over a 5-year period. They found only two instances of fungal corneal infection, but the same organism was found in the lens growths and eye lesions in both events. One fungus was *Fusarium verticilloides* and the other *Curvularia lunata.* Several additional patients experienced ocular injection, SPS, and irritation while wearing contaminated

lenses, and these authors[101] believe it likely that liberated fungal toxins were involved. Other fungi commonly identified in human corneal ulcers but not specific to contact lens wear are both *Candida* (a yeast) and *Aspergillus.* Penley et al.[74] suggest that either heat disinfection or at least 45 minutes of soaking in 3% hydrogen peroxide is necessary to eliminate viable fungi from hydrogel contact lenses.

Fungal ulcers can appear chronic and indolent or acute and severe, depending on the exact organism and host status. They are often difficult to diagnose clinically because cultures are frequently negative. Biopsy can be helpful. Fungal corneal infections may demonstrate feathery borders (hyphate edges), raised infiltrates, endothelial plaque, and "satellite" lesions (Fig 12–8). Several antifungal agents are available, such as amphotericin B, natamycin, and miconazole. Treatment is often difficult and results unpredictable.

Viruses

Both herpetic and adenoviral corneal infections are not uncommon occurrences in ophthalmic practice. Herpetic infection is considered a major cause of corneal blindness around the world. Herpes simplex is known as the "great imitator" of corneal infection and should be considered in the differential diagnosis of most corneal diseases, especially if a dendritic lesion or loss of corneal sensitivity is observed. Corneal disease related to adenoviral infection, whether explosive epidemic keratoconjunctivits or milder varieties, is self-limiting. Although transient subepithelial infiltrates and punctate subepithelial scars are common sequelae, this infection rarely results in any severe permanent visual loss. Both of these viral infections are occasionally encountered in patients concomitantly wearing contact lenses, but neither has been etiologically linked to any form of contact lens wear.

The human immunodeficiency virus has been isolated from the tears, conjunctiva, and corneas of infected individuals,[34] but there have been no documented cases suggesting that this disease can be transmitted through any form of ocular contact or contact lens wear.

Protozoa *Acanthamoeba*

Acanthamoeba is a genus of free-living protozoa found ubiquitously in soil, water, and air. They exist in two forms: mobile trophozoites and cysts, the latter of which is double walled and therefore responsible for this microorganism's impressive resistance. *Acanthamoeba* species tolerate a broad range of climate ($-20°$ C–$42°$ C) and pH (3.9–9.75) and have been found in saltwater, freshwater, chlorinated water, hot tubs, and beneath frozen lakes. It

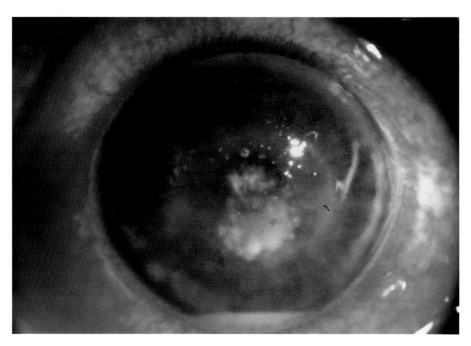

FIG 12–8.
Fungal corneal infection (*Fusarium* species by culture). (Courtesy of J.E. Levenson.)

may even be isolated from the air. *Acanthamoeba astronyxis, Acanthamoeba castellani, Acanthamoeba culbertsoni, Acanthamoeba hatchetti, Acanthamoeba polyphaga,* and *Acanthamoeba rysodes* appear to be the principal ocular pathogenic species.

Corneal infection associated with *Acanthamoeba* was first reported in 1974,[69] and although only a small number were reported through 1981 (none in association with contact lens wear), a dramatic increase began in the middle of that decade. From 1984 through 1987, 62 instances of *Acanthamoeba*-associated corneal infection were reported, and 82% of these occurred in contact lens wearers (Fig 12–9).[68] The increase in incidence might be the result of better recognition of this disease. A retrospective study of eight penetrating keratoplasties performed for "idiopathic" corneal ulceration revealed two instances in which *Acanthamoeba* infection had been missed.[16] The observation that *Acantamoeba* keratitis occurs in patients who had previously healthy eyes but used homemade saline solution as part of their contact lens care was made in 1985.[67] Infection was subsequently attributed to nonsterile water sources, including tap water, well water, water from a home "purification kit," saline solution intended for intravenous use, and even saliva.[16, 66] Daily wear of hydrogel contact lenses appears to be the primary predisposing mode of lens use, but several other types of contact lens wear have also been associated with this infection, including extended wear of hydrogel lenses, rigid gas-permeable (RGP) and hard lenses, and the Saturn II.[53, 68]

The presumed etiology of infection is through amoebic contamination of the lens during cleaning, rinsing, and storage or during swimming. Subsequent chemical disinfection is often ineffective.[58] Silvany et al.[84–86] challenged several contact lens disinfection systems with *A. castellani* and *A. polyphaga* cysts and trophozoites. Effective systems included heat disinfection (70° C–80° C for 10 minutes), 3% hydrogen peroxide for 2 to 3 hours, 0.001% thimerosal with edetate for 4 hours, 0.005% benzalkonimum chloride with edetate and reagent for 4 hours, and either 0.001% chlorhexidine for 4 hours or 0.004% chlorhexidine for 1 hour. Several chemical systems (including 0.001% thimerosal without edetate, 0.13% potassium sorbate with edetate, and 0.00005% polyaminopropyl biguanide with edetate) and a 3% hydrogen peroxide system wherein neutralization is achieved with a metal catalyst were ineffective.

Epithelial trauma associated with lens manipulation (insertion and removal) or overwear may be involved because there are patients with *Acanthamoeba* contamination of their care systems who suffer no corneal infection.[26] Of interest, contact lens cases contaminated with *Acanthamoeba* have other contaminents as well, namely, fungi and gram-negative bacteria,[25] perhaps as food sources.

The epidemiology of this severe corneal infection in the United States was recently reviewed.[90] Two hundred and eight cases were studied, of which 189 had information regarding risk factors. Contact lenses of all types were worn by 85% of these patients, and 64% of these contact lens wearers had a history of use of salt tablet–prepared saline solution. Patients aged 50 years and older were more likely to have a concomitant history of ocular trauma than younger patients.

Clinical features of an *Acanthamoeba* infection include a history of severe pain and photophobia, central or

A

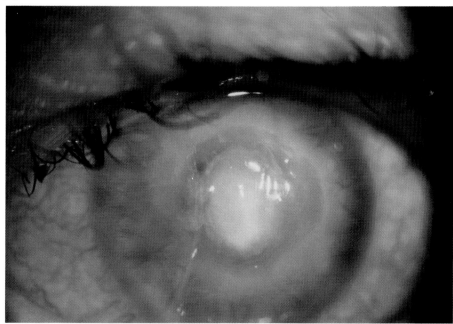

B

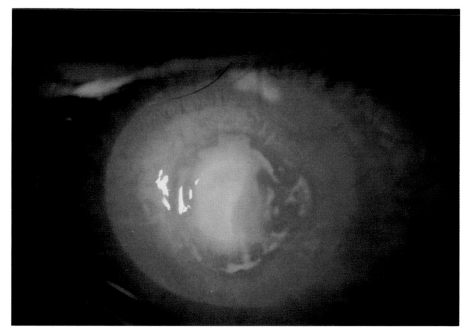

FIG 12–9.
Culture-proved *Acanthamoeba* central corneal infection, seen with both white **(A)** and blue **(B)** (with fluorescein) illumination.

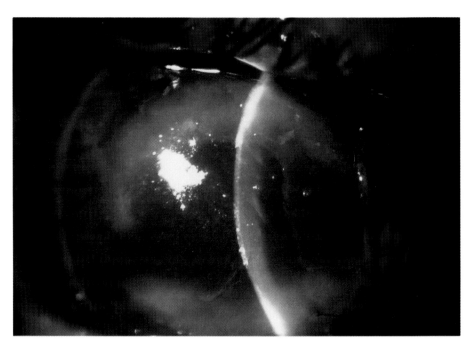

FIG 12–10.
Recurrence of *Acanthamoeba* infection in a corneal graft. Note ring infiltrate.

paracentral infiltrates (early in the disease course), and ring infiltrates (late in the disease course) (Fig 12–10). Additional signs include a dendriform epithelial lesion (clinically suggestive of herpetic keratitis), recurrent epithelial breakdown, radial keratoneuritis, chemosis, usually mild anterior chamber reaction, and sclerokeratitis.

Initial cultures and smears are often negative unless special techniques (e.g., calcofluor white stain or culturing on nonnutrient agar with an *Escherichia coli* overlay) and deeper biopsy are used.

Although early cases appeared refractory to vigorous antibiotic medical treatment,[17] more recently management with a collection of antimicrobial agents (including topical dibromopropamidine isethionate, neomycin-polymyxin B-gramicidin, propamidine isethionate, miconazole nitrate, clotrimazole, corticosteroids, and oral ketoconazole and itraconazole) has proved more successful. Epithelial debridement may be a successful adjunct as well.[45] Berger

et al.[7] reported curing six of seven patients with documented *Acanthamoeba* keratitis after prolonged and intensive treatment with a specific combination of three of these topical agents.

Distribution of Microbial Keratitis

When corneal infections in the general population are considered, different patterns of microbial keratitis have been reported at various referral centers both in North America and Europe. Gram-positive culture results dominate the overall results of these microbiological studies. The principal regional differences appear to be an increased prevalence of pseudomonal and fungal infections in warmer southern latitudes and the predominance of staphylococcal and streptococcal infections in cooler northern climates (see Table 12–3).[70] Systemic associations include alcoholism, diabetes, psychological disturbances, and coma or stupor

TABLE 12–3.

Geographical Comparison of Microbial Keratitis in General (Not Specifically Contact Lens–Wearing) Populations*

Microorganism	San Francisco, Ostler et al.[72] (1947–1976), 134	New York, Asbell and Stenson[3] (1950–1976), 494	Miami, Liesegang and Forster[57] (1969–1977), 371	Houston, Jones[48] (1972–1979), 232	Los Angeles, Ormerod et al.[70] (1972–1983), 186	Total No.	Total (%)
Staphylococcus	27	239	70	79	95	510	(33)
Other gram-positive	57	30	70	136	64	357	(23)
Pseudomonas	18	40	74	57	37	226	(15)
Other gram-negative	22	104	39	46	46	257	(17)
Fungi	—	5	134	40	20	199	(13)

*Column headings list city, study (year), and number of positive cultures. These numbers of positive cultures in the table are the best possible values found in the various cited studies, but some inconsistencies and inaccuracies may exist, probably related to conversion of data from numbers to percentage and back and to instances of mixed culture results.

that lead to corneal exposure. Ocular predisposing factors include trauma, corneal surgery, use of topical corticosteroids, dry eye and exposure keratitis, and, of course, contact lens use (most particularly extended wear).[23, 54, 83]

For cosmetic contact lens users, when cultures are positive, *Pseudomonas* has been noted to account for one half to three fourths of the associated corneal ulcers across a broad range of studies (Table 12–4[1]). It appears that contact lens wear may selectively alter the susceptibility of the normally resistant healthy cornea to infection by this gram-negative bacteria.[32, 52] Of interest, several authors comment that infections associated with the extended or continuous use of hydrogel lenses as bandages (i.e., therapeutic use) where the epithelial surface may be presumed to be altered or diseased appear to be more associated with cultures of gram-positive bacteria and unusual microorganisms than with the gram-negative bacteria (e.g., *Pseudomonas*) seen in cosmetic contact lens use. *Staphylococcus* species are the second most commonly isolated bacterial group. Other bacteria, fungi, and protozoa are less common but clearly possible additional microbes to be considered with infection associated with contact lens wear (Table 12–5).

MANAGEMENT

Management of corneal infection with contact lens wear includes (1) prevention, (2) rapid diagnosis, and (3) appropriate treatment.

Prevention

We believe the two principal risk factors in corneal infection associated with cosmetic contact lens wear are (1) extended wear use of contact lenses and (2) poor contact lens care techniques. A third risk factor is the use of hydrogel contact lenses as a bandage for some corneal disease, but here the risks are often unavoidable. Prevention consists of minimizing the risk to patients by *avoiding the use of contact lenses on extended wear as much as possible*. In cases where such use is necessary (e.g., in the management of pediatric aphakia or hydrogel lenses as bandages), patients should be alerted to the risks of this mode of wear (so that they will be seen without delay if any signs or symptoms occur), and the number of successive nights of use should be reduced, when medically possible, to 1 week or less in agreement with current FDA protocol.

Both RGP lenses and disposable hydrogel lenses have recently been proposed for extended wear, with the implied suggestion that they offer improved physiological results and will reduce the rate of infection. Our experience suggests this is not the case,[28, 29] and Grant and Holden[36] report a persistent incidence of 1% peripheral corneal ulcers with at least one brand of disposable hydrogel contact lens (Fig 12–11). Technical study indicates that the oxygen permeability of all disposable hydrogel materials is identical to that of "reusable" materials of the same chemistry and water content.[99]

Compliant and hygienic use of contact lens care regimens and eliminating exposure to nonsterile water (e.g., swimming with contact lenses on the eyes) or any home-

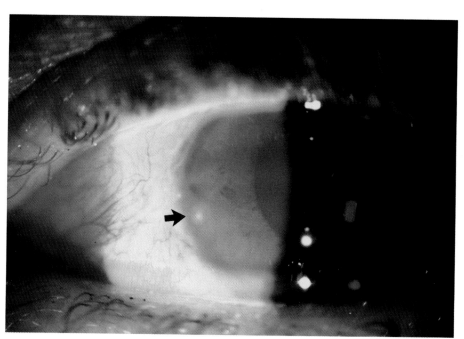

FIG 12–11.
Small peripheral infiltrate *(arrow),* with staining, associated with extended wear of disposable hydrogel lenses (myopic correction). This lesion could be early microbial ulceration. (Courtesy of R.T. Kame.)

TABLE 12–4.

Distribution of Bacterial Keratitis Among Contact Lens Wearers From Various Studies*

Microorganism	Los Angeles, Weissman et al.[97] (1984), 13/18	Philadelphia, Galantine et al.[35] (1984), 29/56	Houston, Patrinely et al.[73] (1985) 14/14	Los Angeles, Ormerod and Smith[71] (1986) 36/42	Miami, Alfonso et al.[2] (1986) 64/118	Los Angeles, Mondino et al.[65] (1986) 29/40
Staphylococcus	2	11	6	12	5	14
Other gram-positive	1	0	2	8	4	5
Pseudomonas	9	13	6	17	40	12
Other gram-negative	1	0	0	6	10	3
Fungi	0	1	0	2	2	0
Protozoa *(Acanthamoeba)*	0	0	0	1	0	0

*Column headings list city, study (year), and number of positive cultures/number of infections. Because of differences in methods of reporting among the several studies and the fact that some cultures may yield more than one positive result, the numbers in the table do not always add up to the numbers of total positive cultures.

TABLE 12–5.

Microbes of Concern Regarding Corneal Infection Associated With Contact Lens Wear in the Major Studies Cited in the Chapter*

Bacteria
  Gram-negative
    Bacilli (rods)
      *Pseudomonas aeruginosa**
      Other *Pseudomonas* sp
      *Serratia marcescens**
      Proteus sp
      Klebsiella sp
      Escherichia coli
      Enterobacter aerogenes
      Morganella morgagnii
    Diplococci
      Moraxella sp
  Gram-positive
    Cocci
      *Staphylococcus aureus**
      *Staphylococcus epidermidis** (coagulase-negative
        staphylococci)
      *Streptococcus pneumoniae**
      Other *Streptococcus* sp
      Enterococcus
      Micrococcus sp
    Bacilli
      Bacillus sp
      Propionibacterium acnes
      Corynebacterium sp
      Mycobacterium sp
Fungi
  *Fusarium**
  Aspergillus
  Penicillium
  Curvularia
  Candida (yeast)
Protozoa
  Acanthamoeba sp*
Viruses
  Herpes simplex
  Herpes zoster
  Adenoviruses
  Human immunodeficiency virus

*The list is roughly in order of frequency of positive cultures, with microbes of specific concern identified with an asterisk. sp = species.

made solutions are important in decreasing the risk of infection (particularly *Acanthamoeba*). Contact lens wear should be discontinued during illness (colds and flus), episodes of ocular irritation, and in the face of contralateral ocular or adnexal infection.

Yet a third additional preventative measure is *routine professional care and supervision.* We believe contact lens–wearing patients should obtain professional evaluations at scheduled intervals of 6 to 9 months under normal conditions and more frequently if any increased risk is suspected (e.g., perhaps 2 to 4 months in instances of extended wear, therapeutic lens use, and after corneal grafts).

Early Recognition

Here the patient must participate in his or her own care. Every contact lens wearer, particularly those who sleep with their lenses in place on occasion or regularly, should know the signs and symptoms of corneal infection: ocular pain and conjunctival injection, tearing, and perhaps discharge or decreased vision. Should any of these occur, contact lenses should be immediately removed. Because these signs and symptoms can be associated with many nonserious complications as well, some of which may have nothing to do with lens wear specifically, the patient should be aware that if these changes persist or worsen after lenses have been removed, they should immediately report to a ophthalmic professional.

The ophthalmic clinician must be able to identify an early or potential corneal infection. Any acutely inflamed and painful eye in a patient wearing a contact lens must be considered a medical emergency, and the patient should be examined as soon as possible. The observation of an epithelial defect with associated infiltrate and discharge should immediately suggest infectious keratitis. All contact lens wear (both eyes) should be discontinued and the patient managed appropriately.

Microorganism	Gothenberg, Chalupa et al.[13] (1987), 28/55	Miami, Koidou-Tsiligianni et al.[54] (1989), 103/196	Philadelphia, Donnefeld et al.[23] (1989), 34/60	Boston, Schein et al.[83] (1989), 53/136	Total No.	(%)
Staphylococcus	1	16	4	17	88	(22)
Other gram-positive	0	5	5	13	43	(11)
Pseudomonas	27	63	20	15	222	(54)
Other gram-negative	0	16	5	6	47	(11)
Fungi	0	0	0	1	6	(2)
Protozoa (*Acanthamoeba*)	0	0	0	2	3	(1)

Treatment

Corneal scrapings should be taken for stains and cultures to identify the offending pathogen. After cultures have been taken, immediate broad-spectrum antibiotic therapy should be initiated. It is important to mention that the use of topical corticosteroids[13] and patching[15] for corneal abrasion in the setting of contact lens wear are not currently considered an initial management option. Both appear to worsen the course of any infectious process, especially those of *Pseudomonas* and fungi.

Treatment of infectious keratitis can involve both medical and surgical intervention and is probably best managed by a corneal specialist.[27] Medical management of microbial keratitis includes broad-spectrum fortified antibiotics, perhaps delivered topically or by subconjunctival depot (where the medicine slowly leaks back out through the needle tract to bathe the anterior segment of the eye). Initial treatment is often modified by the clinical course and the identification and sensitivity of causative microbes isolated by culture. Some patients, especially those with severe infections or who are suspected of being potentially noncompliant, should be hospitalized.

Patients who respond well to antimicrobial treatment are usually considered healed when the epithelial defect closes and other signs and symptoms decline. With improvments in lens design, use, and care to reduce the risk of recurrence, refitting of contact lenses may be considered perhaps 6 weeks after the eye is stable and quiet.

SUMMARY

Corneal infection is a rare but potentially serious complication of contact lens wear. Bacteria (particularly *Pseudomonas* and *Staphylococcus*) are the most common causative agents, followed by fungi and protozoa (*Acantha-*moeba). Viral corneal infections also occur concommitant with contact lens wear, but there does not appear to be any etiological linkage. Clinically, observation of a corneal epithelial defect and associated infiltrate in a setting of pain and discharge and with a history of contact lens wear must be presumed to be a microbial corneal infection until proved otherwise and must be treated as a medical emergency. Clinical management consists of prevention and, in the event of signs or symptoms, immediate response, rapid diagnosis, and appropriate therapeutic actions.

REFERENCES

1. Adams CP, Cohen EJ, Laibson PR, et al: Corneal ulcers in patients with cosmetic extended wear contact lenses. *Am J Ophthalmol* 1983; 96:705–709.
2. Alfonso E, Mandelbaum S, Fox MJ et al: Ulcerative keratitis associated with contact lens wear. *Am J Ophthalmol* 1986; 101:429–433.
3. Asbell P, Stenson S: Ulcerative keratitis: Survey of 30 years' laboratory experience. *Arch Ophthalmol* 1982; 100:77–80.
4. Baum JL, Jones DB: Initial therapy of suspected microbial corneal ulcers. *Surv Ophthalmol* 1979; 24:97–116.
5. Baum JL, Panjwani N: Adherence of *Pseudomonas* to soft contact lenses and cornea: Mechanisms and prophylaxis, in Cavanaugh H (ed): *The Cornea: Transactions of the World Congress on the Cornea III.* New York, Raven Press, 1988.
6. Belmont JB, Ostler HB, Dawson CR, et al: Non-infectious ring-shaped keratitis associated with *Pseudomonas aeruginosa*. *Am J Ophthalmol* 1982; 93:338–341.
7. Berger ST, Mondino BJ, Hoft RH, et al: Successful medical management of *Acanthamoeba* keratitis. *Am J Ophthalmol* 1990; 110:395–403.
8. Bergmanson JPG, Ruben CM, Chu LWF: Epithelial morphological response to soft hydrogel contact lenses. *Br J Ophthalmol* 1985; 69:373–379.
9. Binder PS: The extended wear of soft contact lenses. *J Clin Exp Ophthalmol* 1979; pp 15–32.

10. Binder PS: Extended wear Hydrocurve and Sauflon contact lenses. *Am J Ophthalmol* 1980; 90:309–316.

11. Brown SI, Bloomfield S, Pierce DB, et al: Infections with the therapeutic soft contact lens. *Arch Ophthalmol* 1974; 91:274–277.

12. Campbell RC, Caroline PJ: Inefficacy of soft contact lens disinfection techniques in the home environment. *Contact Lens Forum* 1990; 15:17–26.

13. Chalupa E, Swarbrick HA, Holden BA et al: Severe corneal infections associated with contact lens wear. *Ophthalmology* 1987; 94:17–22.

14. Chun MW, Weissman BA: Compliance in contact lens care. *Am J Optom Physiol Opt* 1987; 64:274–276.

15. Clemons CS, Cohen EJ, Arentsen JJ, et al: *Pseudomonas* ulcers following patching of corneal abrasions associated with contact lens wear. *CLAO J* 1987; 13:161–164.

16. Cohen EJ, Buchanan HW, Laughrea PA, et al: Diagnosis and management of *Acanthamoeba* keratitis. *Am J Ophthalmol* 1985; 100:389–395.

17. Cohen EJ, Parlato CJ, Arentsen JJ, et al: Medical and surgical treatment of *Acanthamoeba* keratitis. *Am J Ophthalmol* 1987; 103:615–625.

18. Collins MJ, Carney LG: Patient compliance and its influence on contact lens wearing problems. *Am J Optom Physiol Opt* 1986; 63:952–956.

19. Cooper RL, Constable IJ: Infective keratitis in soft contact lens wearers. *Br J Ophthalmol* 1977; 61:250–254.

20. Dixon JM, Young CA, Baldone JA, et al: Complications associated with the wearing of contact lenses. *JAMA* 1966; 195:901–903.

21. Dohlman CH: The function of the epithelium in health and disease. *Invest Ophthalmol* 1971; 10:383–407.

22. Dohlman CH, Boruchoff SA, Mobilia EF: Complications in use of soft contact lenses in corneal disease. *Arch Ophthalmol* 1973; 90:367–371.

23. Donnefield ED, Cohen EJ, Arentsen JJ, et al: Changing trends in contact lens associated corneal ulcers. *CLAO J* 1986; 12:145–149.

24. Donzis PB, Mondino BJ, Weissman BA: *Bacillus* keratitis associated with contaminated contact lens care systems. *Am J Ophthalmol* 1988; 105:195–197.

25. Donzis PB, Mondino BJ, Weissman BA, et al: Microbial analysis of contact lens care systems contaminated with *Acanthamoeba*. *Am J Ophthalmol* 1989; 108:53–56.

26. Donzis PB, Mondino BJ, Weissman BA, et al: Microbial contamination of contact lens care systems. *Am J Ophthalmol* 1987; 104:325–333.

27. Dunn JP, Mondino BJ, Weissman BA: Infectious keratitis in contact lens wear, in Bennett ES, Weissman BA (eds): *Clinical Contact Lens Practice*. Philadelphia, JB Lippincott Co, 1991.

28. Dunn JP, Mondino BJ, Weissman BA, et al: Corneal ulcers associated with disposable hydrogel contact lenses. *Am J Ophthalmol* 1989; 108:113–117.

29. Ehrlich M, Weissman BA, Mondino BJ: *Pseudomonas* corneal ulcer after use of extended wear rigid gas permeable contact lens. *Cornea* 1989; 8:225–226.

30. Eichenbaum JW, Feldstein M, Podos SM: Extended wear aphakic soft contact lenses and corneal ulcers. *Br J Ophthalmol* 1982; 66:663–666.

31. Farris RL: Is your office safe? No. *Cornea* 1990; 9(suppl):S44–S46.

32. Fleiszig SMJ: *The Pathogenesis of Contact Lens Related Infectious Keratitis*. Doctoral thesis, Melbourne, University of Melbourne, 1990.

33. Freedman H, Sugar J: *Pseudomonas* keratitis following cosmetic soft contact lens wear. *Contact Lens J* 1976; 10:21–25.

34. Fujikawa LS, Salahuddin SZ, Ablashi D, et al: HTLV-III in the tears of AIDS patients. *Ophthalmology* 1986; 93:1479–1481.

35. Galantine PG, Cohen EJ, Laibson PR, et al: Corneal ulcers associated with contact lens wear. *Arch Ophthalmol* 1984; 102:891–894.

36. Grant T, Holden BA: The clinical performance of disposable (58%) extended wear lenses. Transactions of the British Contact Lens Association International Conference, 1988, pp 63–64.

37. Hamano H, Hori M, Hamano T, et al: Effects of contact lens wear on the mitosis of corneal epithelium and lactate content in the aqueous humor of rabbits. *Jpn J Ophthalmol* 1983; 27:451–458.

38. Hartstein J (ed): *Extended Wear Contact Lenses for Aphakia and Myopia*. St Louis, CV Mosby Co, 1982.

39. Hassman G, Sugar J: *Pseudomonas* corneal ulcer with extended soft contact lenses for myopia. *Arch Ophthalmol* 1983; 101:1549–1550.

40. Hirji NK, Larke JR: Corneal thickness in extended wear of soft contact lenses. *Br J Ophthalmol* 1979; 63:274–276.

41. Holden BA, Kotow M, Grant T, et al: The Cornea and Contact Lens Research Unit of the University of New South Wales position on hydrogel extended wear. New South Wales, Australia, March 4, 1986.

42. Holden BA, Mertz GW: Critical oxygen levels to avoid corneal edema for daily and extended wear contact lenses. *Invest Ophthalmol Vis Sci* 1984; 25:1161–1167.

43. Holden BA, Sweeney DF, Sanderson G: The minimum precorneal oxygen tension to avoid corneal edema. *Invest Ophthalmol Vis Sci* 1984; 25:476–480.

44. Holden BA, Sweeney DF, Vannas A, et al: Effects of long-term extended contact lens wear on the human cornea. *Invest Ophthalmol Vis Sci* 1985; 26:1489–1501.

45. Holland GN, Donzis PB: Rapid resolution of early *Acanthamoeba* keratitis after epithelial debridement. *Am J Ophthalmol* 1987; 104:87–89.

46. Jones DB: Early diagnosis and therapy of bacterial corneal ulcers. *Int Ophthalmol Clin* 1973; 13:1–29.

47. Jones DB: Pathogenesis of bacterial and fungal keratitis. *Trans Ophthalmol Soc UK* 1978; 98:367–371.

48. Jones DB: Initial therapy of suspected microbial corneal ulcers: II. Specific antibiotic therapy based on corneal smears. *Surv Ophthalmol* 1979; 24:105–116.

49. Jones DB: Strategy for the initial management of sus-

pected microbial keratitis, in *Symposium on Medical and Surgical Diseases of the Cornea.* St Louis, CV Mosby Co, 1980.

50. Kent HD, Cohen EJ, Laibson PR, et al: Microbial keratitis and corneal ulceration associated with therapeutic soft contact lenses. *CLAO J* 1990; 16:49–52.

51. Kenyon E, Polse KA, Seger RG: Influence of wearing schedule on extended wear complications. *Ophthalmology* 1986; 93:321–326.

52. Klotz SA, Misra RP, Butrus SI: Contact lens wear enhances adherence of *Pseudomonas aeruginosa* and binding of lectins to the cornea. *Cornea* 1990; 9:266–270.

53. Koenig SB, Solomon JM, Hyndiuk RA, et al: *Acanthamoeba* keratitis associated with gas permeable contact lens wear. *Am J Ophthalmol* 1987; 103:832.

54. Koidou-Tsiligianni A, Alfonso E, Forster RK: Ulcerative keratitis associated with contact lens wear. *Am J Ophthalmol* 1989; 108:64–67.

55. Krachmer JH, Purcel JJ: Bacterial corneal ulcers in cosmetic soft contact lens wearers. *Arch Ophthalmol* 1978; 96:57–61.

56. Larke JR, Hirji NK: Some clinically observed phenomena in extended contact lens wear. *Br J Ophthalmol* 1979; 63:475–477.

57. Liesegang TJ, Forster RK: Spectrum of microbial keratitis in South Florida. *Am J Ophthalmol* 1980; 90:39–40.

58. Ludwig IH, Meisler DM, Rutherford I, et al: Susceptibility of *Acanthamoeba* to soft contact lens disinfection systems. *Invest Ophthalmol Vis Sci* 1986; 27:626–628.

59. MacRae S: Contact lens as a corneal "time bomb," in *Eye Research Seminar.* New York, Research to Prevent Blindness, 1988.

60. Mandell RB, Farrell R: Corneal swelling at low atmospheric oxygen pressures. *Invest Ophthalmol Vis Sci* 1971; 19:697–701.

61. Masters BR: Oxygen tensions of rabbit corneal epithelium measured by non-invasive redox fluorometry. *Invest Ophthalmol Vis Sci* 1984; 25(suppl):102.

62. Millidot M, O'Leary DJ: Effect of oxygen deprivation on corneal sensitivity. *Acta Ophthalmol* 1980; 58:434–439.

63. Millidot M, O'Leary DJ: Abnormal epithelial fragility in diabetes and contact lens wear. *Acta Ophthalmol* 1981; 59:827–833.

64. Mondino BJ, Dethlefs B: Occurrence of phlyctenules after immunization with ribitol teichoic acid of *Staphylococcus aureus. Arch Ophthalmol* 1984; 102:461–463.

65. Mondino BJ, Weissman BA, Farb MD, et al: Corneal ulcers associated with daily wear and extended wear contact lenses. *Am J Ophthalmol* 1986; 102:58–65.

66. Moore MB: *Acanthamoeba* keratitis. *Arch Ophthalmol* 1988; 106:1181–1183.

67. Moore MB, McCulley JP, Luckenbach M, et al: *Acanthamoeba* keratitis associated with soft contact lenses. *Am J Ophthalmol* 1985; 100:396–403.

68. Moore MB, McCulley JP, Newton C, et al: *Acanthamoeba* keratitis. A growing problem in soft and hard

contact lens wearers. *Ophthalmology* 1987; 94:1654–1661.

69. Naginton J, Watson PG, Playfair TJ, et al: Amoebic infection of the eye. *Lancet* 1974; 2:1537–1540.

70. Ormerod LD, Hertzmark E, Gomez DS, et al: Epidemiology of microbial keratitis in southern California. *Ophthalmology* 1987; 94:1322–1333.

71. Ormerod LD, Smith RE: Contact lens associated microbial keratitis. *Arch Ophthalmol* 1986; 104:79–83.

72. Ostler HB, Okumoto M, Wiley C: The changing pattern of the etiology of central bacterial corneal (hypopyon) ulcer. *Trans Pac Coast Otolaryngol Ophthalmol Soc* 1976; 57:235–246.

73. Patrinely JR, Wilhelmus KR, Rubin JM, et al: Bacterial keratitis associated with extended wear soft contact lenses. *CLAO J* 1985; 11:234–236.

74. Penley CA, Llabres C, Wilson LA, et al: Efficacy of hydrogen peroxide disinfection systems for soft contact lenses. *CLAO J* 1985; 11:65–68.

75. Pitts RE, Krachmer JH: Evaluation of soft contact lens disinfection in the home environment. *Arch Ophthalmol* 1979; 97:470–472.

76. Poggio ED, Glynn RJ, Schein OD, et al: The incidence of ulcerative keratitis among users of daily wear and extended wear soft contact lenses. *N Engl J Med* 1989; 312:779–783.

77. Polse KA, Mandell RB: Critical oxygen tension at the corneal surface. *Arch Ophthalmol* 1971; 84:505–508.

78. Ramphal R, McNiece MT, Polack F: Adherence of *Pseudomonas aeruginosa* to the injured cornea. A step in the pathogenesis of corneal infections. *Ann Ophthalmol* 1981; 13:421–425.

79. Roth HW, Iwasaki W, Takayama M, et al: Complication caused by silicon elastomer lenses in West Germany and Japan. *Contacto* 1980; 19:28–36.

80. Ruben M: Acute eye disease secondary to contact lens wear. *Lancet* 1976; 1(7951):138–140.

81. Salz JJ, Schlanger JL: Complications of aphakic extended wear lenses encountered during a seven year period in 100 eyes. *CLAO J* 1983; 9:241–244.

82. Schein OD, Glynn RJ, Poggio ED, et al: The relative risk of ulcerative keratitis among users of daily wear and extended wear soft contact lenses. *N Engl J Med* 1989; 321:773–778.

83. Schein OD, Ormerod LD, Barraquer E, et al: Microbiology of contact lens related keratitis. *Cornea* 1989; 8:281–285.

84. Silvaney RE, Moore MB, McCulley JP: The effect of less than 4 hour exposures of thimerosal, benzalkonium chloride and chlorhexidine on *Acanthamoeba castellani* and *Acanthamoeba polyphaga. Invest Ophthalmol Vis Sci* 1989; 30(suppl):41.

85. Silvaney RE, Wood TS, Bowman RW, et al: The effect of preservatives in contact lens solutions on two species of *Acanthamoeba. Invest Ophthalmol Vis Sci* 1987; 28(suppl):371.

86. Silvaney RE, Wood TS, Bowman RW, et al: The effect of

contact lens solutions on two species of *Acanthamoeba*. *Invest Ophthalmol Vis Sci* 1988; 29(suppl):253.

87. Spoor TC, Hartel WC, Wynn P, et al: Complications of continuous wear soft contact lenses in a non-referral population. *Arch Ophthalmol* 1984; 102:1312–1313.

88. Stark WJ, Kracher GP, Cowan CL, et al: Extended wear contact lenses and intraocular lenses for aphakic correction. *Am J Ophthalmol* 1979; 88:535–542.

89. Stark WJ, Martin N: Extended wear contact lenses for myopic correction. *Arch Ophthalmol* 1981; 99:1963–1966.

90. Stehr-Green JK, Bailey TM, Visvesvara GS: The epidemiology of *Acanthamoeba* keratitis in the United States. *Am J Ophthalmol* 1989; 107:331–336.

91. Stein RM, Clinch TE, Cohen EJ, et al: Infected versus sterile corneal infiltrates in contact lens wearers. *Am J Ophthalmol* 1988; 105:632–636.

92. Stern GA, Lubniewski A, Allen C: The interaction between *Pseudomonas aeruginosa* and the corneal epithelium. *Arch Ophthalmol* 1985; 103:1221–1225.

93. Stern GA, Weitzenkorn D, Valenti J: Adherence of *Pseudomonas aeruginosa* to the mouse cornea. Epithelial v stromal adherence. *Arch Ophthalmol* 1982; 100:1956–1958.

94. Uniacke CA, Hill RM, Greenberg M, et al: Physiological tests for new contact lens materials: 1. Quantitative effects of selected oxygen atmospheres on glycogen storage, LDH concentration and thickness of the corneal epithelium. *Am J Optom Arch Am Acad Optom* 1972; 49:329–332.

95. Weissman BA, Donzis PB, Hoft RH: Keratitis and contact lens wear: A review. *J Am Optom Assoc* 1987; 58:799–803.

96. Weissman BA, Mondino BJ: Is daily wear better than extended wear? Arguments in favor of daily wear. *Cornea* 1990; 9(suppl):S25–S27.

97. Weissman BA, Mondino BJ, Pettit TH, et al: Corneal ulcers associated with extended wear soft contact lenses. *Am J Ophthalmol* 1984; 97:476–481.

98. Weissman BA, Remba MJ, Fugedy E: Results of the extended wear contact lens survey of the Contact Lens Section of the AOA. *J Am Optom Assoc* 1987; 58:166–171.

99. Weissman BA, Schwartz SD, Gottschalk-Katsev N, et al: Oxygen permeability of disposable soft contact lenses. *Am J Ophthalmol* 1990; 110:269–273.

100. Wilhelmus KR: Review of clinical experience with microbial keratitis associated with contact lens wear. *CLAO J* 1987; 13:211–214.

101. Wilson LA, Ahearn DG: Association of fungi with extended wear soft contact lenses. *Am J Ophthalmol* 1986; 101:434–436.

102. Wilson LA, Schlitzer RL, Ahearn DG: *Pseudomonas* corneal ulcers associated with soft contact lens wear. *Am J Ophthalmol* 1981; 92:546–554.

103. Zantos SD, Holden BA: Ocular changes associated with continuous wear of contact lenses. *Aust J Optom* 1978; 61:418–426.

Index

A

Abrasion, 103–156,
  123–156
  adhesion of rigid contact
    lenses causing,
    149–150
  benzalkonium chloride,
    144
  brick dust, 145
  chemical, 140–144
    summary of factors
      related to, 140
  contact lenses causing,
    123–156
  cosmetics causing,
    146–148, 149
  DMV device causing, 131
  electron microscopy of,
    154
  enzyme exposure and,
    143
  finger scrape, 132
  finger squeeze, 132
  fingernail, 133
  foreign body, 144–146
    under contact lens, 145
    diffuse, 146
    summary of, 145
  form of, diagnosis,
    124
  healing of wound,
    152–155
  hydrogen peroxide
    causing, 140–142
  hypoxia causing,
    128–131
    summary of, 128
  investigation, 123–126
  with keratotomy, radial,
    151
  lens calculi causing,
    145–146
  from lens cracks, chips,
    nicks and tears,
    133–137
  lens edge design causing,
    poor, 132–133
  lens film causing, 147
  lens removal causing,
    131–132
  mechanical, 131–140
    summary of, 131

observation, 126–128
  perspective on, 155
  polymethylmethacrylate
    overwear
  position, diagnosis, 124
stain
  blotch, 151
  chemical, summary of
    factors related to,
    140
  conjunctival
    compression, 149,
    151
  smile, under soft
    contact lenses, 137
  superior arc, 137–138
staining
  arcuate, superior, due
    to contact lenses,
    rigid, 138
  blotch, 148
  bubble, 139–140
  chemical, 127
  dimple veil, 141
  dry streak, 145, 148
  epithelial, superior, 140
  epithelial, superior
    limbal, 138
  epithelial microcysts,
    131
  furrow, 138, 139
  hydrogel microcystic,
    130–131
  keratoconus, 151–152
  mechanical, 131
  methods, 126–128
  postkeratoplasty, 151
  sensitivity to preserved
    solutions, 143
  swirl, of keratoconic
    cornea, 153
  surfactant cleaner,
    142–143
  tear film residues, 145
  ultraviolet, 152, 153
Acanthamoeba: in corneal
  infection, 265–268
Acetate butyrate, cellulose
  (see Cellulose acetate
  butyrate)
Adenosine triphosphate:
  production and
  corneal cell, 25

Aesthesiometer of
  Cochet-Bonnet, 90
  clinical use, 90
Age
  corneal sensitivity in
    non-contact lens
    wearers and, 91
  corneal touch threshold as
    function of, 92
Alcian blue dye: in dry eye,
  210
Allergic
  inflammation, 225
  reaction
    giant conjunctivitis as,
      237–240
  in keratitis, 109
Altitude: corneal swelling
  and, 8
Anaerobic isoenzyme
  patterns, 174
Anaphylaxis (see
  Inflammation,
  hypersensitivity type
  I in)
Anesthesia of cornea,
  89–101
  measurement method,
    90–91
Anomalies: ring, impression,
  138
Anoxia, 1–102
  contact lens-induced
    relative, corneal
    sequelae of, 4 (See
    also Hypoxia)
Anti-inflammatory agents: in
  conjunctivitis, giant
  papillary, 250
Antigens: in conjunctivitis,
  giant, proposed
  antigens, 239–240
Aphakia
  with cataract extraction
    earlier, 53
  with diabetes, 256
  with keratopathy, bullous,
    49
Astigmatism: contact lenses
  causing, 76
Atopy: and giant
  keratoconjunctivitis,
  238–239

Atrophy: iris, essential, 51

B

Bacteria
  in corneal infection,
    263–265
  keratitis due to, 270
Bacterial
  exotoxins, chemotic
    conjunctiva after, 116
  ulcer, 116
BAK
  corneal disruption due to,
    108
  epithelial disruption due
    to, 107
Basement membrane: and
  endothelium, 43–44
Benzalkonium chloride
  abrasion, 144
  epithelial punctate
    staining, 231
  hypersensitivity and
    toxicity of, 231
Biomicroscopy: of eye by
  Vogt's, 45
Bleb
  endothelial, due to
    hypoxia, 29–31
  Zantos-Holden response,
    55
Blink
  change in dry eye, 196–197
  rate, 171
Blinking
  and contact lenses, 171
  poor, in 3 and 9 o'clock
    staining, 200
Blotch stain, 151
Blotch staining, 148
Brick dust: causing abrasion,
  145
Bubble staining, 139–140
Bullous keratopathy: with
  aphakia, 49

C

Calcium
  carbonate tear film
    deposits on hydrogel,
    182–184

Calcium (cont.)
    phosphate tear film
        deposits on hydrogel,
        183
Calculi of lens
    causing abrasion, 145–146
    tear film deposits on
        hydrogel and, 181
Capillary permeability:
    increase in
    inflammation, 222
Carbon dioxide: cornea and,
    31
Cataract: extraction, aphakia
    after, 53
Cell
    cornea (See Cornea, cell)
    endothelial (see
        Endothelium, cell)
    mast (see Mast cell)
Cellulose acetate butyrate
    lipid tear film deposits on,
        188
    tear film deposits on, 187
Chandler's syndrome, 51
Chemical
    abrasion (see Abrasion,
        chemical)
    staining, 127
Chemistry
    of lens surface, 184–186
    of tear and hydrogel,
        186–187
Chemosis: chlorhexidine
    toxicity and, 232
Chemotic conjunctiva after
    bacterial exdotoxins,
    116
Chlorhexidine:
    hypersensitivity and
    toxicity, 231–232
Cleaners: of lenses,
    alteration in, in
    conjunctivitis,
    247–248
CO₂ (see Carbon dioxide)
Cochet-Bonnet
    aesthesiometer, 90
    clinical use, 90
Collagen layer: posterior,
    endothelial, 48
Color fringe pattern: of tear
    film, 163
Complement cascade: in
    inflammation, 222
Conjunctiva
    chemotic, after bacterial
        exotoxins, 116
    compression stain, 149
    hemorrhage due to contact
        lenses, 132
    hyperemia, 116
        after thimerosal, 232

stain, compression, 151
staining in dry eye,
    208–210
Conjunctivitis
    giant papillary, 237–252
        allergic reaction,
            evidence for,
            237–240
        anti-inflammatory
            agents in, 250
        antigens in, proposed,
            239–240
        atopy and, 238–239
        cause as an open
            question, 237–240
        cessation of lens wear,
            248
        diagnosis, 240–247
        disposable lenses in,
            248–249
        drugs in, 249–251
        gas-permeable lenses
            in, rigid, 248
        hyperemia in, 243
        IgE-mediated
            hypersensitivity in,
            238
        lens solution or cleaner
            alteration, 247–248
        lens type and, 248–249
        mast cell stabilizers in,
            249–250
        papilla in, 241
        pasrameter changes in,
            248–249
        replacement of lens,
            248
        replacement of lenses,
            programmed,
            248–249
        seasonal occurrence,
            239
        signs of, 246
        soft contact lens in,
            traditional, 248
        stage 4, deposits in,
            247
        stages 2, 3 and 4,
            244–245
        symptoms of, 246
        trauma in, mechanical,
            240
        treatment, 247–251
        treatment
            recommendations,
            250–251
        treatment
            recommendations,
            summary, 250
        treatment summary,
            250–251
        types of, upper tarsal,
            242

vitamin A drops in, 250
Contact lenses
    abrasions due to (see
        Abrasion)
    anoxia due to, corneal
        sequelae of, 4
    blinking and, 171
    chips causing abrasions,
        133–137
    in conjunctivitis (see
        under Conjunctivitis,
        giant papillary)
    corneal topography
        changes due to,
        69–87
    cracks causing abrasion,
        133–137
    extended wear and
        infection, 258–259
    gas-permeable (see Gas
        permeable)
    hard
        effects of, short-term,
            92–93
        long-term, 94–95
        long-term, recovery
            from effects, 95
    hydrogel (see Hydrogel)
    hypersensitivity reactions
        to, 113–116
    keratoconjunctivitis due
        to, superior limbic,
        117–118
    materials
        oxygen flux
            measurement
            through, 11
        oxygen transmissibility
            measurement, 9–11
    methylmethacrylate (see
        Methylmethacrylate)
    nicks causing abrasions,
        133–137
    refractive error changes
        due to, 69–87
    rigid
        adhesion causing
            abrasion, 149–150
        chisel-shaped edge, 134
        comparison with
            hydrogel, 77–78
        cracked-chipped, 135
        vision quality with, 80
    soft
        clear pupil, tinted,
            causing corneal
            impression, 138
        in conjunctivitis, giant
            papillary, 248
        effects of, short-term,
            93–94
        filaments associated
            with, 150

long-term, 95–96
    nicked, 137
    smile stain under, 137
    torn, 136
    tears causing abrasions,
        133–137
    therapeutic, corneal
        infection and, 261
    vision quality and (see
        Vision quality and
        contact lenses)
    wear
        anesthesia of cornea
            after (see Anesthesia
            of cornea)
        effects of, 79–80
        effects of, short-term,
            92–94
        effects of, short-term,
            recovery from, 93
        hypoxic effects on
            corneal endothelium,
            54–64
        long-term, 94–96
        oxygen availability
            during, 9–18
        oxygen availability
            during, resolution,
            17–18
        soft, hypoxic changes
            in corneal
            endothelium, 57
Contrast sensitivity function
    testing, 78–79
Cornea
    abrasion (see Abrasion)
    anesthesia (see Anesthesia
        of cornea)
    area, sensitivity in
        non-contact lens
        wearers, 91
    blotting, 130–131, 131
    carbon dioxide and, 31
    cell
        adenosine triphosphate
            production and, 25
        function, hypoxia and,
            26–27
        function and oxygen,
            23–27
        glucose source for,
            25–26
        homeostasis, 23–25
        ion concentrations, 24
        lactate efflux and,
            25–26
    clouding due to
        polymethylmethacry-
        late, 128
    curvature
        orthokeratology and, 82
        vs. base curve-corneal
            relationship, 82

curvature changes
with contact lenses,
69–80
deliberate, 80–83
polymethylmethacrylate
causing, 69–70
dehydration in dry eye,
196
desiccation
with hydrogel,
203–204
with hydrogel, causes,
204
with hydrogel,
description, 203–204
with hydrogel,
management, 204
management
nomogram, 202
peripheral, 133
peripheral, extreme
form, 200
disruption, BAK causing,
108
distortion due to
polymethylmethacry-
late, 70
in dry eye (*see* Dry eye,
cornea in)
eccentricity, corneal touch
threshold as function
of, 91
edematous formation,
129–130
diagnosis, differential,
130
endothelium (*see*
Endothelium of
cornea)
epithelium (*see* Epithelium
of cornea)
exhaustion syndrome, 69
farinata, 52
guttatae, 48
H⁺ and, 26
hydration, pump-leak
hypothesis for
maintenance, 23
hyperemia, 118
infection (*see* Infection,
corneal)
infiltrates
after contact lens, 257
etiologies, common,
258
with hydrogel, 257
multiple subepithelial,
257
infiltration by inflammation,
225–226
laceration, 132
broken glass causing,
146

healed, electron
microscopy of, 155
metabolism, and oxygen,
3–5
mosaic, anterior, 137
neovascularization of,
228–229
hydrogel and, 229
oxygen and (*see under*
Oxygen)
oxygen needs of, 5
oxygen pathways to, 23
oxygen requirements of,
3–20
oxygen tension (*see*
Oxygen tension of
cornea)
pH and hypoxia, 29–31
redox fluorometry, 174
rehabilitation, 33–34
rose bengal staining of, 125
scar, postkeratoplasty, 152
sensitivity
effect of various types
of contact lenses on,
93
as function of eye
color, 92
hypoxia and, 32–33
loss mechanism, 96–97
measurement of, 89–90
neurotransmitter for,
98–99
in non-contact lens
wearers, 91–92
in non-contact lens
wearers, age and, 91
in non-contact lens
wearers, iris color in,
91
recovery after long-term
hard lenses, 96
sequelae of contact
lens-induced relative
anoxia, 4
striae with stromal
swelling, 30
stroma (*see* Stroma)
surface, oxygen tension
at, 98
swelling (*see* Swelling of
cornea)
topography changes due to
contact lenses,
69–87
touch threshold, 91
after hard contact
lenses, 94
change with soft contact
lenses, 96
changes as function of
oxygen mixtures,
partial, 97

as function of age, 92
as function of eyelid
closure, 97
as function of hard
contact lens wear
length, 95
transparency of, 21–23
ulcer (*see* Ulcer)
warpage syndrome,
70–71
wrinkling, 137
Corticosteroid use: and
corneal infection, 261
Cosmetics: causing abrasion,
146–148, 149
Cotton thread phenol red
test: in dry eye, 205
CTT (*see* Cornea touch
threshold)
Cytology, impression
cell formations obtained
by, 208
in dry eye, 207

D

Deadaptation: in
polymethylmethacry-
late complications,
72–73
Degranulation: of mast cell,
239
Dehydration: through lens,
256
Dellen: with stromal
thinning, 201
Dendriform lesions,
112–113
epithelial, diagnosis,
differential, 113
Dendrite, true, 114
in herpes simplex
keratitis, 113
Dendritic ulcer: herpes
simplex, 130
Diabetes mellitus
with aphakia, 256
corneal infection and, 261
Dimple
veil staining, 141
veiling, 139–140
DK/L, 9–11
DMV device: causing
abrasion, 131
Drugs
in conjunctivitis, giant
papillary, 249–251
intervention in
inflammatory
process, 224
systemic, in dry eye and
ocular surface
disease, 196

Dry eye, 195–218
blink change in, 196–197
borderline, management,
212
causes, 196
with contact lenses,
195–218
cornea in, 197–204
3 and 9 o'clock
staining, 197–204
3 and 9 o'clock
staining, causes,
198–200
3 and 9 o'clock
staining, description,
197
3 and 9 o'clock
staining, grades 1
and 2, 198
3 and 9 o'clock
staining, grades 3
and 4, 199
3 and 9 o'clock
staining, incidence,
198
3 and 9 o'clock
staining,
management,
200–203
3 and 9 o'clock
staining, Schnider
grading system, 198
dehydration in, 196
staining in, 208–210
drugs associated with,
systemic, 196
education of patients in,
211
environmental factors in,
212
eyelid
conformity loss in, 196
scrubs in, 212
grading with Latin square
diagram, 215
hot compresses in, 212
incidence, 195
lens material selection in,
211–212
lipid layer rupture in, 196
lubrication in, 212–213
management, 210–215
marginal, in 3 and 9
o'clock staining, 200
prediction tests, 204–210
punctal plugs in, 214–215
installation procedure,
214
questionnaires, 210, 211
reasons for contact lenses
inducing, 196
selection of patients in,
211

Dry eye (*cont.*)
  symptoms, 195
  tear film thinning in, 196
  types, 196
Dry streak staining, 145,
    148
Dystrophy
  combined
      epithelial-endothelial,
      48
  endothelial, 48–54
    congenital hereditary,
        50
    late hereditary, 48
    Fuchs', 48–49
      early, 49
    polymorphous, posterior,
        50
    pre-Descemet's, 52–54

                E

Edema
  corneal edematous
      formation, 129–130
    diagnosis, differential,
        130
    epithelial, due to hypoxia,
        28–29
    polymethylmethacrylate
        causing, 69
  (*See also* Swelling)
Education: of patients in dry
    eye, 211
Electron microscopy
  of corneal abrasion, 154
  of epithelial cell
      migration, 154
  of epithelial microvillae,
      154
  of healed corneal
      laceration, 155
  scanning, of endothelim,
      46
  transmission, of
      endothelium, 46
Embryology: of corneal
    endothelium, 37–38
Endothelium
  basement membrane and,
      43–44
  bedewing after contact
      lens wear, 56
  blebs due to hypoxia,
      29–31
  cell
    areas, calculated, 58,
        59, 60
    density, 47
    density after contact
        lens wear, 56
    function, 48
    shape, 47–48

sides, distribution of
    number, 60–61
  terminology definition,
      47
confocal microscopy of,
    46–47
of cornea
  changes in, 47–54
  description of, 37–44
  embryology, 37–38
  hydrogel lenses, 6 years
      wear and, 58
  hypoxic changes after,
      37–64
  hypoxic changes after
      soft contact lens
      wear, 57
  hypoxic effects of
      contact lens wear on,
      54–64
  morphology, 38–41
  physiology, 41–43
  polymethylmethacrylate
      contact lens wear
      and, 57
  polymethylmethacrylate
      lenses, 9 years wear,
      58
  polymethylmethacrylate
      lenses, 23 years
      wear, 59
  posterior, 38
dystrophy (*see* Dystrophy,
    endothelial)
electron microscopy of
  scanning, 46
  transmission, 46
examination, 44–47
  clinical techniques,
      44–45
  histological techniques,
      45–46
  laboratory techniques,
      45–47
function, 42–43
  reduction and hypoxia,
      33
  temperature reversal
      experiment of
      Davson, 42
hypoxia complicating,
    29–31, 33
intercellular vacuole, 62
interface between
    posterior limiting
    lamina and
    endothelium, 41
junctional complex, 41
lamina, posterior limiting,
    48
light microscopy of, 46
mosaic, 40, 54, 55
  with polymegethism, 62

nutrition and, 42
pathologic conditions
  acquired, 50–51
  associated with,
      48–54
polymegethism
  due to contact lens,
      formation theory, 63
  and hypoxia, 33
posterior limiting lamina,
    43–44
senescent, 47–48
Environmental factors: in
    dry eye, 212
Enzyme exposure: and
    abrasion, 143
Epithelium, 21–36
  arcuate lesions, superior,
      119–120
  cell migration, electron
      microscopy of, 154
  of cornea, hypoxic
      changes in, 21–36
  debridement
    accidental, 133
    contact lens removal
        causing, soft, 134
  dendriform lesions,
      diagnosis,
      differential, 113
  disruption
    BAK causing, 107
    hydrogen peroxide
        causing, 107
  DMV device pulling off,
      131
  downgrowth, 51
  dystrophy, with
      endothelial
      dystrophy, 48
  edema to hypoxia, 28–29
  healing and hypoxia, 29
  hypoxia
    chronic effects, 31–33
    complicating, 27–29
  microcysts (*see*
      Microcysts)
  microvillae, electron
      microscopy of, 154
  necrosis after hair curling
      device, 150
  pseudodendrite, 129–130
  punctate lesions after
      hydrogel, 110
  splitting, 119, 139, 140
  staining
    punctate, with
        benzalkonium
        chloride, 231
    superior, 140
    superior limbal, 138
  thinning and hypoxia,
      31–32

trauma and infection, 261
vacuoles, 111
Exotoxins: bacterial,
    chemotic conjunctiva
    after, 116
Eye
  color, corneal sensitivity
      as function of, 92
  dry (*see* Dry eye)
  inflammation (*see*
      Inflammation)
  red (*see* Red eye)
  surface disease, drugs
      associated with,
      systemic, 196
  Vogt's biomicroscopy of,
      45
Eyelid
  closure
    corneal oxygen tension
        and, 8–9
    corneal touch threshold
        as function of, 97
  conformity loss in dry
      eye, 196
  gap enlargement causing 3
      and 9 o'clock
      staining, 199
  scrubs in dry eye, 212

                F

Fingernail abrasion, 133
Fluorescein
  diagnostic, various forms
      of, 126
  dye staining in dry eye,
      208–209, 210
  in tear breakup time in
      dry eye, 205
  for tear breakup time test,
      169
Fluoro-silicone acrylates:
    tear film deposits on,
    189
Fluorometry: corneal redox,
    174
Fluorophotometric technique:
    for tear production
    measurement, 172
Fluorophotometry, in dry
    eye, 205
Fluorotron: for tear
    production
    measurement, 172
Foreign body abrasions (*see*
    Abrasion, foreign
    body)
Fuchs' dystrophy, 48–49
  early, 49
Fungi: in corneal infection,
    265, 266
Furrow staining, 138, 139

G

Gas-permeable
  lenses
    adhesion substance
      under, 152
    HSU values and, 17
    materials for,
      appropriate, 13
    oxygen percentage,
      equivalent, 15
    oxygen transmissibility
      of, 14
    rigid, 3 and 9 o'clock
      staining in, 201
    rigid, changes due to,
      76–78
    rigid, fingernail
      abrasion due to, 133
    rigid, in conjunctivitis,
      giant papillary, 248
    rigid, meibomian gland
      dysfunction due to,
      209
    rigid, myopia
      progression with, 83
    rigid, tear film over,
      165
    rigid, tear film thinning
      due to, 197
  materials
    rigid, immediate
      refitting in
      polymethylmethacry-
      late complications,
      73–74
Giant conjunctivitis (*see*
  Conjunctivitis, giant)
Glass: broken, causing
  corneal laceration,
  146
Glucose: source of corneal
  cell, 25–26

H

H⁺: and cornea, 26
Hair curling device:
  epithelial necrosis
  after, 150
Healing
  of abrasion, 152–155
  epithelial, and hypoxia,
  29
HEMA lenses, 184
Hemorrhage: conjunctiva,
  due to contact lenses,
  132
Herpes simplex
  dendritic ulcer, 130
  diagnosis, differential,
  130
  infections, 112–113

keratitis, true dendrite in,
  113
Homeostasis: of corneal cell,
  23–25
Hot compresses: in dry eye,
  212
HSU values: and
  gas-permeable lenses,
  17
Hydration: of cornea,
  pump-leak hypothesis
  for maintenance, 23
Hydrogel
  corneal desiccation with
    (*see* Cornea,
    desiccation with
    hydrogel)
  corneal infiltrate with, 257
  lens surface chemistry
    and, 185
  microbubbles, 130–131
  microcystic staining,
    130–131
  microdeposits, 130–131
  myopia progression with,
    83
  neovascularization of
    cornea and, 229
  red eye and, acute,
    syndrome of, 230
  staining with, punctate
    superficial, 256
  *Staphylococcus
    epidermidis* on, 183
  surface irregularities,
    formation of deposits
    in, 187
  tear evaporation rate and,
    179
  tear film and, 164
  tear film deposits on (*see*
    Tear film deposits on
    hydrogel)
  vascularization and, 229
Hydrogel lenses
  changes due to, 77–78
    comparison with rigid
      lenses, 77–78
    mode of lens, 77
  endothelium after 6 years
    wear, 58
  oxygen levels and,
    critical, 9
  oxygen percentages,
    equivalent, 15
  oxygen transmissibility of,
    14
  stromal pH decrease with,
    30
  vision quality and, 79–80
Hydrogen: epithelial
  punctate lesions after,
  110

Hydrogen peroxide
  abrasion due to, 140–142
  causing epithelial
    disruption, 107
Hyperemia
  chlorhexidine toxicity in,
    232
  conjunctival, 116
    after thimerosal, 232
  in conjunctivitis, giant,
    243
  cornea, 118
Hypersensitivity
  to chlorhexidine, 231–232
  IgE-mediated, in giant
    conjunctivitis, 238
  to preservatives, 231–233
  reactions
    to contact lenses,
      113–116
    in keratitis, 109
  skin basophilic, in giant
    conjunctivitis,
    237–238
  thimerosal, 232–233
    causing pseudodentrite,
      129
  type I, in inflammation
    (*see* Inflammation,
    hypersensitivity in,
    type)
Hypertrophy: limbal, 138,
  139, 151
Hypoxia
  abrasions due to, 128–131
    summary of, 128
  complications
    acute, 27–33
    epithelium, 27–29
  corneal cell function and,
    26–27
  corneal sensitivity and,
    32–33
  effects of, chronic, 31–33
  endothelial blebs due to,
    29–31
  endothelial function
    reduction and, 33
  endothelial polymegathism
    and, 33
  endothelium complicated
    by, 29–31, 33
  epithelial edema due to,
    28–29
  epithelial healing and, 29
  epithelial thinning and,
    31–32
  epithelium and, chronic
    effects, 31–33
  in keratitis, 111–112
  superficial punctate,
    27–28
  microcysts and, 31, 32

neovascularization and, 33
pH and, corneal, 29–31
polymegethism due to, 63
stroma complicated by,
  29–31, 33
stromal swelling due to,
  29
stromal thickness
  reduction and, 33
(*See also* Anoxia)
Hypoxic
  changes
    in corneal endothelium,
      37–64
    in corneal epithelium,
      21–36
    in stroma, 21–36
  effects on corneal
    endothelium after
    contact lens wear,
    54–64
  stress measurement of
    oxygen availability
    under contact lenses,
    18

I

Immunoglobulin: E-mediated
  hypersensitivity in
  conjunctivitis, 238
Impression ring anomaly,
  138
Infection, 253–274
  corneal, 255–273
    bacteria in, 263–265
  contact lens care
    regimens in,
    269–270
  corticosteroid use and,
    261
  definition, 255–258
  diabetes and, 261
  early recognition, 270
  epithelial trauma and,
    261
  extended wear lenses
    in, 258–259
  fungal, 266
  historical perspectives,
    258
  incidence, 262
  incidence, estimated,
    with various contact
    lenses, 263
  management, 269–271
  microbes of concern in,
    270
  microorganisms in,
    263–269
  noncompliance with
    contact lens care
    techniques, 260–261

Infection (*cont.*)
    oxygen and, 259–260
    protozoa *Acanthamoeba*
        in, 265–268
    risk factors, 258–262
    smoking and, 261–262
    *Streptococcus
        pneumoniae,* 263
    therapeutic contact lens
        and, 261
    treatment, 271
    viruses, 265
    inflammatory
        consequences of,
        226–227
Inflammation, 219–252,
    221–235
    allergic, 225
    capillary permeability
        increase in, 222
    complement cascade in,
        222
    as consequence of
        infection, 226–227
    corneal infiltration by,
        225–226
    hypersensitivity in, type I,
        222–223
    inflammatory mediators
        released by, 223
    mechanism of, 223
    mechanism of, 222–224
    with pannus and
        phlyctenule, 227
    process of, pharmacologic
        intervention in, 224
    prostaglandins in, 223–224
    "snowball" infiltrative
        opacities, 226
    viral, 225
Ion concentrations: for
    corneal cell, 24
Iris
    atrophy, essential, 51
    color and corneal
        sensitivity in
        non-contact lens
        wearers, 91
Isoenzyme patterns:
    anaerobic, 174

K

Keratic precipitate, 50, 52
Keratitis, 105–122
    allergic reactions in, 109
    bacterial, distribution of,
        270
    filamentary, 148
    herpes simplex virus, true
        dendrite in, 113
    hypersensitivity reactions
        in, 109

hypoxia in, 111–112
marginal, 117–120
microbial
    distribution of,
        268–269
    geographical
        comparison of
        populations, 268
    nummular, 113–117
    punctate superficial,
        109–112
        due to hypoxia, 27–28
        lens dehydration in,
        109–112
        Thygeson's, 109
    punctate superior, contact
        lenses causing, soft,
        144
    toxic reactions in,
        106–109
Keratoconjunctivitis
    epidemic, 116–117
    limbic, 117
        contact lenses causing,
            117–118, 233
        superior, due to contact
            lenses, 117–118,
            144
Keratoconus
    contact lenses causing,
        76
    polymethylmethacrylate in
        etiology of, 75–76
    staining, 151–152
    swirl, 153
Keratology
    efficacy, 81–82
    myopia and, 81
Keratopathy
    bullous aphakic, 49
    Thygeson's, 148
Keratoplasty: corneal scar
    after, 152
Keratotomy, radial
    abrasion and, 151
    scars, 152

L

Lactate
    dehydrogenase/malate
        dehydrogenase ratio,
        175
    efflux of corneal cell,
        25–26
Lactoferrin assay: in dry
    eye, 207
Lamina, posterior limiting
    endothelium and, 43–44,
        48
    transverse section through,
        43–44
LDH/MDH ratio, 175, 176

Lenses
    binding in 3 and 9 o'clock
        staining, 200, 202
    calculi (*see* Calculi of lens)
    chemistry of surface,
        184–186
    chemistry of surface,
        hydrogel and, 185
    contact (*see* Contact
        lenses)
    dehydration
        in keratitis, superficial
            punctate, 109–112
        through lens, 256
    edge
        abrasion causing 3 and
            9 o'clock staining,
            198–199
        chafing causing 3 and 9
            o'clock staining,
            198–199
    gas-permeable (*see*
        Gas-permeable
        lenses)
    HEMA, 184
    hydrogel (*see* Hydrogel
        lenses)
    integrity of surface, 187
    water content of, 184
Leukocyte esterase test: in
    dry eye, 206
Lid (*see* Eyelid)
Light microscopy: of
    endothelium, 46
Limbal hypertrophy, 138,
    139, 151
Limbic keratoconjunctivitis
    (*see*
    Keratoconjunctivitis,
    limbic)
Lipid layer rupture: in dry
    eye, 196
Lipid tear film deposits
    on cellulose acetate
        butyrate, 188
    on hydrogel, 181
    on silicone, 189
Lubrication: in dry eye,
    212–213
Lysozyme test: in dry eye,
    206–207

M

Makeup abrasion, 149
Marmoreal interference
    fringe pattern, 161
    contaminated, 162
Mast cell
    degranulation, 239
    stabilizers in
        conjunctivitis, giant
        papillary, 249–250

Mechanical trauma: in giant
    conjunctivitis, 240
Medications: systemic, in
    dry eye and ocular
    surface disease, 196
Meibomian gland dysfunction
    in dry eye, 207
    with gas-permeable
        lenses, rigid, 209
Microbes: of concern in
    corneal infection, 270
Microbial
    keratitis (*see* Keratitis,
        microbial)
    ulcer, 269
Microcysts
    epithelial, 111
        staining, 131
    eruption, epithelium after,
        110
    grading system, 32
    hydrogel staining, 130–131
    and hypoxia, 31, 32
Micrograph: specular, 56
Microorganisms: and cornea,
    263–269
Microscopy
    electron (*see* Electron
        microscopy)
    light, of endothelium, 46
Model
    of oxygen available to
        eye, progressive
        reduction, 8
    of oxygen percentages,
        equivalent, 16
Mosaic
    cornea, anterior, 137
    endothelial, 54, 55
        in ploymegethism, 62
    shagreen, posterior,
        51–52
Myopia
    keratology and, 81
    progression
        with gas-permeable
            lenses, rigid, 83
        with hydrogel, 83
        with polymethylmetha-
            crylate, 83
        in young people, 83
Myopic creep, 77

N

Necrosis: epithelial, after
    hair curling device,
    150
Necrotizing corneal ulcer,
    228
Neovascularization
    of cornea, 228–229
    hypoxia and, 33

Neurotransmitter: for corneal sensitivity, 98–99
Nitrogen goggle leads, 27
Nomogram: for management of long-term polymethylmethacrylate wearers, 74
Nutrition: and endothelium, 42

O

Ocular (*see* Eye)
Ortho-K 60 lens, 80
Orthokeratology, 80–83
  contact lens position, 82
  corneal curvature and, 82
  definition, 80
  fitting philosophies, 81
  refractive changes and, 82
  sphericalization, 82–83
    adverse effects, 83
    temporal effects, 82
Osmolality: of tears with contact lenses, 178
Osmolarity: of tear in dry eye, 206
Oxygen
  availability
    during contact lens wear, 9–18
    during contact lens wear, resolution, 17–18
    hypoxic stress measurement of, 18
  available to eye, reduction of, model of, 8
  corneal infection and, 259–260
  corneal metabolism and, 3–5
  demands of cornea, mean, 12
  flux measurement through contact lens materials, 11
  levels, critical, and lens thicknesses for hydrogel lenses, 9
  mixtures, partial, and corneal touch threshold, 97
  needs of cornea, 5
  pathways to cornea, 23
  percentage, equivalent determination, general concept, 15
    measurements, 14–17
    model for, 16
    for various thicknesses of contact lenses, 15
  performances, calculated, 10

requirements of cornea, 3–20
sensor assembly for oxygen tension measurement, 11
tension of cornea
  eyelid closure and, 8-9
  levels, critical, criteria for, 6-9
  measurement with oxygen sensor assembly, 11
  profiles, 4, 5, 6
  surface, 98
transmissibility
  of contact lens materials, 9-11
  of gas-permeable lenses, 14
  of hydrogel contact lenses, 14
transmissivities, 10
uptake rates, relationships of, 16

P

Pannus: inflammatory, and phlyctenule, 227
pH
  corneal, and hypoxia, 29–31
  stromal
    decrease with hydrogel lenses, 30
    nitrogen goggle leads and, 27
  in tear film, 177
Pharmacologic intervention: in inflammatory process, 224
Phenol red cotton thread test: in dry eye, 205
Phlyctenule: and inflammatory pannus, 227
Pleomorphism: definition, 47
PMMA (*see* Polymethylmethacrylate)
Polygonal: definition, 47
Polymegethism
  after contact lens wear, 56–64
  definition, 47
  endothelial
    contact lens causing, formation theory, 63
    hypoxia and, 33
    mosaic in, 62
  hypoxia causing, 63
Polymethylmethacrylate
  abrasion, overwear, 128–129

changes due to, 69–76
communications of patients, 71–72
complications, 69–76
  cold turkey technique with, 72
  continued use after, 75
  deadaptation in, 72–73
  management, 71
  management methods, 72–74
  refitting, immediate, with rigid gas-permeable materials, 73–74
contact lens wear, corneal endothelium after, 57
corneal clouding due to, 128
corneal curvature changes due to, 69–70
corneal distortion due to, 70
edema due to, 69
evaluation by patient, 71–72
in keratoconus etiology, 75–76
lenses
  23 years wear, 59
  9 years wear, endothelium after, 58
  continued use after complications, 75
  long-term, management nomogram, 74
  myopia progression with, 83
  oxygen uptake rates and, 16
  refitting procedure, 74–75
  refractive changes due to, 69–70
  refractive state after discontinuing, 73
  tear film deposits on, 187
Polymorphism: definition, 47
Polymorphous dystrophy: posterior, 50
Postkeratoplasty staining, 151
Pre-Descemet's dystrophy, 52–54
Preservatives
  hypersensitivity to, 231–233
  toxicity to, 231–233
Preserved solutions: staining due to sensitivity to, 143
Prostaglandins: in inflammation, 223–224

Protein
  concentrations in tears, graphical representation, 173
  tear film deposits
    on hydrogel, 180–181
    on silicone, 189
    on silicone-acrylate, 188
Protozoa *Acanthamoeba:* in corneal infection, 265–268
Pseudodendrite, 112
  diagnosis, differential, 130
  epithelial, 129–130
  thimerasol hypersensitivity causing, 129
Pseudomonas aeruginosa: in corneal infection, 264
Pump-leak hypothesis: in transparency maintenance, 22–23
Punctal plug in dry eye, 214–215
  installation procedure, 214

Q

Questionnaires: in dry eye, 210, 211

R

Red eye
  acute, syndrome of, 229–231
    hydrogel and, 230
    stromal infiltrates in, 230
Refractive
  changes
    accidental with contact lenses, 69–80
    orthokeratology and, 82
    polymethylmethacrylate causing, 69–70
  error
    changes, deliberate, 80–83
    changes due to contact lenses, 69–87
    state after discontinuing polymethylmethacrylate lenses, 73
Rehabilitation: of cornea, 33–34
Rengstorff curve, 71
Ring anomaly: impression, 138
Rose bengal staining
  of cornea, 125
  in dry eye, 209–210

Rupture
  lipid layer, in dry eye,
    196
  of tear film, mechanism
    of, 166, 167

S

Scar
  corneal, postkeratoplasty,
    152
  ketatotomy, radial, 152
Schirmer test: in dry eye,
  204–205
Schnider grading: of 3 and 9
  o'clock staining, 198
Senescent endothelium,
  47–48
Sensitivity
  of cornea (*see* Cornea,
    sensitivity)
  to preserved solutions
    causing staining, 143
Shagreen: posterior mosaic,
  51–52
Silicone
  acrylates
    fluoro-, tear film
      deposits on, 189
    protein tear film
      deposits on, 188
    tear film deposits on,
      187–189
    lipid tear film deposits on,
      189
    protein tear film deposits
      on, 189
    tear film deposits on, 189
Skin hypersensitivity:
  basophilic, and
    conjunctivitis, 237–238
Smile stain: under soft
  contact lenses, 137
Smoking: and corneal
  infection, 261–262
Snellen Chart Visual Acuity,
  78
"Snowball" infiltrative
  opacities, 226
Specular micrograph, 56
Sphericalization in
  orthokeratology,
  82–83
Stain, abrasion (*see*
  Abrasion stain)
Staining
  3 and 9 o'clock (*see* Dry
    eye, cornea in, 3 and
    9 o'clock staining)
  of abrasion (*see* Abrasion
    staining)
  of conjunctiva in dry eye,
    208–210

of cornea in dry eye,
  208–210
epithelial punctate, to
  benzalkonium
  chloride, 231
punctate superficial
  in aphakia in diabetes,
  256
  with hydrogel, 256
rose bengal, of cornea, 125
Staphylococcal toxins: and
  ulcer, 226
Staphylococcus aureus:
  causing corneal ulcer,
  227
Staphylococcus epidermidis:
  on hydrogel, 183
Streptococcus pneumoniae in
  corneal infection, 263
Stress: hypoxic,
  measurement of
  oxygen availability
  under contact lens, 18
Stroma
  hypoxia complicating,
    29–31, 33
  infiltrates in acute red eye
    syndrome, 230
Silicone
  acrylates
    fluoro-, tear film
      deposits on, 189
    protein tear film
      deposits on, 188
    tear film deposits on,
      187–189
    lipid tear film deposits on,
      189
    protein tear film deposits
      on, 189
    tear film deposits on, 189
Skin hypersensitivity:
  basophilic, and
    conjunctivitis,
    237–238
Smile stain: under soft
  contact lenses, 137
Smoking: and corneal
  infection, 261–262
Snellen Chart Visual Acuity,
  78
"Snowball" infiltrative
  opacities, 226
Specular micrograph, 56
Sphericalization in
  orthokeratology,
  82–83
Stain, abrasion (see
  Abrasion stain)
Staining
  3 and 9 o'clock (see Dry
    eye, cornea in, 3 and
    9 o'clock staining)

of abrasion (see Abrasion
  staining)
of conjunctiva in dry eye,
  208–210
of cornea in dry eye,
  208–210
epithelial punctate, to
  benzalkonium
  chloride, 231
punctate superficial
  in aphakia in diabetes,
  256
  with hydrogel, 256
rose bengal, of cornea, 125
Staphylococcal toxins: and
  ulcer, 226
Smoking: and corneal
  infection, 261–262
Snellen Chart Visual Acuity,
  78
"Snowball" infiltrative
  opacities, 226
Specular micrograph, 56
Sphericalization in
  orthokeratology,
  82–83
Stain, abrasion (*see*
  Abrasion stain)
Staining
  3 and 9 o'clock (*see* Dry
    eye, cornea in, 3 and
    9 o'clock staining)
  of abrasion (*see* Abrasion
    staining)
  of conjunctiva in dry eye,
    208–210
  of cornea in dry eye,
    208–210
  epithelial punctate, to
    benzalkonium
    chloride, 231
  punctate superficial
    in aphakia in diabetes,
    256
    with hydrogel, 256
  rose bengal, of cornea,
    125
Staphylococcal toxins: and
  ulcer, 226
Staphylococcus aureus:
  causing corneal ulcer,
  227
Staphylococcus epidermidis:
  on hydrogel, 183
Streptococcus pneumoniae in
  corneal infection, 263
Stress: hypoxic,
  measurement of
  oxygen availability
  under contact lens 18
Stroma
  hypoxia complicating,
    29–31, 33

infiltrates in acute red eye
  syndrome, 230
pH
  decrease with hydrogel
    lenses, 30
  nitrogen goggle leads
    and, 27
swelling
  corneal striae in, 30
  hypoxia causing, 29
  thickness reduction and
    hypoxia, 33
  thinning with dellen, 201
Surfactant cleaner abrasion,
  142–143
Swelling
  of cornea, 6–7
    altitude and, 8
    average, 7
    recording, 7
    response, 11–14
    mean, 14
  stromal (*see* Stroma,
    swelling)
  (*See also* Edema)

T

Tear
  breakup time
    with contact lenses,
      170, 171
    in dry eye, 205
    noninvasive, in dry eye,
      205–206
  chemistry and hydrogel,
    186–187
  of contact lenses causing
    abrasion, 133–137
  evaporation
    contact lenses,
      177–180
    in dry eye, 206
    rate, 179
    rate with hydrogel, 179
  fern patterns in dry eye,
    206
  film (*see below*)
  osmolality with contact
    lenses, 178
  osmolarity in dry eye, 206
  physicochemical
    properties with
    contact lenses,
    175–177
  prism height in dry eye,
    207–208, 209
  production
    contact lenses and,
      171–172
    measurement,
      fluorophotometric
      technique, 172

Tear *(cont.)*
  tests in dry eye,
      204–205
  protein concentrations,
      graphical
      representation, 173
  substitutes
      composition of, 213
      properties of, 213
Tear film, 159–194
  breakup, 170
      in 3 and 9 o'clock
          staining, 200
      in tear breakup time
          test, 169
      tests in dry eye,
          205–206
  changes with contact
      lenses, 159–194
  composition with contact
      lenses, 172–180
  deposits
      on cellulose acetate
          butyrate, 187
      with contact lenses,
          180–189
      factors affecting amount
          of, 184–187
      on fluoro-silicone
          acrylates, 189
      on hydrogel, 180–189
      on hydrogel, calcium
          carbonate, 182–184
      on hydrogel, calcium
          phosphate, 183
      on hydrogel, lens
          calculi, 181–182
      on hydrogel, lipids, 181
      on hydrogel, protein,
          180–181
      on hydrogel, surface
          irregularities and
          deposit formation,
          187

  lipid *(see* Lipid tear
      film deposits)
  on polymethylmethacry-
      late, 187
  protein *(see* Protein tear
      film deposits)
  on silicone, 189
  on silicone-acrylates,
      187–189
disjoining pressure, 168
dry spot formation
  mechanism, 166
gas-permeable lenses and,
  rigid, 165
on hydrogel, 164
interference fringe pattern
  amorphous pattern, 162
  color fringe pattern, 163
  flow pattern, 163
  marmoreal, 161
  marmoreal,
      contaminated, 162
normal, disruption of,
  166–169
pH in, 177
residues, 145
rupture, mechanism of,
  166, 167
stability
  with contact lenses, 165
  measurements, 169–170
structure, 159–160
  with contact lenses,
      160–165
  drawn to scale, 160
  in dry eye, 206
thinning
  in dry eye, 196
  with gas-permeable
      contact lenses, 197
Thimerosal
  hypersensitivity, 232–233
  causing pseudodentrite,
      129

preserved solution,
  causing
  pseudodendrite, 112
  toxicity of, 232–233
Thygeson's
  keratopathy, 148
  superficial punctate
      keratitis, 109
Tiffen yellow no. 2, 126
Toxic reactions: in keratitis,
  106–109
Toxicity
  of chlorhexidine,
      231–232
  of preservatives,
      231–233
  of thimerosal, 232–233
Toxins: staphylococcal, and
  ulcer, 226
Transparency
  of cornea, 21–23
  maintenance, pump-leak,
      hypothesis, 22–23
Trauma
  epithelial, and infection,
      261
  mechanical, in giant
      conjunctivitis, 240

U

Ulcer
  bacterial, 116
  corneal
      necrotizing, 228
      Staphylococcus aureus,
          227
  herpes simplex, dendritic,
      130
  microbial, 269
  staphylococcal toxins and,
      226
Ultraviolet abrasion, 152,
  153

V

Vacuoles: epithelial, 111
Vascularization: and
  hydrogel, 229
Veil, dimple, 139–140
  staining, 141
Virus(es)
  in corneal infection, 265
  in inflammations, 225
Vision
  contrast test system
      contrast sensitivity
          chart, 74
  quality and contact lenses,
      78–80
      hydrogel lenses, 79–80
      measurement methods,
          78–79
      rigid lenses, 80
Visual acuity
  Snellen Chart, 78
  variable-contrast charts,
      78
Vitamin A drops: in
  conjunctivitis, giant
  papillary, 250
Vogt's biomicroscopy: of
  eye, 45

W

Water content: of lens, 184
Wound healing: of abrasion,
  152–155

X

Xerosis, 157–218

Z

Zantos-Holden bleb
  response, 55